53

Bone Disease
Fifth Series

Test and Syllabus

Jon A. Jacobson, MD
Editor

Marnix T. van Holsbeeck, MD
Editor

Harris L. Cohen, MD
Editor

Elaine S. Gould, MD
Assistant Editor

Gerson E. Alvarez, MD
Kirkland W. Davis, MD
David P. Fessell, MD
Mark J. Kransdorf, MD
Kenneth S. Lee, MD
William B. Morrison, MD
Teik C. Oh, MB
Hollis G. Potter, MD
Cesare Romagnoli, MD
Brandon M. Schooley, MD
Mark E. Schweitzer, MD
Lynne S. Steinbach, MD
Geert M. Vanderschueren, MD, PhD
Adam C. Zoga, MD

Library of Congress Data

Bone Disease (fifth series) test and syllabus: Harris L. Cohen, Jon A. Jacobson, Marnix
T. van Holsbeeck [editors]; Gerson E. Alvarez, Kirkland W. Davis, David P. Fessell, Mark
J. Kransdorf, Kenneth S. Lee, William B. Morrison, Teik C. Oh, Hollis G. Potter, Cesare
Romagnoli, Brandon M. Schooley, Mark E. Schweitzer, Lynne S. Steinbach, Geert M.
Vanderschueren, Adam C. Zoga [co-authors].
   p. cm. — (Professional self-evaluation program; set 53)
   "Committee on Professional Self-Evaluation, Commission on Education"—Cover.
   Includes bibliographical references and index.
   ISBN 978-1-55903-053-3 — ISBN 1-55903-000-3 (series) Library of Congress
   Control Number: 2010906735

Note: While the American College of Radiology and the editors of the publication have attempted to
include the most current and accurate information possible, errors may inadvertently appear. Diagnostic
and interventional decisions should be based on the individual circumstances of each case.

Volume 53

Bone Disease

Fifth Series
Test and Syllabus

Section Editors

Jon A. Jacobson, M.D
Professor of Radiology and Director, Division of Musculoskeletal Radiology, University of Michigan, Ann Arbor, Michigan

Marnix T. van Holsbeeck, M.D.
Professor of Radiology, Wayne State University Medical School. Division Director and Fellowship Program Director for Musculoskeletal Radiology, Henry Ford Hospital, Detroit, Michigan.

Series Editor in Chief

Harris L. Cohen, M.D., FACR
Professor of Radiology, Pediatrics, Obstetrics and Gynecology, and Chairman, Department of Radiology, University of Tennessee Health Science Center. Medical Director, LeBonheur Children's Medical Center, Memphis, Tennessee.

Assistant Editor

Elaine S. Gould, M.D.
Associate Professor of Clinical Radiology and Orthopedic Surgery, Chief of Musculoskeletal Radiology, and Director, Musculoskeletal Fellowship Program, State University of New York, Stony Brook University Medical Center, Stony Brook, New York.

Authors

Gerson E. Alvarez, M.D. Attending Staff of Radiology, Division of Musculoskeletal Radiology, Henry Ford Hospital, Detroit, Michigan.

Kirkland W. Davis, M.D. Associate Professor of Radiology, Division of Musculoskeletal Radiology, University of Wisconsin School of Medicine and Public Health, Madison, Wisconsin.

David P. Fessell, M.D. Associate Professor of Radiology, Division of Musculoskeletal Radiology, University of Michigan Medical Center, Ann Arbor, Michigan.

Mark J. Kransdorf, M.D., FACR Professor of Radiology, Mayo Clinic College of Medicine, and Consultant, Musculoskeletal Imaging, Mayo Clinic, Jacksonville, Florida.

Kenneth S. Lee, M.D. Assistant Professor of Radiology, University of Wisconsin School of Medicine & Public Health, and Director of Musculoskeletal Ultrasound, University of Wisconsin Hospital & Clinics, Madison, Wisconsin.

William B. Morrison, M.D. Professor of Radiology, and Director, Musculoskeletal Radiology Division, Thomas Jefferson University Hospital, Philadelphia, Pennsylvania.

Teik C. Oh, M.B., AFRCSI, FRCR Consultant Musculoskeletal Radiologist, Department of Imaging, Royal Preston Hospital, Lancashire, United Kingdom.

Hollis G. Potter, M.D. Chief of Magnetic Resonance Imaging, Hospital for Special Surgery, and Professor of Radiology, Weill Medical College of Cornell University, New York, New York.

Cesare Romagnoli, M.D., FRCPC Associate Professor, Department of Medical Imaging, The University of Western Ontario. Staff Radiologist and Director of Ultrasound, London Health Sciences Centre, University Hospital, London, Ontario.

Brandon M. Schooley, M.D. Musculoskeletal Radiologist, Allegheny Radiology Associates, Pittsburgh, Pennsylvania.

Mark E. Schweitzer, M.D. Chief of Radiology, The Ottawa Hospital. Chair of Diagnostic Imaging and Professor of Radiology, The University of Ottawa, Ontario, Canada.

Lynne S. Steinbach, M.D., FACR Professor of Radiology and Orthopaedic Surgery and Director, Musculoskeletal Imaging Fellowship, University of California, San Francisco, California.

Geert M. Vanderschueren, M.D., Ph.D. Professor of Radiology, Department of Radiology, Musculoskeletal Radiology Section, University Hospitals of Leuven, Leuven, Belgium (Europe).

Adam C. Zoga, M.D. Associate Professor of Radiology and Director, Musculoskeletal MRI, Thomas Jefferson University Hospital, Philadelphia, Pennsylvania.

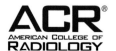

Professional Self-Evaluation Program
Commission on Education
American College of Radiology

PROFESSIONAL SELF-EVALUATION COMMITTEE

Production Manager: Victoria A. Lamb
Copy Editor: Paula R. Ellison, Gainesville, Virginia
Index: EEI Communications, Alexandria, Virginia.
Printing: United Book Press, Baltimore, Maryland

FACULTY DISCLOSURE INFORMATION

The faculty members listed below have indicated they have no relevant financial relationships or potential conflicts of interest related to the material presented. They also do not intend to discuss off-label use in accordance with the ACCME Standards and FDA requirements.

The American College of Radiology has received no commercial support for this activity.

Gerson E. Alvarez, M.D.
Harris L. Cohen, M.D.
Kirkland W. Davis, M.D.
David P. Fessell, M.D.
Elaine P. Gould, M.D.
Jon A. Jacobson, M.D.
Mark J. Kransdorf, M.D.
Kenneth S. Lee, M.D.
William B. Morrison, M.D.
Teik C. Oh, M.B.
Hollis G. Potter, M.D.
Cesare Romagnoli, M.D.
Brandon M. Schooley, M.D.
Mark E. Schweitzer, M.D.
Lynne S. Steinbach, M.D.
Geert M. Vanderschueren, M.D., Ph.D.
Marnix T. van Holsbeeck, M.D.
Adam C. Zoga, M.D.

Editors' Preface

Since the fourth series of the ACR's *Bone Disease Professional Self-evaluation Test and Syllabus* was published in 1989, musculoskeletal imaging has continued to evolve. Examples include the use of ultrasound in evaluation of tendon abnormalities and the routine use of CT-guided radiofrequency ablation of osteoid osteomas. Imaging also plays a role in the diagnosis of complex clinical syndromes, as exemplified by the use of MR arthrography in the evaluation of femoroacetabular impingement. In addition to newer applications of musculoskeletal imaging, timely updates concerning imaging of the more routine musculoskeletal disorders, such as rotator cuff, meniscus, and anterior cruciate ligament tear, are always needed.

In this, the fifth series of the *Bone Disease Test and Syllabus,* cases are presented that encompass a range of musculoskeletal pathologies. We are pleased that a number of excellent authors have agreed to contribute to this work. With regard to the shoulder, Dr. Fessell presents a comprehensive update on rotator cuff and reviews synovial disorders, and Dr. Steinbach provides an excellent discussion of glenohumeral instability and labral abnormalities. At the wrist, Dr. Potter addresses the triangular fibrocartilage complex and finger pulleys along with the corresponding role of MR imaging. With regard to hip and pelvis, Dr. Davis brings the reader up to date on femoroacetabular impingement, a topic that has recently received much attention in both the orthopedic and radiology literature. Dr. Jacobson reviews an approach to classifying acetabular fractures, including CT correlation, Dr. Lee covers pathologic fractures of the hip, and Dr. Zoga discusses adductor injuries. With

regard to the knee, Dr. Morrison reviews insufficiency fracture, Dr. Alvarez discusses meniscal pathology and injury, and Dr. Jacobson examines anterior cruciate ligament tears and related topics such as mucoid degeneration. At the ankle, Drs. Oh and Schweitzer review imaging of posterior tibialis tendon dysfunction. Dr. Morrison discusses foot neuropathy, infections, and related conditions. Under the final categories of metabolic disorders and tumors, Dr. Schooley discusses the role of imaging in diagnosing metabolic disorders, Dr. Kransdorf looks at malignant and benign bone tumors, Dr. Romagnoli further explores soft tissue anomalies, and Dr. Vanderschueren discusses tumor ablation.

As co-editors, we would like to thank the authors of this syllabus for their work and effort. In addition, we would like to acknowledge Dr. Harris Cohen, editor in chief for the Professional Self-Evaluation Series, and Victoria Lamb of the ACR for their hard work in seeing this project to completion. It is with these contributions that we are able to provide an update and review of musculoskeletal imaging topics that will benefit the reader and his or her practice.

Jon A. Jacobson, M.D.
Professor of Radiology
University of Michigan

Marnix T. van Holsbeeck, M.D.
Professor of Radiology
Henry Ford Hospital

April, 2010

Editor in Chief's Preface

This is the 53nd book of the American College of Radiology's illustrious "Syllabus" series (formally known as the Professional Self-Evaluation and Continuing Education Program) and the fifth book of that series that I have had the privilege to edit. The ACR has decided to end the series with this text.

Like many radiologists who trained in the 70s and 80s, I "grew up" with the ACR syllabus series. The books were great tools for continuing education but also served as excellent board preparation tools at a time when few, if any, other texts could make that claim. I took many of the 15 volumes that had been published by the time I took the oral boards with me to Louisville, each with meticulous notes written in the margins. Many volumes have been written since that time. Each volume presents a surprising quantity of helpful information using a case-based format that introduces a key topic via an unknown image and then expands upon that information by exploring associated clinical, pathophysiologic, and imaging information with additional questions and answers. Courses I have taken in medical education suggest this is an ideal method for education. Each text has tried to bring the reader up-to-date information on the new clinical imaging and technological facts and nuances necessary for practicing the fantastic but ever-changing specialty of radiology. This book, *Bone Disease V*, continues in that tradition.

My job as editor-in-chief has presented me with a bonus opportunity to learn from experts outside my subspecialty. I get to keep up with advances in radiology, while serving as a sort of radiologist "Everyman." In that role, I have tried to keep the texts readable and relevant to all radiologists: those who are experts, those who are beginners, and the vast majority of us who are somewhere in between. I hope the reader agrees.

In this volume, as with all others, we sought to recruit "all-star" writers and editors as well as clinicians. Drs. Marnix van Holsbeeck and Jon Jacobson agreed to co-edit the text and assembled a strong musculoskeletal imaging team to help them write it. Dr. Elaine Gould served as my assistant editor, providing excellent and timely work, reviewing and editing various chapters in an area that is her subspecialty. Everyone's efforts were meant to satisfy the need for true, relevant, up-to-date information that is also easy to read and understand. This takes thought, effort, and especially time, which in today's academic world is in ever shorter supply. Each author has given mightily of that limited supply to this effort, and I am grateful for their generosity.

In this volume, *Bone Disease V*, Drs. Gerson Alvarez, Kirkland Davis, David Fessell, Mark Kransdorf, Ken Lee, Teik Oh, Hollis Potter, William Morrison, Cesare Romagnoli, Brandon Schooley, Mark Schweitzer, Lynne Steinbach, Geert Vanderschueren, and Adam Zoga have provided a wide variety of cases with fine images, questions, and a wealth of information.

Many others have been involved in the production of this volume. I particularly appreciate the guidance of Dr. Larry Davis, Chairman of the ACR's Commission on Education, whose advice has been most cogent and helpful.

Vicki Lamb serves as the text's production manager. Her task is immense with an ever-present pressure to get chapters and images out on time and to their next review or layout or printing, as deadlines loom. She is the true glue to the project, and has served the PSE syllabus series and its readers well.

General editing and proofreading was aided by Paula Ellison, who has been providing editing support to the "Syllabi" series for two decades. Susan

Alfarone, my executive assistant at SUNY-Stony Brook and Cynthia Lavender-Owens, my executive assistant at LeBonheur Children's Hospital and the University of Tennessee kept the communications lines open with Vicki Lamb, the editors, and the authors.

Thanks are certainly due those who welcomed us most warmly into our Memphis community, including my colleagues at the University of Tennessee Health Science Center in Memphis, Tennessee, my new academic home. This is particularly true for my Dean, Steve Schwab, my past chairman, Barry Gerald and my LeBonheur colleagues, including Drs. Tom Boulden, Chandrea Smothers, Lynn Magill, and Louis Parvey, all of whom are most helpful to my efforts.

Most important, I must thank my family on the home fronts (which now include both New York and Memphis) who have allowed me the significant time and effort needed for each of the last five syllabi.

My wife, Sandra W. Cohen, M.D., remains tolerant of a husband who "organizes" his work over perhaps too large a swath of our home. Electronic storage and the affordability of bigger homes in Memphis have helped keep the peace. Over the years, my children have helped me with aspects of the books' production: Lauren Elizabeth with manuscripts and Benjamin Adam with computer storage and technical consultations. We are all pulling for Benjamin's recovery. New Rabbi David M. Cohen and his wife Ali help me with edits when I am visiting them overseas. Their children, Leah Baila and Moshe Aharon, provide me with needed "down time," which is always enjoyable but also too short. I thank them all.

My hope is that this syllabus will live up to those that preceded it, written and edited during past decades by outstanding, dedicated radiologists who worked hard to pass on information that was informative and of practical use to their radiology colleagues. It has been an honor to be part of that group and this great body of work.

Enjoy *Bone Disease V* !

Harris L. Cohen, M.D.
April, 2010

Volume 53

Bone Disease

Fifth Series

Test

CME Information

Program Objectives

After completing this program, participants will be able to identify and utilize recent scientific information relating to imaging for diagnosis of the musculoskeletal system. Participants will also be able to select from among the array of imaging modalities and techniques available to the radiologist those most appropriate to diagnose specific musculoskeletal diseases and conditions. In addition, participants will be able to choose the most appropriate current scientific options for differentiating specific disease entities.

CME Credit Award: 20 Credit Hours

The American College of Radiology (ACR) is accredited by the Accreditation Council for Continuing Medical Education (ACCME) to sponsor continuing medical education for physicians.

The ACR designates this educational activity for a maximum of 20 AMA/PRA Category 1 Credits™ towards the AMA's Physician's Recognition Award. Each physician should claim only those hours of credit that he or she actually spent in the educational activity.

The Bone Disease V Test and Syllabus program has been approved for ACR and AMA/PRA Category 1 CME Credit™ for the period from May 2010 to May 2013.*

CME Credit Award Process

To receive the Category 1 credit, participants must complete the accompanying answer sheet and a brief online exercise, at the end of which you will be able to print your CME certificate.

This CME activity was planned and produced in accordance with the ACCME Essentials. The estimated study time is 20 hours. Category 1 CME credit for this program is not transferable. Only the purchaser may apply for and receive Category 1 credit.

At the conclusion of each period, the program is extensively reviewed ensure the validity and timeliness of the content.

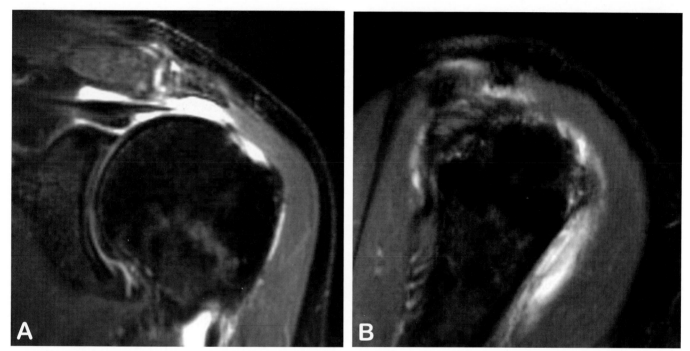

Figure 1-1. Shoulder. MRI. (A) Proton-density, fat-saturated. Coronal oblique plane. (B) Proton-density, fat-saturated. Sagittal oblique plane.

Question 1

You are shown two images (Figure 1-1) from the shoulder MR examination of a 55-year-old man who presented with shoulder pain and decreased range of motion. Which *one* of the following is the MOST likely diagnosis?

(A)   Full-thickness supraspinatus tendon tear
(B)   High-grade, bursal-sided, partial-thickness supraspinatus tendon tear
(C)   Low-grade, bursal-sided, partial-thickness supraspinatus tendon tear
(D)   Intrasubstance type supraspinatus tendon tear
(E)   Tendinosis of the supraspinatus tendon

QUESTIONS 2 and 3:
MARK YOUR ANSWER SHEET WITH THE ONE BEST ANSWER FROM THE OPTIONS PROVIDED

QUESTION 4:
MARK YOUR ANSWER SHEET TRUE (T) OR FALSE (F) FOR EACH OF THE RESPONSE CHOICES.

2. Which *one* of the following is the MOST likely level of accuracy that should be expected for MR imaging of the type of tendon pathology depicted in Question 1?

(A) 50% to 60%
(B) 60% to 70%
(C) 70% to 80%
(D) 80% to 90%
(E) 90% or greater

3. Which *one* of the following is the MOST accurate for detecting full-thickness supraspinatus tendon tears?

(A) MR imaging
(B) Ultrasound
(C) With experienced interpreters, they are equally accurate.

4. The treatment of a supraspinatus tendon tear can be affected by:

(A) Muscle atrophy
(B) Dimensions of the tear (medial to lateral and anterior to posterior)
(C) Thickness of the torn tendon end
(D) Associated pathology in the infraspinatus tendon, biceps brachii long-head tendon, and subscapularis tendon
(E) Presence of an os acromiale

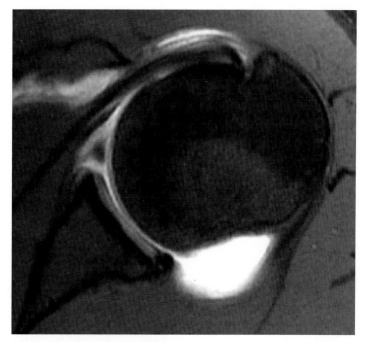

Figure 2-1. Shoulder. MR arthrogram. Lower half of the glenohumeral joint. T1-weighted, fat-suppressed. Axial plane.

Question 5

You are shown an MR image (Figure 2-1) from a 28-year-old man with anterior shoulder instability and pain. The image was obtained at the level of the middle to inferior anterior labrum. Which *one* of the following is the MOST likely diagnosis?

(A)   Anterior labroligamentous periosteal sleeve avulsion (ALPSA lesion)
(B)   Perthes lesion
(C)   Bankart lesion
(D)   Sublabral foramen
(E)   Buford complex

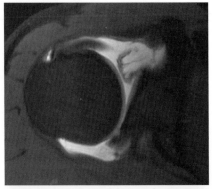

Figure 2-10.
Shoulder. MR
arthrogram.
T1-weighted,
fat-suppressed.
Axial plane.

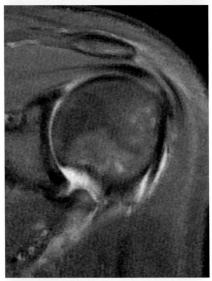

Figure 2-11.
Shoulder. MR
arthrogram.
T1-weighted,
fat-suppressed.
Axial plane.

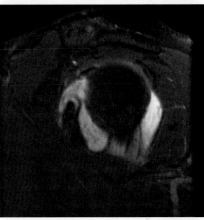

Figure 2-12.
Shoulder. MR.
T1-weighted,
fat-suppressed.
Axial plane.

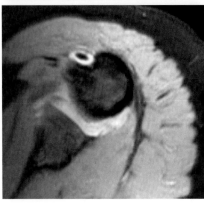

Figure 2-13.
Shoulder. MR.
T2-weighted,
fat-suppressed.
Sagittal plane.

You are shown MR images of four shoulders with a history of instability and a glenohumeral ligament lesion. For each of the numbered images (Figures 2-10 through 2-13 in the test section), select the one lettered diagnosis (A, B, C, D, or E) that is MOST closely associated with it. Each lettered diagnosis may be used once, more than once, or not at all.

6. Figure 2-10
7. Figure 2-11
8. Figure 2-12
9. Figure 2-13

   (A) HAGL lesion
   (B) BHAGL lesion
   (C) RHAGL lesion
   (D) Superior glenohumeral ligament tear
   (E) Middle glenohumeral ligament tear

10. Posterior instability is associated with:

    (A) Posterior labrocapsular periosteal sleeve avulsion (POLPSA) lesion
    (B) Bennett lesion
    (C) Kim lesion
    (D) Osseous Bankart lesion
    (E) Engagement of the humeral head on the anterior glenoid during internal rotation

11. Concerning paralabral cysts:

    (A) They are most commonly associated with anterior labral tears.
    (B) Superior labral cysts often extend into the subscapular notch.
    (C) Cysts in the spinoglenoid notch can denervate the infraspinatus muscle.
    (D) Subacute denervation changes can be seen as both atrophy and fatty infiltration of the muscle.
    (E) Inferior cysts can affect the axillary nerve.

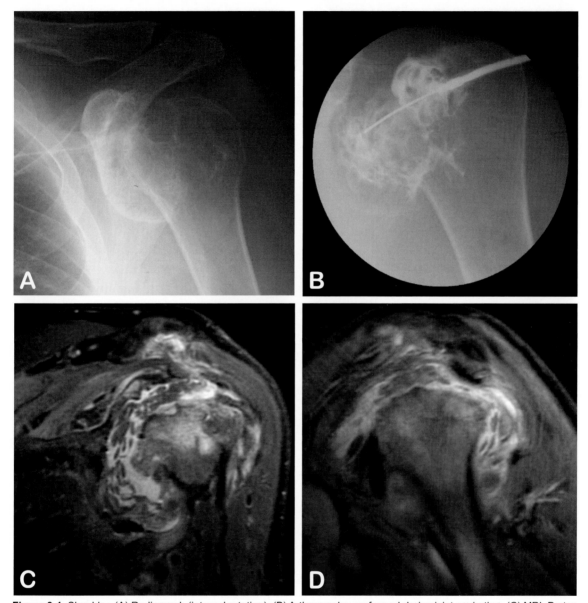

Figure 3-1. Shoulder. (A) Radiograph (internal rotation). (B) Arthrography, performed during joint aspiration. (C) MRI. Proton-density, fat-saturated. Coronal oblique view. (D) MRI. Proton-density, fat-saturated. Sagittal oblique view.

Question 12

You are shown four images (Figure 3-1) from the shoulder MR examination of a 36-year-old man who presents with shoulder pain. Which *one* of the following is the MOST likely diagnosis?

(A)   Rheumatoid arthritis
(B)   Synovial osteochondromatosis
(C)   Pigmented villonodular synovitis
(D)   Lipoma arborescens

QUESTION 13: MARK YOUR ANSWER SHEET TRUE (T) OR FALSE (F) FOR EACH OF THE RESPONSE CHOICES.

QUESTIONS 14 THROUGH 16: MARK YOUR ANSWER SHEET WITH THE ONE BEST ANSWER FROM THE OPTIONS PROVIDED.

13. Regarding synovial chondromatosis of the shoulder:

(A) Treatment may include removal of bodies, synovectomy, or arthroplasty.
(B) It is the same as "rice bodies" in the shoulder.
(C) The shoulder is the most commonly involved joint.
(D) Malignant transformation into chondrosarcoma is uncommon.

14. Which *one* of the following is the MOST sensitive modality for detecting early erosions in rheumatoid arthritis of the shoulder?

(A) Radiography
(B) Ultrasound
(C) MR imaging

15. Regarding pigmented villonodular synovitis of the shoulder,

(A) Radiographs can provide definitive diagnosis.
(B) Erosions are not always present.
(C) MR imaging is the modality of choice for diagnosis and preoperative planning.
(D) Malignant degeneration is rarely associated with this entity.
(E) Recurrence is more common in the shoulder than in the knee.

16. Regarding lipoma arborescens of the shoulder:

(A) The diagnosis can be made with radiographs.
(B) T1-weighted MR imaging is helpful in making the diagnosis.
(C) It only occurs in joints.
(D) It is caused by prior hemarthrosis.
(E) It only occurs in patients over 40.

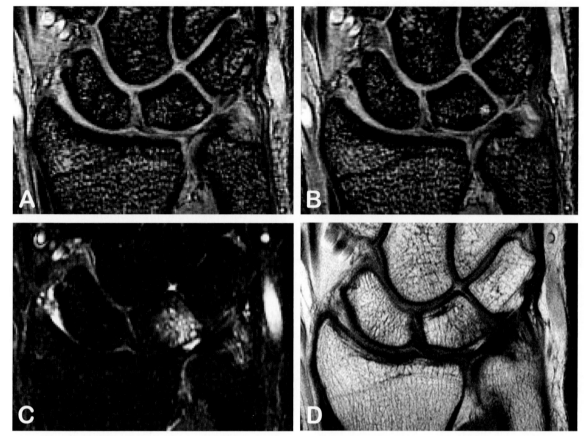

Figure 4-1. Wrist. MRI. (A) T2-weighted, 3-D gradient echo. Coronal plane. (B) T2-weighted, 3-D gradient echo. (C) Fast inversion recovery (FIR). (D) Proton-density-weighted, moderate echo time, fast spin-echo.

Question 17

You are shown four MR images (Figure 4-1) from the right wrist of a right-hand-dominant 36-year-old man. The patient presented with ulnar-sided wrist pain. Which *one* of the following is the MOST likely diagnosis?

(A)   Kienböck's disease
(B)   Giant cell tumor of the lunate
(C)   Ulnar impaction syndrome
(D)   Ulnar styloid abutment syndrome

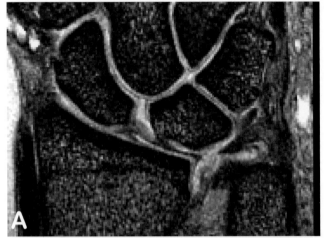

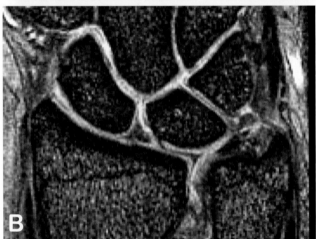

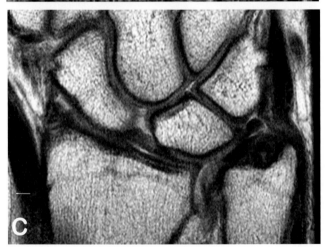

Figure 4-6. Right wrist. MRI. (A & B) T2-weighted, three-dimensional, gradient-echo. Coronal plane. (C) Moderate-echo-time, Proton-density-weighted, fast-spin-echo. Coronal plane.

18. You are shown three MR images (Figure 4-6) of the right wrist in an 18-year-old, right-hand-dominant female gymnast, who presents with ulnar-side wrist pain. This case illustrates which *one* of the following:

    (A) Peripheral detachment of the triangular fibro-cartilage
    (B) Tear of the extensor carpi ulnaris tendon sheath
    (C) Lunotriquetral ligament tear
    (D) Central defect of the triangular fibrocartilage

19. Which *one* of the following is NOT a component of the triangular fibrocartilage complex?

    (A) Ulnolunate ligament
    (B) Ulnotriquetral ligament
    (C) Lunotriquetral ligament
    (D) Meniscal homologue

20. Regarding lesions of the triangular fibrocartilage, which *one* of the following statements is true?

    (A) Only central lesions of the triangular fibro-cartilage can be successfully repaired.
    (B) Peripheral tears are associated with ulnar positive variance.
    (C) Tears are characteristically associated with lesions of the extensor carpi ulnaris tendon.
    (D) Diagnosis requires the presence of dispropor-tionate amount of fluid in the distal radio-ulnar joint.
    (E) None of the above is correct.

21. Which *one* of the following is true regarding imaging of the triangular fibrocartilage?

    (A) Fast spin-echo imaging is useful for assess-ment of cartilage loss adjacent to the TFC.
    (B) Accurate diagnosis requires the use of MR arthrography.
    (C) Optimal positioning is at the isocenter of the magnet in the "Superman" position.
    (D) Slice resolution should be 3 mm.

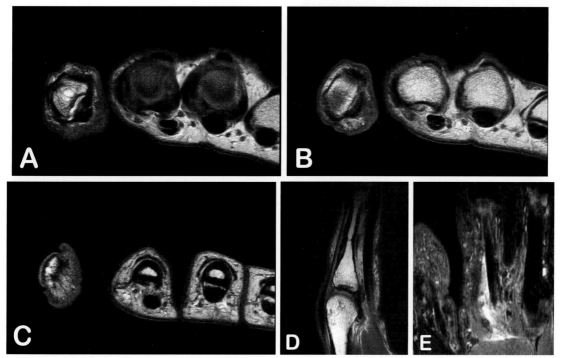

Figure 5-1. Index finger. MRI. (A to C) Proton-density-weighted, fast spin-echo (FSE). Axial plane. (D) Moderate echo time, proton-density-weighted, FSE. Sagittal plane. (E) Fast inversion recovery. Coronal plane.

Question 22

You are shown axial, sagittal, and coronal MR images (Figure 5-1) through the right index finger of a 33-year-old woman with a recent history of trauma. Which *one* of the following is the MOST likely diagnosis?

(A)   Flexor tendon laceration
(B)   Metacarpophalangeal joint subluxation
(C)   Pulley disruption
(D)   Vincula disruption

23. Which *one* of the following sports is most commonly associated with pulley injuries?

(A) Basketball
(B) Football
(C) Rock climbing
(D) Squash

24. Surgical management of pulley disruption typically involves which *one* of the following:

(A) Flexor tendon transfer
(B) Primary repair
(C) Allograft reconstruction
(D) Autograft reconstruction

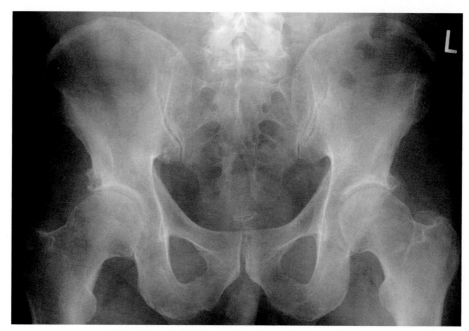

Figure 6-1. Pelvis. Radiograph. Anteroposterior view.

Question 25

This 56-year-old man presented with right hip pain. You are shown a radiograph of his pelvis (Figure 6-1). Which *one* of the following is the MOST likely underlying cause of this patient's advanced degenerative joint disease involving both hips?

(A) Ankylosing spondylitis
(B) Cam femoroacetabular impingement
(C) Pincer femoroacetabular impingement
(D) Osteonecrosis
(E) Rheumatoid arthritis

26. All of the following statements are true
EXCEPT:

(A) Cam femoroacetabular impingement primarily leads to damage of the acetabular
articular cartilage.
(B) Femoroacetabular impingement does not
lead to accelerated degeneration of the hip
joint.
(C) Pincer femoroacetabular impingement first
leads to damage of the acetabular labrum.
(D) Patients with surgically proven femoroacetabular impingement most commonly have
a combination of cam and pincer types.
(E) Patients suffering from slipped capital
femoral epiphysis may develop cam
morphology as adults.

27. Regarding Figure 6-7, what condition does the
patient have that may cause accelerated degenerative joint disease involving the right hip?

(A) Ankylosing spondylitis
(B) Cam femoroacetabular impingement
(C) Pincer femoroacetabular impingement
(D) Osteonecrosis
(E) Rheumatoid arthritis

28. For the patient with a combination of a focal acetabular labral tear, localized articular
cartilage defects, and femoroacetabular impingement, surgical options include all of the
following EXCEPT:

(A) Cartilage treatment techniques, such as
microfracture, chondroplasty, and mosaic-
plasty
(B) Labral debridement or repair
(C) Hip resurfacing
(D) Femoroplasty
(E) Resection of the acetabular rim

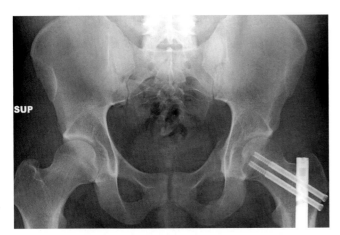

Figure 6-7. Pelvis. Radiograph. Anteroposterior view.

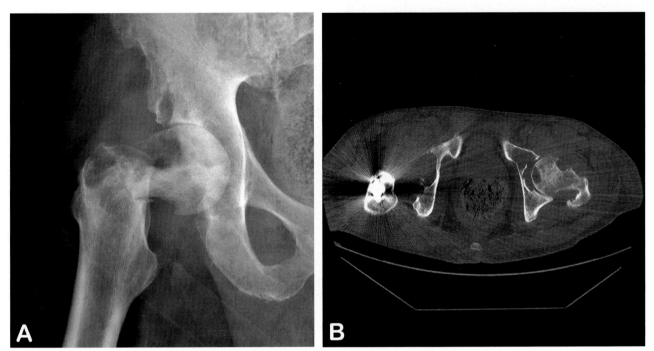

Figure 7-1. (A) Right hip. Radiograph. Anteroposterior view. (B) Pelvis. Thin-section CT. Axial plane.

Question 29

A 78-year-old African-American man presents after falling at his home. You are shown an initial radiograph (Figure 7-1A) and a CT image (Figure 7-1B) obtained later in the workup. The patient has a past medical history of end-stage renal disease secondary to hypertensive nephrosclerosis and is maintained on hemodialysis. His medical history also includes hypertension for more than 15 years, diabetes for more than 30 years, and bowel issues for a few years. What is the *one* MOST likely underlying cause of the patient's pathologic fracture?

(A)   Metastases
(B)   Multiple myeloma
(C)   Pigmented villonodular synovitis
(D)   Amyloidosis
(E)   Rheumatoid arthritis

30. Musculoskeletal manifestations of dialysis-related amyloidosis include all of the following EXCEPT?

(A) Shoulder pad sign
(B) Osteolytic lesions
(C) Carpal tunnel syndrome
(D) Pathologic fractures
(E) Rheumatoid arthritis

31. True or False? Amyloidosis usually presents as a focal disease.

32. What factor or factors affect quality of hemofiltration in preventing or delaying onset of osteoarticular dialysis-related amyloidosis?

(A) Porosity
(B) Membrane thickness
(C) Material composition
(D) All of the above

33. The imaging characteristics of osteoarticular amyloidosis include all of the following EXCEPT:

(A) Erosions or osteolytic lesions with preservation of the joint space
(B) Decreased signal intensity on T1-weighted images
(C) Nondistended joint capsule with sonographic evaluation
(D) Moderate enhancement of bone lesions after gadolinium-based contrast injection
(E) Variable signal intensity on T2-weighted images

34. Which *one* of the following is the BEST method for the treatment of osteoarticular amyloidosis?

(A) Prevention by use of high flux hemodialysis membranes
(B) Surgery involving curettage and bone grafting of bone lesions
(C) Percutaneous cementoplasty of bone lesions to prevent pathologic fracture
(D) Proper insulin therapy to maintain target hemoglobin A1C
(E) None of the above

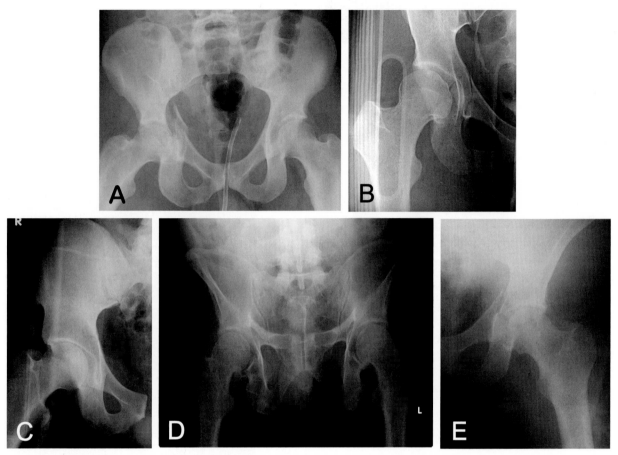

Figure 8-1. Radiographs. (A) Pelvis. Anteroposterior view. (B) Right hip. Anteroposterior view. (C) Right hip. Anteroposterior view. (D) Pelvis. Outlet view. (E) Left hip. Anteroposterior view.

Questions 35 through 39

You are shown five radiographs of the pelvis or hip from *five different patients* (Figures 8-1A through 8-1E), each of whom presented with pain after significant trauma. Select the one lettered diagnosis (A, B, C, D, or E) for each figure. Each lettered diagnosis should be used once.

35.   Figure 8-1A
36.   Figure 8-1B
37.   Figure 8-1C
38.   Figure 8-1D
39.   Figure 8-1E

                (A)   Transverse acetabular fracture
                (B)   Posterior wall acetabular fracture
                (C)   Both-column acetabular fracture
                (D)   T-shaped acetabular fracture
                (E)   Transverse with posterior wall acetabular fracture

(B) Anteroposterior compression
(C) Vertical shear
(D) Complex

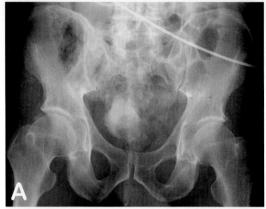

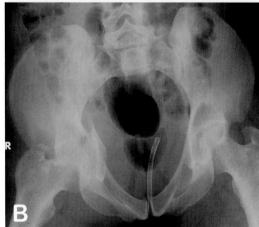

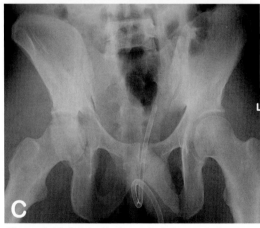

Figure 8-14. Pelvis. Radiograph. Anteroposterior view.

40. Concerning Figure 8-14, which *one* of the following BEST describes the mechanism of injury producing the radiographic findings?

(A) Lateral compression

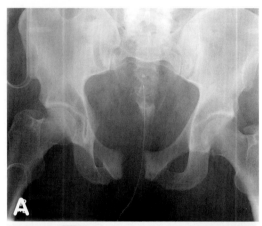

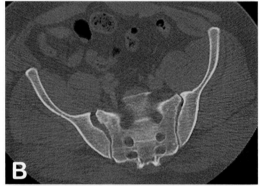

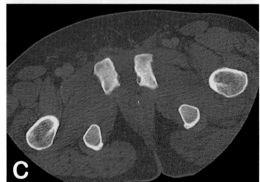

Figure 8-17. Pelvis. (A) Radiograph. Anteroposterior view. (B and C) CT. Axial plane.

41. Concerning Figure 8-17, which *one* of the following BEST describes the mechanism of injury producing the radiographic findings?

(A) Lateral compression
(B) Anteroposterior compression
(C) Vertical shear
(D) Complex

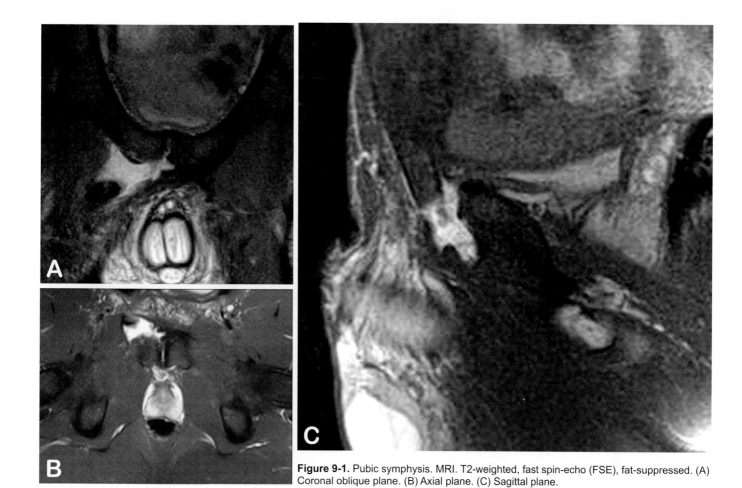

Figure 9-1. Pubic symphysis. MRI. T2-weighted, fast spin-echo (FSE), fat-suppressed. (A) Coronal oblique plane. (B) Axial plane. (C) Sagittal plane.

Question 42

A 24-year-old professional American football player presented with acute onset of left-sided groin pain following a hyperextension and twisting injury at the waist. The patient also suffers from chronic right-sided groin pain. You are shown three images (Figure 9-1) from the patient's T2-weighted, fast spin-echo, fat-suppressed MRI. Which *one* of the following is the MOST likely diagnosis?

(A)   Osteitis pubis
(B)   Traumatic inguinal hernia
(C)   Rectus abdominis / adductor aponeurosis tear
(D)   Adductor tubercle avulsion

44. In the setting of athletic pubalgia, which *one* of the following is the MOST common adductor tendon injured?

(A) Adductor longus
(B) Adductor brevis
(C) Adductor magnus
(D) Gracilis

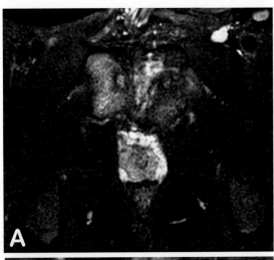
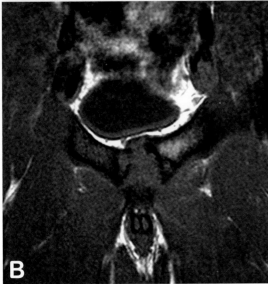

Figure 9-3. MRI. (A) T2-weighted, FSE fat-suppressed. Axial plane. (B) Proton-density-weighted FSE. Coronal oblique plane.

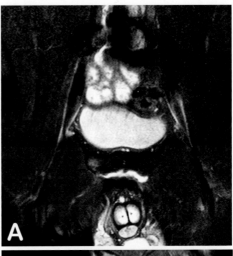
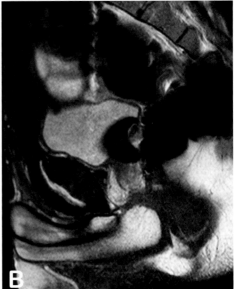

Figure 9-6. MRI. T2-weighted, FSE, fat-suppressed. (A) Coronal oblique plane. (B) Sagittal plane.

43. Based on your evaluation of Figure 9-3, which *one* of the following is the dominant finding in this 18-year-old soccer player with chronic bilateral groin pain?

(A) Osteitis pubis
(B) Traumatic inguinal hernia
(C) Rectus abdominis/adductor aponeurosis tear
(D) Adductor tubercle avulsion

45. The patient in Figure 9-6 is a runner with bilateral groin pain whose MRI findings show a lesion that can be referred to as which *one* of the following?

(A) Adductor longus strain
(B) Rectus abdominis/adductor aponeurotic plate disruption
(C) Bilateral inguinal hernia
(D) Gilmore groin

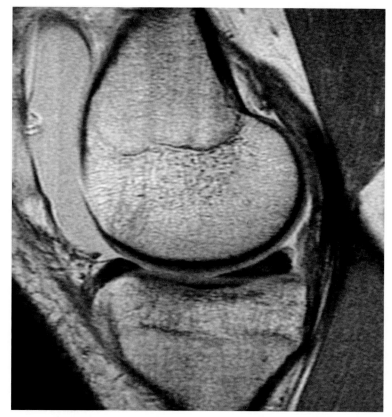

Figure 10-1. Knee. MRI. Fast spin-echo (FSE). Sagittal plane.

Question 46

You are shown a single sagittal fast spin-echo MR image (Figure 10-1) of the knee. The patient is a 33-year-old woman who presented after trauma. Which *one* of the following is the MOST likely diagnosis?

(A)   Meniscocapsular injury/separation
(B)   Parameniscal cyst
(C)   Medial collateral ligament bursitis
(D)   Joint effusion with fluid in the joint recess
(E)   Meniscal flounce

QUESTION 47: MARK YOUR ANSWER
SHEET WITH THE ONE BEST ANSWER
FROM THE OPTIONS PROVIDED.

47. Concerning meniscocapsular separation, which *one* of the following is true?

(A) It is most common on the lateral side.
(B) Prognosis is poor without surgical treatment.
(C) MRI is highly accurate in the diagnosis of meniscocapsular separation.
(D) Fluid between deep and superficial fibers of MCL is diagnostic.
(E) Irregularity of posterior meniscal margin on sagittal images is one sign of meniscocapsular separation on MRI.

QUESTIONS 48 AND 49:
MARK YOUR ANSWER SHEET TRUE
(T) OR FALSE (F) FOR EACH OF THE
RESPONSE CHOICES.

48. Concerning the anatomy of the meniscus:

(A) The lateral meniscus is larger than the medial meniscus.
(B) The circumferential fibers resist hoop stress and are concentrated in the inner third.
(C) The medial meniscus is relatively mobile compared to the lateral meniscus.
(D) The peripheral two thirds of the menisci are supplied by the perimeniscal capillary plexus.
(E) Functions of the menisci include distribution of synovial fluid.

49. Concerning meniscal tears:

(A) The lateral meniscus is most frequently involved.
(B) Grade II signal is linear and extends to the articular surface.
(C) MRI sensitivity is higher for lateral meniscal tears.
(D) Medial meniscal tears are more common in the setting of an acute ACL tear.
(E) The incidence of meniscal tears in asymptomatic patients with radiographic evidence of OA has been found to be as high as 60%.

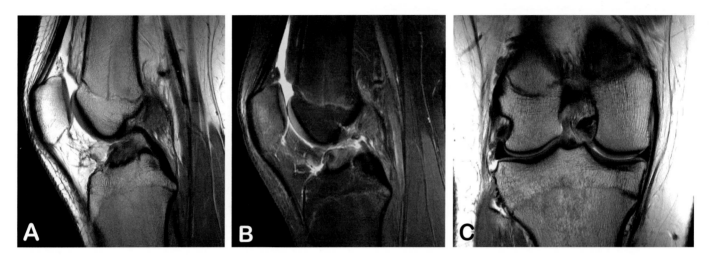

Figure 11-1. Knee. MRI. (A) Intermediate-weighted. Sagittal plane (B) Fluid-sensitive. Sagittal plane. (C) Intermediate-weighted. Coronal plane.

Question 50

A 19-year-old woman presents with knee pain. You are shown (A) sagittal intermediate-weighted, (B) sagittal fluid-sensitive, and (C) coronal intermediate-weighted MR images of her knee (Figure 11-1). Which *one* of the following is the most likely diagnosis?

(A)   Normal anterior cruciate ligament
(B)   Partial-thickness tear of anterior cruciate ligament
(C)   Full-thickness tear of anterior cruciate ligament
(D)   Mucoid degeneration of anterior cruciate ligament
(E)   Cyclops lesion (localized arthrofibrosis)

51. This ancillary finding supports the diagnosis of anterior cruciate ligament tear:

(A) Lateral compartment bone marrow edema
(B) Lateral femoral notch sign
(C) Anterior tibial translation
(D) Buckling of posterior cruciate ligament
(E) Posterior tibial plateau avulsion fracture

52. Concerning mucoid degeneration of the anterior cruciate ligament:

(A) It can be misinterpreted as ligament tear.
(B) It is also called "celery stalk" anterior cruciate ligament.
(C) It is associated with adjacent ganglion cysts.
(D) It is associated with anterior cruciate ligament laxity.
(E) It may be overlooked at arthroscopy.

53. Concerning cyclops lesion (or localized anterior arthrofibrosis):

(A) It is a complication after anterior cruciate ligament repair.
(B) It is asymptomatic.
(C) It characteristically is seen anterior in the intercondylar notch.
(D) It is usually uniformly low signal on MRI.
(E) Synovial sarcoma should be strongly considered in the differential diagnosis.

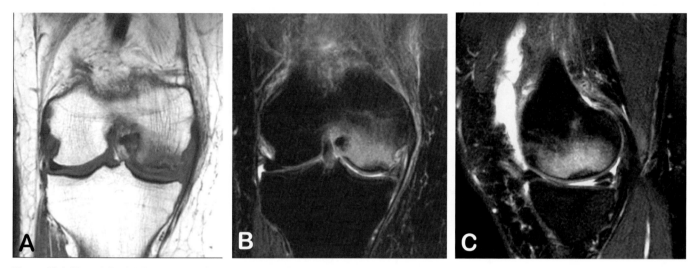

Figure 12-1. Knee. MRI. (A) T1-weighted. Coronal plane. (B) T2-weighted, fat-saturated. Coronal plane. (C) T2-weighted, fat-saturated. Sagittal plane.

Question 54

You are shown coronal T1-weighted, coronal T2-weighted, fat-saturated (FS), and sagittal T2-weighted, fat-saturated MR images of the knee of a 53-year-old woman. With which *one* of the following are the findings MOST consistent?

(A)   Osteomyelitis
(B)   Subchondral insufficiency fracture
(C)   Cartilage loss
(D)   Osteochondritis dissecans
(E)   Acute fracture

55. SONK (spontaneous osteonecrosis of the knee) is an outdated term because:

(A) It is not spontaneous.
(B) It does not necessarily progress to osteo-necrosis.
(C) It does not involve the knee.
(D) Both (A) and (B)

56. Subchondral insufficiency fracture of the knee is associated with:

(A) Lack of osteoarthritis
(B) Meniscal tear
(C) Meniscal debridement
(D) Osteopenia
(E) All of the above

57. Subchondral insufficiency fracture can occur at the tibia as well as the femoral condyle. *True or False?*

58. Subchondral insufficiency fracture at the knee can heal spontaneously. *True or False?*

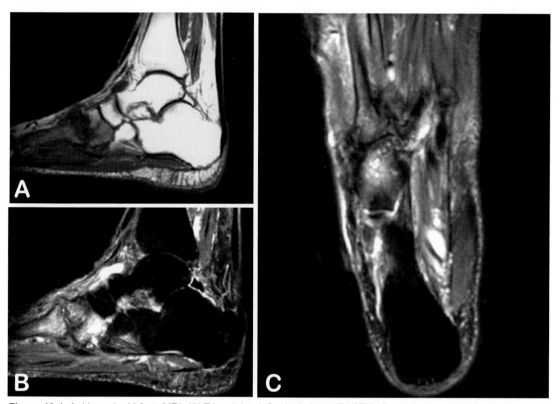

Figure 13-1. Ankle and mid-foot. MRI. (A) T1-weighted. Sagittal plane. (B) STIR. Sagittal plane. (C) T2-weighted, fat-saturated. Axial plane.

Question 59

You are shown three MR images acquired in a diabetic patient who presented with a swollen, erythematous foot. Radiographs were nonspecific. CBC is normal. There is a small skin ulcer. Which *one* of the following is MOST accurate?

(A)   Findings are most consistent with osteomyelitis.
(B)   Findings are most consistent with neuropathic osteoarthropathy.
(C)   MRI cannot differentiate infection from neuropathic disease.
(D)   A bone biopsy should be performed through the ulcer.

60. Findings on MRI that help differentiate neuropathic osteoarthropathy from infection include:

(A) Subchondral cysts
(B) Sinus tract to bone
(C) Fluid collections
(D) Bone marrow edema
(E) Both A and B

61. The BEST single test for evaluation of the foot in a diabetic with ulceration and clinical concern for infection is:

(A) Three-phase bone scan
(B) Radiographs
(C) MRI
(D) Labeled white blood cell scan
(E) Ultrasound

62. Regarding sequences, the *one* LEAST useful for diagnosis of osteomyelitis is:

(A) STIR
(B) T1-weighted, spin-echo
(C) Proton density
(D) T2-weighted, fast spin-echo, fat-suppressed
(E) Gradient-recalled echo (GRE)

63. Regarding use of gadolinium contrast for diagnosis of osteomyelitis on MRI:

(A) It is essential to check creatinine clearance/ glomerular filtration rate prior to contrast administration in diabetic patients and patients over 60.
(B) Contrast should only be given when absolutely necessary.
(C) Contrast can help delineate areas of necrosis, abscesses, and sinus tracts, and can differentiate inflammation from "bland" soft tissue edema.
(D) Contrast is best reserved for preoperative cases.
(E) All of the above.

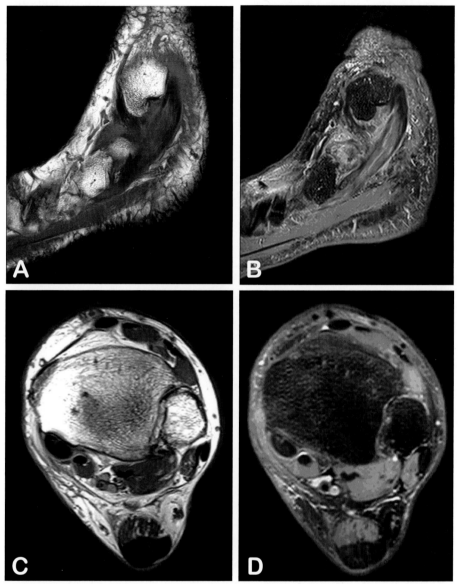

Figure 14-1. Left ankle. MRI. (A) T1-weighted. Sagittal plane. (B) T2-weighted, fat-suppressed. Sagittal plane. (C) T1-weighted. Axial plane. (D) T2-weighted, fat-suppressed. Axial plane.

Question 64

You are shown four images (Figure 14-1) from the left ankle MRI examination of a 56-year-old woman who presented with a history of chronic left ankle pain. Which *one* of the following is the MOST likely diagnosis?

(A)   Medial malleolar fracture
(B)   Flexor hallux longus tear
(C)   Posterior tibialis dysfunction
(D)   Ankle joint arthropathy

65. Regarding MRI use in fractures:

(A) It is useful in detecting stress fractures.

(B) A rim of fluid signal around an osteo-chondral fragment indicates it is a stable fragment.

(C) Signal changes within surrounding bone marrow are due to hemorrhage.

(D) There are no specific distinguishing features of new compared to old fractures.

66. Regarding flexor hallucis longus (FHL) tendon:

(A) Complete tears are common in patients with active lifestyles.

(B) A mechanism of injury is constant repetitive extension movement, which stretches the tendon.

(C) Long-standing inflammation may lead to hallux rigidus.

(D) Fluid in the synovial fluid is always abnormal and indicates that pathology is present.

67. Regarding ankle joint arthropathy:

(A) In neuropathic arthropathy, T1-weighted images demonstrate high signal intensity.

(B) It is a more common site of involvement by rheumatoid arthritis than is the fore-foot.

(C) Hemophilic arthropathy results in low signal foci throughout the synovium.

(D) Most cases due to osteoarthritis do not have a specific cause.

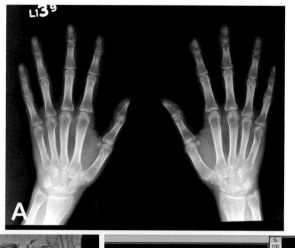

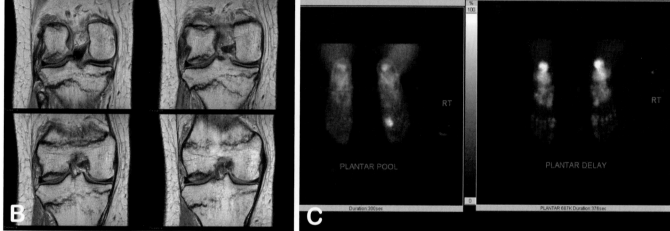

Figure 15-1. (A) Radiograph. Right and left hands. Posteroanterior view. (B) MRI. Right knee. Proton-density-weighted. Coronal view. (C) Three-phase Tc-99m methylene diphosphonate bone scan. Plantar view. Pool- and delayed-phase images.

Question 68

This 44-year-old woman had a 3-year history of pain in her back and throughout the lower extremities. She used a walker and had been on disability for 2 years. Evaluation included an electromyogram and a thigh muscle biopsy, both of which yielded negative results You are shown a posteroanterior radiograph of both hands (Figure 15-1A), a coronal MR image of the knee (Figure 15-1B), and a bone scan (Figure 15-1C). Which *one* of the following is the MOST likely diagnosis?

(A)   X-linked hypophosphatemia
(B)   Fanconi syndrome
(C)   Oncogenic osteomalacia
(D)   Autosomal dominant hypophosphatemic rickets
(E)   Hypophosphatasia

69. Which *one* of the following is the BEST next step in the workup for a patient with osteomalacia with low serum phosphate levels, evidence of renal phosphate wasting, no family history of a metabolic bone disorder, and no identifiable nutritional etiology?

(A) Whole-body delayed-phase bone scan
(B) Whole-body CT
(C) "Whole-body" MRI
(D) In-111 pentetreotide imaging

70. Which *one* of the following is the MOST commonly diagnosed tumor or process in a patient with oncogenic osteomalacia?

(A) Giant cell tumor of tendon sheath, bone, or soft tissues
(B) Angiofibroma
(C) Osteosarcoma
(D) Hemangiopericytoma
(E) Fibrous dysplasia

71. Which *one* of the following is the gold standard for the diagnosis of osteomalacia?

(A) Radiographic skeletal survey
(B) Nuclear medicine bone scan
(C) Bone biopsy
(D) Bone densitometry

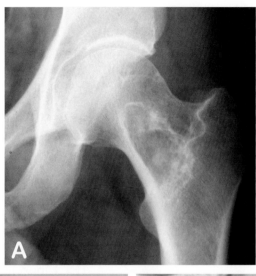

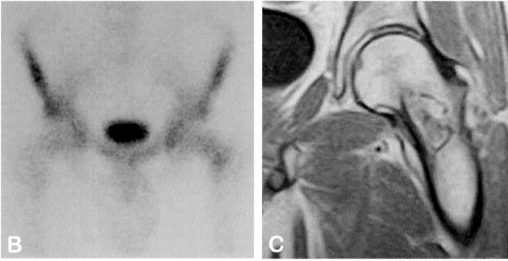

Figure 16-1. (A) Left femur. Radiograph. Anteroposterior position. (B) Pelvis. Technetium-99m MDP bone scan. Anteroposterior position. (C) Left femur. MRI. T1-weighted (TR/TE; 650/25). Coronal plane.

Question 72

A 48-year-old man presented with a 2-month history of vague groin pain. You are shown an anteroposterior radiograph of his left femur, a corresponding image from a technetium-99m MDP bone scan, and an MR image (Figure 16-1). Which *one* of the following is the MOST likely diagnosis for the lesion shown in Figure 16-1?

(A)   Fibrous dysplasia
(B)   Nonossifying fibroma (fibroxanthoma)
(C)   Intraosseous lipoma
(D)   Osteoblastoma
(E)   Lymphoma

73. Regarding intraosseous lipoma:

(A) It is often perceived as a rare lesion.
(B) It is likely a congenital lesion.
(C) It is a precursor to liposarcoma.
(D) It is a simple histological diagnosis for the pathologist.
(E) Patients are invariably symptomatic.

74. Imaging findings in intraosseous lipoma:

(A) Must show the lesion to be entirely adipose tissue
(B) Must show the majority of the lesion to be adipose tissue
(C) May show no or almost no adipose tissue in the lesion
(D) May show cysts within the lesion
(E) May show varying amounts of calcification/ossification

75. Regarding intraosseous lipoma:

(A) It is most common in the calcaneus.
(B) It is almost invariably seen in children.
(C) Stage 3 lesions are the least common.
(D) The radiographic appearance is always specific for a benign mass.
(E) Calcaneal lesions typically have thin sclerotic margins with central calcification or ossification.

76. The differential diagnosis for the radiographic findings of intraosseous lipoma would include:

(A) Fibrous dysplasia
(B) Simple bone cyst
(C) Nonossifying fibroma (fibroxanthoma)
(D) Enchondroma
(E) Liposclerosing myxofibrous tumor (LSMFT)

77. Regarding intraosseous lipoma:

(A) Patients typically have multiple lesions.
(B) Upper extremity lesions are most common.
(C) Metaphyseal involvement is typical.
(D) MR imaging of Stage 2 lesions will often show cysts within lesions.
(E) Lesions are histologically identical to soft tissue lipoma.

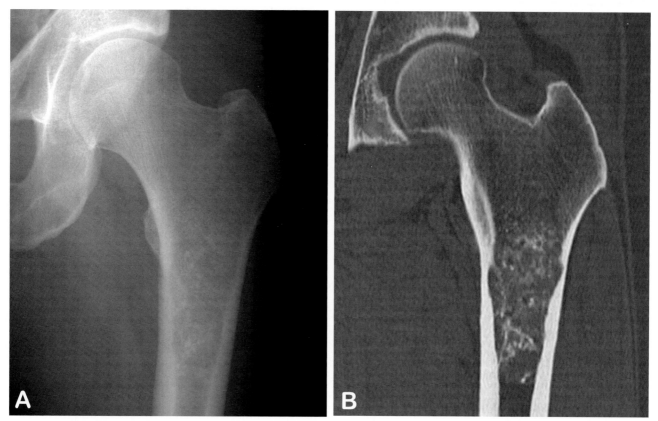

Figure 17-1. Left femur. (A) Radiograph. Anteroposterior view. (B) CT. Reformatted in coronal plane. No IV contrast.

Question 78

A 44-year-old man presented with increasing, vague groin pain of several months duration. You are shown a radiograph and a reformatted coronal CT, without contrast (Figure 17-1). Which *one* of the following is the MOST likely diagnosis for the lesion shown in Figure 17-1?

(A)   Enchondroma
(B)   Bone infarct
(C)   Dedifferentiated chondrosarcoma
(D)   Chondrosarcoma
(E)   Fibrocartilagenous dysplasia

79. Regarding intramedullary chondrosarcoma:

(A) It is common in children.
(B) Most patients will present with pain.
(C) Pathologic fracture is not uncommon.
(D) It is most common in the small bones of the hands.
(E) Long bone involvement is usually limited to the diaphysis.

80. Regarding the distinction between enchondroma and chondrosarcoma:

(A) It is usually made easily based on percutaneous biopsy.
(B) It is usually made easily on clinical grounds.
(C) It is often a difficult distinction for pathologists.
(D) In general, chondrosarcomas are larger than enchondromas.
(E) Epiphyseal involvement is not a useful discriminating feature.

81. On radiographs of patients with long bone cartilage tumors:

(A) Chondrosarcomas usually demonstrate mineralization.
(B) In general, high-grade chondrosarcomas have more extensive matrix mineralization than low-grade chondrosarcomas.
(C) The presence of scalloping is more important than the depth of scalloping in determining malignancy.
(D) The longitudinal extent of scalloping is more important than the depth of scalloping in determining malignancy.

(E) The same criteria used for analyzing lesions of the small bones of the hands and feet can be used for assessing lesions of the long bones.

82. Regarding the imaging of intramedullary chondrosarcoma:

(A) Lesions generally do not show increased radionuclide accumulation on scintigraphy.
(B) CT is especially useful in determining the extent and depth of endosteal scalloping.
(C) The presence and pattern of mineralization on CT imaging is useful in distinguishing enchondroma from chondrosarcoma.
(D) The nonmineralized portions of low-grade chondrosarcoma will demonstrate a low attenuation on CT imaging.
(E) The nonmineralized portions will show peripheral and septal contrast enhancement on CT imaging.

83. Regarding the MR imaging of intramedullary chondrosarcoma:

(A) Identification of entrapped foci of yellow marrow on T1-weighted images within a cartilage lesion virtually excludes the diagnosis of chondrosarcoma.
(B) The nonmineralized hyaline cartilage within a chondrosarcoma may show a cyst-like signal intensity.
(C) The extent and depth of endosteal scalloping cannot be adequately assessed on MR imaging.
(D) The pattern of contrast enhancement on MR imaging can reliably distinguish enchondroma from chondrosarcoma.
(E) The rate of contrast enhancement on MR imaging has been accepted as a standard method to distinguish enchondroma from chondrosarcoma.

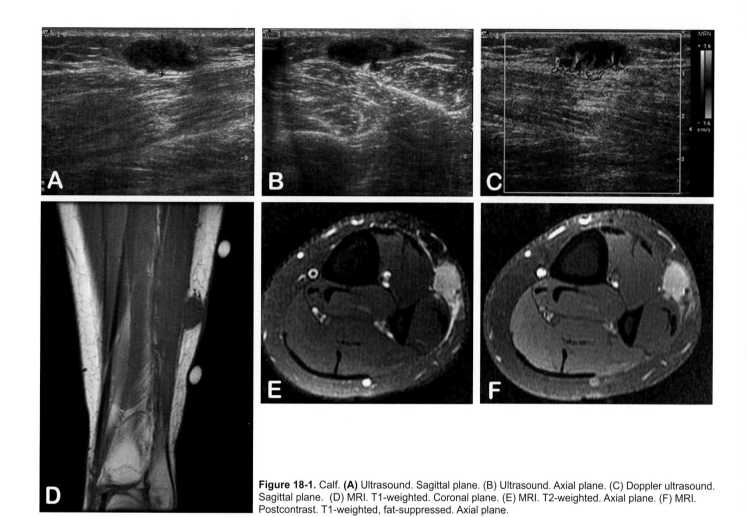

Figure 18-1. Calf. **(A)** Ultrasound. Sagittal plane. (B) Ultrasound. Axial plane. (C) Doppler ultrasound. Sagittal plane. (D) MRI. T1-weighted. Coronal plane. (E) MRI. T2-weighted. Axial plane. (F) MRI. Postcontrast. T1-weighted, fat-suppressed. Axial plane.

Question 84

A 19-year-old woman presented with a lump at the lateral aspect of the distal lower limb. It was slightly tender on palpation, and there was no redness or discoloration of the overlying skin. You are shown three ultrasound images and three MR images (Figure 19-1). Which *one* of the following is the MOST likely diagnosis?

(A)   Soft tissue sarcoma
(B)   Foreign body granuloma
(C)   Fibromatosis
(D)   Granular cell tumor
(E)   Hematoma

85. Regarding fibromatosis:

(A) It can cause metastasis.

(B) The superficial form is more aggressive than the deep form.

(C) Palmar fibromatosis causes retraction more often than plantar fibromatosis.

(D) Plantar fibromatosis is a synonym for plantar fasciitis.

(E) Palmar fibromatosis and plantar fibromatosis are often bilateral.

86. Regarding subcutaneous lipomas:

(A) They represent the most common subcutaneous mass.

(B) At least two-thirds of superficial lipomas have a characteristic ultrasound pattern and do not require further workup.

(C) Marked vascular flow on Doppler virtually excludes the diagnosis of lipoma.

(D) Follow-up of subcutaneous lipomas is recommended to rule out malignant transformation.

87. Regarding benign/malignant characterization of subcutaneous nodules:

(A) Subcutaneous benign nodules are 5 times more common than subcutaneous malignant nodules.

(B) Absence of fat in a mass virtually excludes liposarcoma.

(C) Posterior enhancement of a subcutaneous nodule on ultrasound is not a reliable sign that it is benign.

(D) Malignant peripheral nerve sheath tumors are 10 times more common in patients with neurofibromatosis 1 than in the general population.

(E) Neurofibromatosis 1 is associated with numerous neoplasms, including gastrointestinal stromal tumors.

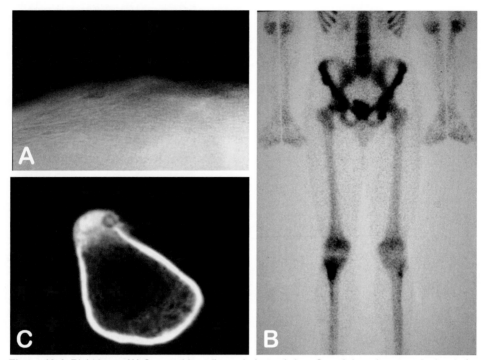

Figure 19-1. Right knee. (A) Cross-table radiograph. Lateral view. Coned-down image at the level of the tibial tuberosity. (B) Delayed-phase technetium bone scan. Increased uptake is identified in the region of the right tibial tuberosity. (C) CT. Axial plane at the proximal tibia.

Question 88

This 20-year-old man presented with knee pain. You are shown a lateral radiograph of the knee (Figure 19-1A), a technetium bone scan delayed image (Figure 19-1B) and an unenhanced axial CT scan (Figure 19-1C). Which *one* of the following is the MOST likely diagnosis?

(A)   Cortical abscess
(B)   Stress fracture
(C)   Cortical hemangioma
(D)   Osteoid osteoma

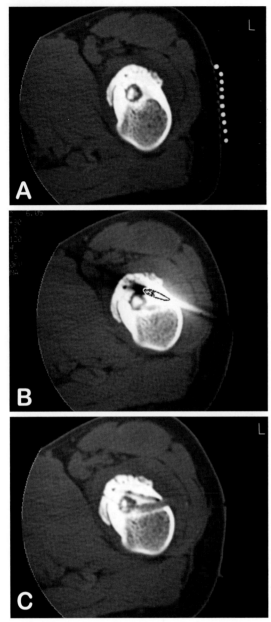

Figure 19-6. CT. Left proximal femur. Axial plane.

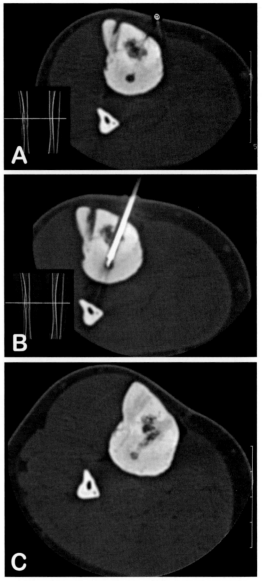

Figure 19-8. CT. Axial plane through the right mid-tibia.

89. The diagnosis of osteoid osteoma in this 25-year-old woman with left hip pain was made based upon clinical and radiological criteria. Thermocoagulation was performed successfully through a lateral approach (two electrode positions were used, corresponding to the "double track" present after thermocoagulation). Which *one* of the following is the MOST likely routine heating time for the thermocoagulation of an osteoid osteoma per electrode position (the electrode is placed in different positions across the osteoid osteoma to ensure complete ablation)?

(A) Four minutes at 90° C
(B) Two minutes at 90° C
(C) Four minutes at 150° C
(D) Ten minutes at 45° C

90. In this 19-year-old woman successful thermocoagulation of an osteoid osteoma in the right mid-tibia was performed. Axial CT images before and after successful thermocoagulation (Figure19-8) are shown. Select the *one* MOST appropriate answer to the question below. After successful thermocoagulation for osteoid osteoma with a routine noncooled tip (5mm exposed tip) the likelihood of advanced bone healing (complete to near-complete ossification of the nidus) on CT scan 6 to 12 months later, is around:

(A) 0 percent for successfully treated patients
(B) 20 percent for successfully treated patients
(C) 50 percent for successfully treated patients
(D) 75 percent for successfully treated patients

Bone Disease

Fifth Series

Test and Syllabus

TABLE OF CONTENTS

The Table of Contents is placed in this unusual location so that the reader will not be distracted by information that helps to answer the questions before completing the test. A detailed index of the topics considered in this syllabus is provided (beginning on page 203) for further reference.

Bone Disease

Fifth Series

Syllabus

Case 1

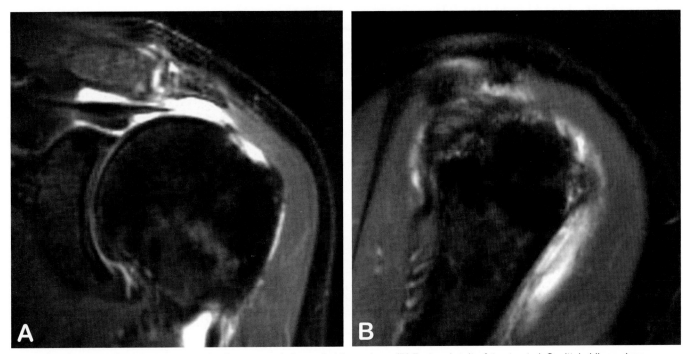

Figure 1-1. Shoulder. MRI. (A) Proton-density, fat-saturated. Coronal oblique plane. (B) Proton-density, fat-saturated. Sagittal oblique plane.

Question 1

You are shown two images (Figure 1-1) from the shoulder MR examination of a 55-year-old man who presented with shoulder pain and decreased range of motion. Which *one* of the following is the MOST likely diagnosis?

(A) Full-thickness supraspinatus tendon tear
(B) High-grade, bursal-sided, partial-thickness supraspinatus tendon tear
(C) Low-grade, bursal-sided, partial-thickness supraspinatus tendon tear
(D) Intrasubstance type supraspinatus tendon tear
(E) Tendinosis of the supraspinatus tendon

David P. Fessell, M.D.

Rotator Cuff Injury

Question 1

Which *one* of the following is the MOST likely diagnosis?

(A) Full-thickness supraspinatus tendon tear
(B) High-grade, bursal-sided, partial-thickness supraspinatus tendon tear
(C) Low-grade, bursal-sided, partial-thickness supraspinatus tendon tear
(D) Intrasubstance type supraspinatus tendon tear
(E) Tendinosis of the supraspinatus tendon

This patient's coronal oblique proton-density, fat-saturated MRI of the shoulder (Figure 1-2) shows abnormal fluid intensity signal in the expected location of the distal supraspinatus tendon in both the coronal oblique and sagittal oblique planes. The tendon is disrupted from the bursal surface to the articular surface. The findings are consistent with a full-thickness supraspinatus tendon tear **(Option (A) is correct).**

In the United States, failure of the rotator cuff results in over 4.5 million physician visits per year. While

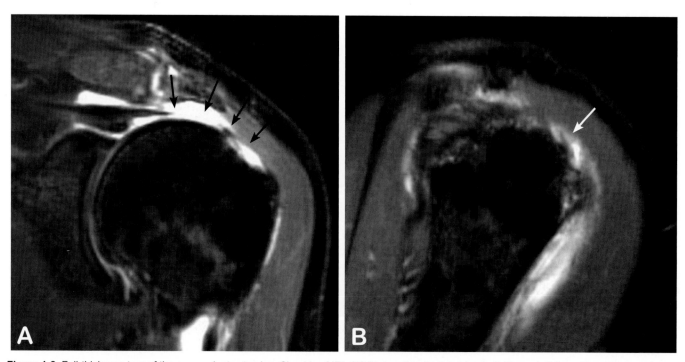

Figure 1-2. Full-thickness tear of the supraspinatus tendon. Shoulder. MRI. (A) Proton-density, fat-saturated. Coronal oblique view. There is abnormal fluid intensity signal (arrows) in the expected location of the distal supraspinatus tendon. The tendon is disrupted from the bursal surface to the articular surface. (B) Proton-density, fat-saturated. Sagittal oblique view. There is abnormal fluid intensity signal (white arrow) in the expected location of the distal supraspinatus tendon with absence of the tendon noted when compared to the adjacent infraspinatus tendon.

tears can be from acute trauma, the more common etiology is age-related wear and tear, typically starting at the anterior aspect of the articular surface of the supraspinatus tendon. If untreated, the natural history is one of gradual progression. The tendons (supraspinatus, infraspinatus, subscapularis, and teres minor) of the rotator cuff work together to produce "balanced compressive forces," which provide stability and optimal function. Tears can lead to pain and loss of strength, mobility, and stability.

Radiographs can be helpful in detecting chronic full-thickness tears of the supraspinatus and infraspinatus tendons, if marked narrowing of the acromiohumeral distance is noted. In adults, the normal acromiohumeral distance is greater than 6 mm and usually closer to 1 cm. In cases of long-standing tears of the supraspinatus and infraspinatus tendons, the humeral head articulates with the acromion, with coexisting degenerative change. This condition is called rotator cuff arthropathy.

MR imaging is commonly used to evaluate the rotator cuff of the shoulder (Figure 1-3A). It provides global imaging of the anatomy and pathology of the shoulder, including the tendons, muscles, joint, and bone marrow. With MR imaging, a tendon tear is seen as tendon discontinuity or fluid intensity signal, involving the tendon on proton density-, T2-, or other fluid-weighted sequences in which fluid appears bright or high signal.

MR imaging is by far the most expensive modality used to evaluate the rotator cuff and its availability is variable. Most patients can tolerate MR imaging; however, some patients experience claustrophobia and require premedication. Open MR magnets may also help such patients complete the MR imaging sequences. Some patients, however, may also have pacemakers, aneurysm clips, or other contraindications to MR imaging. An additional limitation for MR is the fact that dynamic imaging during joint motion, which can be helpful in evaluating for impingement or for biceps subluxation or dislocation, cannot be used with conventional MR imaging.

Ultrasound is increasingly being used to evaluate the supraspinatus and rotator cuff tendons of the shoulder (Figure 1-3B). Ultrasound excels at imaging superficial tendons and has higher resolution than MR imaging for superficial structures. Advantages of ultrasound include direct correlation with the site of symptoms and pain, the opportunity to perform dynamic maneuvers during joint motion, considerably lower cost compared to MR imaging, and widely available equipment. Disadvantages include the learning curve and a current lack of diagnostic medical sonographers experienced in performing shoulder sonography and radiologists who are familiar with musculoskeletal sonography. At sonography, a tear is seen as anechoic or hypoechoic discontinuity of the normally echogenic and fibrillar tendon fibers (Figure 1-4).

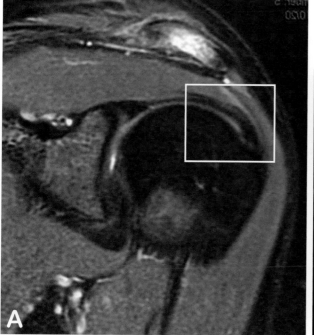
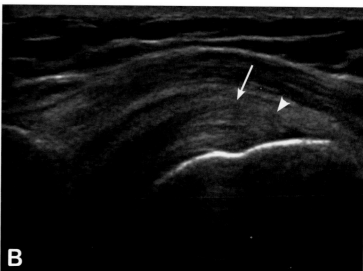

Figure 1-3. Normal supraspinatus tendon. MRI. Shoulder. (A) Proton-density, fat-saturated. Coronal oblique view. The supraspinatus tendon is low signal and is intact at its insertion on the greater tuberosity. (B) Longitudinal ultrasound image (along the long axis of the tendon) corresponding to the region in the box in panel A. The supraspinatus tendon is fibrillar, linear and echogenic (arrow). It is intact at its insertion (arrowhead) on the greater tuberosity.

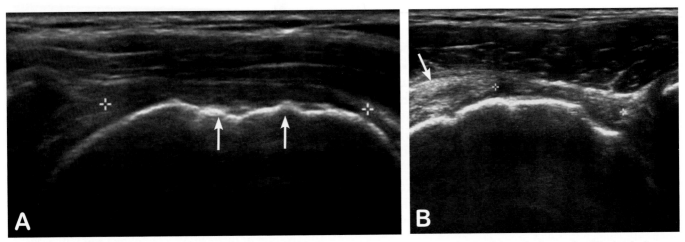

Figure 1-4. Full-thickness tear of the supraspinatus tendon. Ultrasound. Shoulder. (A) Longitudinal image (along the long axis of the tendon), equivalent to the coronal oblique image in Figure 1-1. There is absence of the tendon, with echogenic debris noted (between the + cursors) as well as cortical irregularity at the expected location of the distal supraspinatus tendon (arrows). The tendon is disrupted from the bursal surface to the articular surface. (B) Transverse image (along the short axis of the tendon) equivalent to the sagittal image in Figure 1-1. There is abnormal, mixed echogenicity debris in the expected location of the distal supraspinatus tendon (between the + cursors). The tendon is absent. This area may be compared to the image of the adjacent infraspinatus tendon (arrow).

With standard shoulder arthrography, contrast is injected into the glenohumeral joint, and radiographs are obtained after injection to assess for a rotator cuff tear. Standard arthrography only places contrast in the glenohumeral joint and cannot detect bursal-sided, partial-thickness tears. The procedure is invasive and provides very limited assessment of the shoulder compared to MR imaging or ultrasound. With the advent of MR imaging and ultrasound, standard arthrography has essentially been superseded. With MR arthrography of the shoulder, routine shoulder arthrography is performed with injection of a dilute gadolinium solution, followed immediately by MR imaging of the shoulder. MR arthrography is most often used when a labral abnormality is of clinical concern. MR arthrography may also be helpful to visualize more subtle articular-sided, partial-thickness tears of the supraspinatus tendon.

Partial-thickness supraspinatus tendon tears can be bursal-sided or articular-sided. Such tears can be low-grade (involving less than 50% of the tendon thickness) or high-grade (involving greater than 50% of the tendon thickness). With a bursal-sided, partial-thickness tear, the articular-sided tendon fibers are intact **(Option (B) is incorrect)**. If a distal bursal-sided tear is

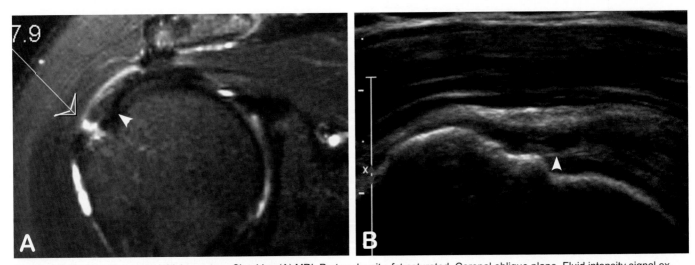

Figure 1-5. Bursal-sided, partial-thickness tear. Shoulder. (A) MRI. Proton-density, fat-saturated. Coronal oblique plane. Fluid intensity signal extends from the bursal surface to the cortex of the greater tuberosity (arrow). Intact fibers on the articular side are noted (arrowhead), consistent with a partial-thickness tear. A small amount of bursal fluid is also present. (B) Ultrasound (different patient). Longitudinal view along the long axis of the tendon. There is a hypoechoic defect noted in the distal supraspinatus tendon (arrow), at the supraspinatus insertion. Volume loss is noted, and the tendon is disrupted from the bursal surface toward the articular surface with a few articular-sided fibers (arrowhead) remaining intact. Findings are consistent with a very high-grade, bursal-sided, partial-thickness tear.

noted, the medial aspect of the supraspinatus insertion ("footprint") must be scrutinized to determine if any articular-sided fibers are present. If such fibers are present, the tear is a partial-thickness, bursal-sided tear (Figure 1-5). If the tendon defect extends from the bursal surface through the articular surface of the tendon, a full-thickness tear is present. Orthopedic surgeons are increasingly more often treating partial-thickness tears that show disruption of as little as 25% to 30% of the tendon thickness, i.e. partial-thickness tears.

If a tendon defect extends from the articular surface of the supraspinatus tendon toward the bursal surface with intact bursal-sided fibers, then an articular-sided,

partial-thickness tear is present (Figure 1-6). No intact bursal-sided fibers are present in the test case (**Option (C) is incorrect**). Articular-sided partial tears are more common than bursal-sided partial-thickness tears. A "rim rent" tear is a unique type of articular-sided tear located at the extreme anterior aspect of the supraspinatus tendon at the most medial aspect of the insertion on the greater tuberosity (Figure 1-7). This "leading edge" of the supraspinatus tendon should be given extra attention and scrutiny when evaluating the rotator cuff. Special patient positions (modified Crass) with the palm of the hand on the hip can aid ultrasound evaluation of this region (see Suggested Reading #12).

On proton-density or T2-weighted images, fluid intensity signal that is located in the substance of the supraspinatus tendon but does not extend to the bursal or articular surface is consistent with an intrasubstance or interstitial tear. In the test case, no normal distal supraspinatus tendon is seen, and the tendon is discontinuous (**Option (D) is incorrect**). At ultrasound, an interstitial tear is noted as a hypoechoic or anechoic region within the substance of the tendon, without extension to the bursal or articular surfaces.

On proton-density or T2-weighted MR sequences, increased tendon signal that does not reach the intensity of fluid signal may be due to tendinosis (Figure 1-8A). At ultrasound, there is loss of the normal, fibrillar echotexture of the tendon (Figure 1-8B). Such tendons may also demonstrate tendon thickening without

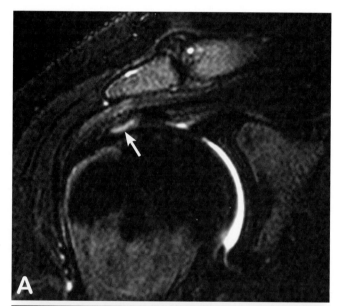

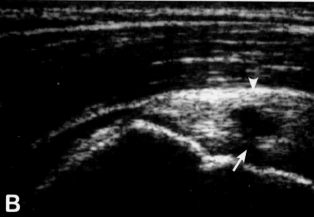

Figure 1-6. Articular-sided, partial-thickness tears. (A) MRI. Proton-density, fat-saturated. Coronal oblique view. A low-to-moderate-grade, articular-sided, partial-thickness tear is seen (arrow). (B) Ultrasound (different patient). Longitudinal view along the long axis of the tendon, equivalent to the imaging plane in Figure 1-4A. There is a hypoechoic defect noted in the distal supraspinatus tendon (arrow). The tendon is disrupted from the articular surface toward the bursal surface with intact fibers at the most superficial aspect of the bursal surface (arrowhead), consistent with a high-grade, articular-sided, partial-thickness tear.

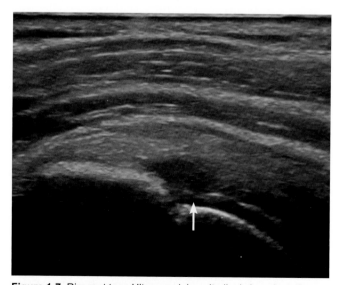

Figure 1-7. Rim-rent tear. Ultrasound. Longitudinal view along the long axis of the tendon. There is a hypoechoic defect noted in the distal supraspinatus tendon (arrow), at the very anterior and medial aspect of the supraspinatus insertion. The tendon is disrupted from the articular surface toward the bursal surface with less than 50% of the tendon thickness involved. Findings are consistent with a low- to moderate-grade, articular-sided, partial-thickness tear. At this location the tear is also called a "rim-rent tear."

a defect or discontinuity of the tendon **(Option (E) is incorrect).** "Tendinosis," is the preferred term for what used to be called "tendonitis," since inflammatory cells are not present in these tendons at pathology. Increased signal on T1 images, or with sequences using a TE of less than 60, can be due to magic angle artifact. This artifact can occur when imaging curved structures such as the tendons of the shoulder or ankle and can be noted when the main magnetic field is at

55 degrees to the structure being imaged. Lack of fluid signal on T2-weighted sequences (TE of greater than 60), and lack of tendon thickening helps prevent misinterpretation magic angle artifact with the pathologic tendinosis.

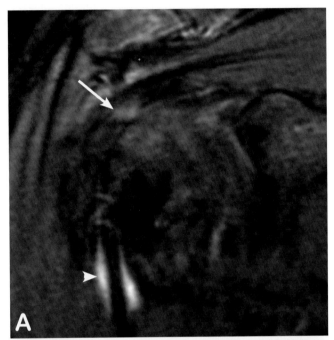

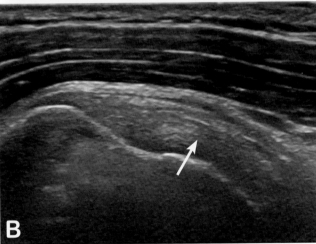

Figure 1-8. Tendinosis. Shoulder. (A) MRI. Proton-density, fat-saturated. Coronal oblique view. A vague region of mildly increased signal is noted in the distal supraspinatus tendon (arrow). Signal intensity is lower than that of the fluid in the biceps tendon sheath (arrowhead). At arthroscopy (performed for acromioplasty) the tendon was inspected, and no tear was noted. Findings are consistent with tendinosis. (B) Ultrasound (different patient). Longitudinal image along the long axis of the tendon. There is loss of much of the normal linear, echogenic, fibrillar architecture without volume loss or tendon disruption (arrow). Findings are consistent with tendinosis.

Question 2

Which *one* of the following is the MOST likely level of accuracy that should be expected for MR imaging of the type of tendon pathology depicted in Question 1?

(A) 50% to 60%
(B) 60% to 70%
(C) 70% to 80%
(D) 80% to 90%
(E) 90% or greater

MR imaging utilizing a 1.5T magnet, a dedicated shoulder coil, coronal oblique and sagittal oblique proton density- or T2-weighted sequences with fat saturation, and an experienced interpreter should routinely yield accuracies of greater than 90% for full-thickness tears of the supraspinatus tendon **(Option (E) is correct).** Accuracies of 50% to 90% are lower than those that have been shown in the literature and lower than the accuracies that should be obtained by an experienced interpreter **(Options (A-D) are incorrect).** Experience of the interpreter, familiarity with pitfalls, and technically optimal images are needed to obtain optimal diagnostic accuracy with MR imaging. Partial thickness tears are more variable in their pathologic presentation, ranging from very low-grade tears with minimal tendon disruption to very high-grade tears with only a few wispy fibers remaining intact. Thus the imaging accuracy for partial tears would also be expected to be more variable. MR imaging has a lower accuracy for detecting partial-thickness tears than for full-thickness tears.

Question 3

Which *one* of the following is the MOST accurate modality for detecting full-thickness supraspinatus tendon tears?

(A) MR imaging
(B) Ultrasound
(C) With experienced interpreters, they are equally accurate.

Several recent studies demonstrate equivalent accuracy for MR imaging and ultrasound in the detection of full-thickness tears of the supraspinatus **(Option (C) is correct).** As with MR imaging, absence of the tendon is noted with sonography of a full-thickness tear (Figure 1-4). To achieve the best accuracy for either MR imaging or ultrasound, technical factors must be optimized. Technical factors for ultrasound include high-requency ultrasound transducers, (12 MHz or higher, depending on the patient's body habitus), optimal gain and focal zone settings, and an experienced sonographer. Experience of the MR and ultrasound interpreters cannot be underestimated. In head-to-head comparison studies with both modalities examining the same patients, using surgical correlation, experienced sonographers, and experienced MR interpreters, the accuracies were equivalent for full-thickness tears **(Options (A) and (B) are incorrect).** Variable accuracy has been reported for both MR imaging and sonographic evaluation of partial-thickness supraspinatus tendon tears. In more recent studies, however, accuracies for both modalities have improved.

ing superior to a line which connects the tips of the scapula on a sagittal image (Figure 1-9). Ultrasound can easily and quickly assess the rotator cuff muscles, including the muscles of the opposite shoulder, which aids assessment of subtle atrophy (Figure 1-10).

The size of a rotator cuff tear has implications for the decision to perform surgery, the type of surgery, and rate of tear recurrence. Larger tears have a poorer prognosis, especially if the largest dimension of the tear exceeds 4 cm **(Option (B) is true).** Primary repair may not be possible with large or massive tears (greater than 4 cm in greatest dimension). Recovery of strength is also slower with these larger tears. Dimensions of the tear should be measured in medial to lateral dimension (measured on the oblique coronal plane), and in the anterior to posterior dimension (measured on the oblique sagittal plane).

Associated biceps brachii or subscapularis tendon pathology is often present in the setting of rotator cuff tears (Figure 1-11). Such pathology would be treated during the same surgery as the supraspinatus tendon tear, and its presence may affect the decision to perform open or arthroscopic surgery. Thus, preoperative imaging diagnosis aids operative planning and treatment

Question 4

The treatment of a supraspinatus tendon tear can be affected by:

(A) Muscle atrophy
(B) Dimensions of the tear (medial to lateral and anterior to posterior)
(C) Thickness of the torn tendon end
(D) Associated pathology in the infraspinatus tendon, biceps brachii long-head tendon, and subscapularis tendon
(E) Presence of an os acromiale

Muscle atrophy is an important factor in the outcome of rotator cuff tears. A poorer outcome (including increased likelihood that the tear will recur) after cuff repair can be expected if muscle atrophy is present. Some surgeons will not operate if high-grade muscle atrophy is noted **(Option (A) is true).** Many classifications exist for determining muscle atrophy. These include the tangent line method and the Goutallier classification. The Goutallier classification is commonly used in orthopedics. A Goutallier Grade 0 has no fatty deposits, Grade 1 has some fatty streaks, Grade 2 has more muscle than fat, Grade 3 has equal muscle and fat, and Grade 4 has more fat than muscle. The tangent line method is commonly used in radiology, with the supraspinatus muscle normally extend-

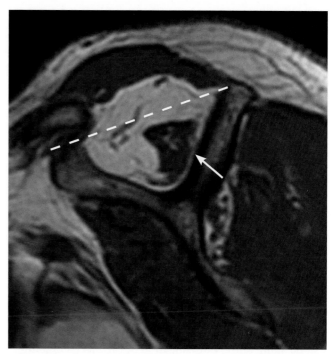

Figure 1-9. Marked volume loss of the supraspinatus muscle. MRI. Shoulder. (A) T1-weighted, without fat saturation. Sagittal oblique view. The supraspinatus muscle normally fills the fossa of the scapula and extends superficial to a line connecting the tips of the scapula (dotted line). In this case the fossa (arrow) is not filled, consistent with marked supraspinatus muscle atrophy, secondary to a chronic full-thickness tear of the supraspinatus tendon (not shown).

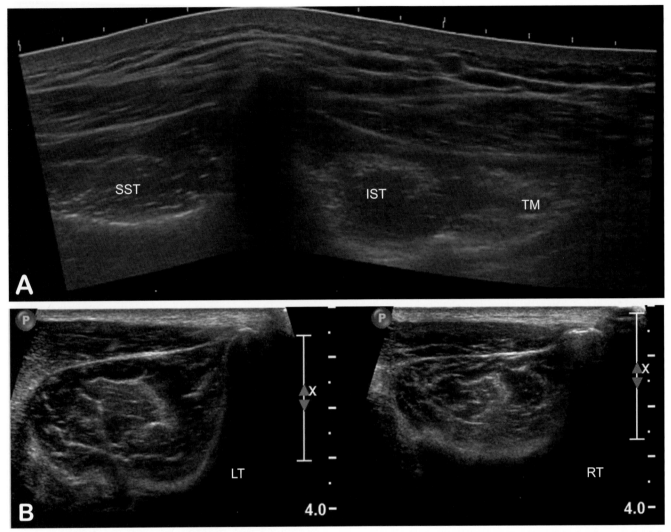

Figure 1-10. Normal and atrophic supraspinatus muscle. Ultrasound. Shoulder. (A) Extended field of view from the supraspinatus fossa to the inferior aspect of the teres minor shows normal rotator cuff muscle volume and echogenicity. (B) Sonography of a normal left supraspinatus muscle (for comparison) and an atrophic right supraspinatus muscle in a patient with a full-thickness tear of the right supraspinatus tendon. SST = supraspinatus, IST = infraspinatus tendon, TM = teres minor, LT = left, RT = right.

(Option (D) is true). In some cases, biceps pathology may be the source of pain, even more so than a rotator cuff tear. There can be a poorer outcome for rotator cuff tears if the biceps tendon is abnormal and if the supraspinatus tear extends to involve the coracohumeral ligament and superior fibers of the subscapularis tendon. The subscapularis tendon is incompletely visualized at arthroscopy. Preoperative imaging can help alert the surgeon to pathology of this tendon and thus aid treatment. If the superior fibers of the subscapularis are torn, there can be subluxation or dislocation of the biceps brachii long head tendon, also contributing to pain or symptoms. Although MR imaging is a static examination, ultrasound can be preformed dynamically during internal and external rotation of the shoulder to assess for biceps brachii subluxation or dislocation as well as impinge-

ment of the supraspinatus tendon during arm abduction.

Os acromiale is the term used when there is no osseous fusion of the acromial apophysis (Figure 1-12). This apophysis has been reported to fuse late, up to age 25 in some patients. It can be a source of impingement for the rotator cuff and can potentially be a source of symptoms after rotator cuff repair if it is not recognized and its existence addressed. In some cases an os acromiale may require surgical fixation prior to rotator cuff repair, especially if it is mobile or impinging on the rotator cuff **(Option (E) is true).** When an os acromiale is present its size should be described (anterior to posterior dimension) along with the amount of displacement from the acromion. Any step-off between the os and the acromion at the bursal surface of the rotator cuff (noted in the sagittal oblique plane) should also be reported. When an os acromiale is noted, the presence of such a step-off may be the most important factor for predicting underlying rotator cuff pathology.

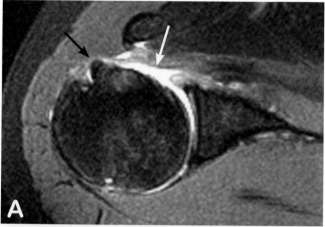

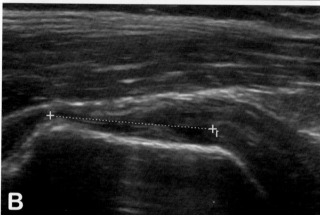

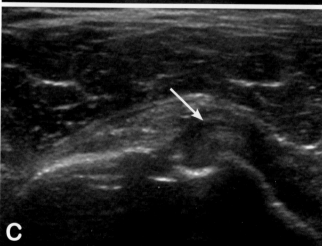

Figure 1-11. Full-thickness subscapularis tendon tear. Shoulder. (A) MRI. Proton- density, fat-saturated. Axial view. Fluid intensity signal is noted at the expected location of the subscapularis tendon (white arrow). Medial subluxation of the biceps tendon is also noted (black arrow). (B) Ultrasound. Longitudinal view along the long axis of the subscapularis tendon. Absence of the tendon is noted with fluid and debris at the expected location of the tendon. (C) Transverse view of the bicipital groove. There is medial subluxation of the tendon (arrow). Such medial subluxation of the biceps tendon can be a source of pain and cause wear, or potentially tear, of the tendon.

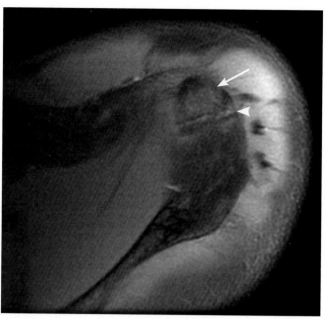

Figure 1-12. Os acromiale. Shoulder. MRI. Proton-density, fat saturated. Axial plane. An os acromiale is present (arrow) with minimal displacement from the acromion (arrowhead).

Suggested Readings

ROTATOR CUFF: GENERAL

1. Morag Y, Jacobson JA, Miller B, De Maeseneer M, Girish G, Jamadar D. MR imaging of rotator cuff injury: what the clinician needs to know. RadioGraphics 2006; 26:1045–1065.

ROTATOR CUFF: MR IMAGING AND ULTRASOUND

2. Dinnes J, Loveman E, McIntyre L, Waugh N. The effectiveness of diagnostic tests for the assessment of shoulder pain due to soft tissue disorders: a systematic review. Health Technol Assess. 2003;7: 1–166.
3. Khoury V, Cardinal E, Brassard P. Atrophy and fatty infiltration of the supraspinatus muscle: sonography versus MRI. AJR Am J Roentgenol. 2008;190:1105–1111.
4. Matsen FA, 3rd. Clinical practice. Rotator-cuff failure. N Engl J Med. 2008;358:2138–2147.
5. Teefey SA, Rubin DA, Middleton WD, Hildebolt CF, Leibold RA, Yamaguchi K. Detection and quantification of rotator cuff tears. Comparison of ultrasonographic, magnetic resonance imaging, and arthroscopic findings in seventy-one consecutive cases. J Bone Joint Surg Am. 2004;86-A:708–716.
6. Vlychou M, Dailiana Z, Fotiadou A, Papanagiotou M, Fezouli-

dis IV, Malizos K. Symptomatic partial rotator cuff tears: diagnostic performance of ultrasound and magnetic resonance imaging with surgical correlation. Acta Radiol. 2009;50:101–105.

ROTATOR CUFF: MR IMAGING

7. Goutallier D, Postel JM, Gleyze P, Leguilloux P, Van Driessche S. Influence of cuff muscle fatty degeneration on anatomic and functional outcomes after simple suture of full-thickness tears. J Shoulder Elbow Surg. 2003;12:550–554.
8. Iannotti JP, Zlatkin MB, Esterhai JL, Kressel HY, Dalinka MK, Spindler KP. Magnetic resonance imaging of the shoulder. Sensitivity, specificity, and predictive value. J Bone Joint Surg Am. 1991;73:17–29.
9. Morag Y, Jacobson JA, Shields G, et al. MR arthrography of rotator interval, long head of the biceps brachii, and biceps pulley of the shoulder. Radiology. 2005;235:21–30.
10. Reinus WR, Shady KL, Mirowitz SA, Totty WG. MR diagnosis of rotator cuff tears of the shoulder: value of using T2-weighted fat-saturated images. AJR Am J Roentgenol. 1995;164:1451–1455.
11. Spencer EE, Jr., Dunn WR, Wright RW, et al. Interobserver agreement in the classification of rotator cuff tears using magnetic resonance imaging. Am J Sports Med. 2008;36:99–103.
12. Vinson EN, Helms CA, Higgins LD. Rim-rent tear of the rotator cuff: a common and easily overlooked partial tear. AJR Am J Roentgenol. 2007;189:943–946.

MUSCULOSKELETAL ULTRASOUND: GENERAL

13. Jacobson, JA. Fundamentals of Musculoskeletal Ultrasound. Saunders. 2007.
14. Nazarian LN. The top 10 reasons musculoskeletal sonography is an important complementary or alternative technique to MRI. AJR Am J Roentgenol. 2008;190:1621–1626.

OS ACROMIALE

15. Ouellette H, Thomas BJ, Kassarjian A, et al. Re-examining the association of os acromiale with supraspinatus and infraspinatus tears. Skeletal Radiol. 2007;36:835–839.
16. Sahajpal D, Strauss EJ, Ishak C, Keyes JM, Joseph G, Jazrawi LM. Surgical management of os acromiale: a case report and review of the literature. Bull NYU Hosp Jt Dis. 2007; 65:312–316.

Case 2

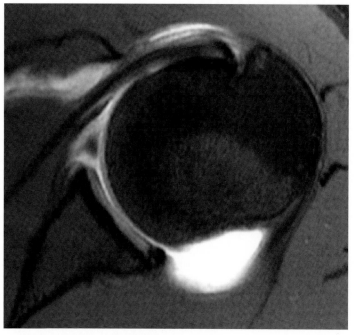

Figure 2-1. Shoulder. MR arthrogram. Lower half of the glenohumeral joint. T1-weighted, fat-suppressed. Axial plane.

Question 5

You are shown an MR image from a 28-year-old man with anterior shoulder instability and pain. The image was obtained at the level of the middle to inferior anterior labrum (Figure 2-1). Which *one* of the following is the MOST likely diagnosis?

(A) Anterior labroligamentous periosteal sleeve avulsion (ALPSA lesion)
(B) Perthes lesion
(C) Bankart lesion
(D) Sublabral foramen
(E) Buford complex

Lynne S. Steinbach, M.D.

Glenohumeral Instability and Associated Labral Pathology

Question 5

Which *one* of the following is the MOST likely diagnosis?

(A) Anterior labroligamentous periosteal sleeve avulsion (ALPSA lesion)
(B) Perthes lesion
(C) Bankart lesion
(D) Sublabral foramen
(E) Buford complex

An axial T2-weighted, fat-suppressed image of the glenohumeral joint at the level of the anteroinferior labrum (Figure 2-2) shows a detached anteroinferior labrum, consistent with a Bankart lesion **(Option (C) is correct).** A Bankart lesion results from anterior shoulder dislocation. The lesion in this case is an avulsion of the anteroinferior labrum from the glenoid rim with detachment from the scapular periosteum. Other Bankart variants of the anteroinferior labrum can be seen (Table 2-1).

Instability of the glenohumeral joint can be functional or anatomic. With functional instability, the shoulder is clinically stable, but there is subjective instability. The patient has shoulder pain, clicking and locking, and the shoulder feels unstable, but no subluxation or dislocation is noted on physical examination. In such situations, a labral tear is often present.

Anatomic shoulder instability is related to subluxation or dislocation and can be atraumatic or traumatic. In the atraumatic form, there can be congenital causes, such as a hypoplastic or shallow glenoid or a lax capsule. The traumatic form can be acute and related to dislocation or more chronic and related to repetitive microtrauma like that seen in throwing athletes. Compo-

nents of the joint that contribute to stability include the osseous structures comprising the glenoid surface and humeral head, the labrum surrounding the glenoid, the capsule, and the three (superior, middle, and inferior) glenohumeral ligaments.

Anterior instability is the most common form of instability, comprising approximately 95% of cases. Anterior dislocation often results in lesions of the inferior glenohumeral ligament-labral complex (IGHLLC).

The fibrocartilaginous labrum surrounds the glenoid and attaches to the bone with a hyaline cartilage

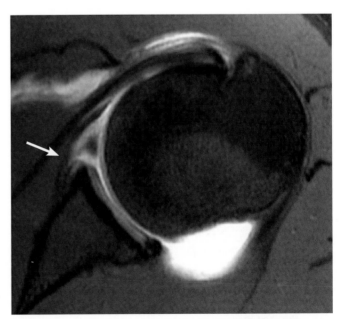

Figure 2-2 (same as Figure 2-1). Bankart lesion. Shoulder. MR arthrogram. Lower half of the glenohumeral joint. T1-weighted, fat-suppressed. Axial plane. A tear of the anterior inferior labrum with disruption of the scapular periosteum (arrow), termed a Bankart lesion, is seen.

Table 2-1. Anteroinferior labral lesions associated with anterior shoulder dislocation	
Name	*Morphologic Characteristics*
Bankart lesion	Tear with disruption of periosteal attachment
Anterior labroligamentous periosteal sleeve avulsion (ALPSA) lesion	Tear with inferomedial displacement and preservation of attachment to scapular periosteum
Perthes lesion	Tear with no displacement and with preservation of attachment to scapular periosteum

interface. It also attaches to the glenoid rim through a periosteal attachment. Tears of the anteroinferior labrum that are related to anterior instability are called Bankart lesions and their variants. It is important to describe the various characteristics of the labral tears, whether anterior, posterior, superior, or inferior. They have been given different names and acronyms in the literature. The acronyms are used here because they are well known in the orthopedic literature. As long as the pathology is correctly identified and described, there is no need for the imager to memorize these terms, although it is helpful to be familiar with them.

The Bankart lesion is the most common labral lesion related to anterior instability. It results from anterior dislocation of the shoulder with the humeral head extending below the coracoid anterior to the anteroinferior glenoid rim. The labrum avulses from the rim and has no scapular periosteal attachment, so that it extends into the joint while still attached to the inferior glenohumeral ligament (IGHL) (Figure 2-3A). The lack of scapular periosteal attachment allows the labrum to move in the joint away from the inferior glenoid rim. Sometimes, but not often, the labrum retracts to the top of the joint, forming a glenoid labrum ovoid mass, or GLOM sign (Figure 2-3B). Many of these anterior labral lesions are associated with Hill Sachs

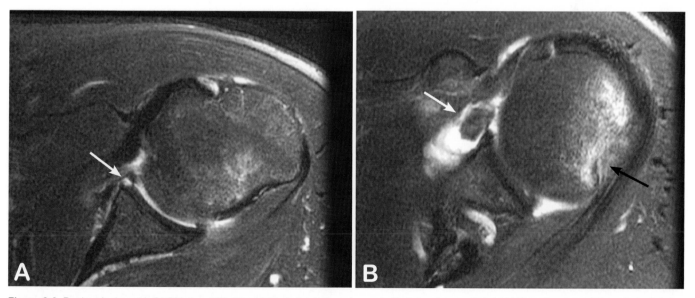

Figure 2-3. Bankart lesion with GLOM sign. MR. T2-weighted. Axial plane. Lower half of glenohumeral joint. (A) There is a tear of the anterior inferior labrum with disruption of the scapular periosteum (arrow), termed a Bankart lesion. (B) Plane at a level of the rotator interval superior to that in panel A. With no periosteal attachment, most of the labrum has retracted superiorly (arrow). The presence of a glenoid labrum ovoid mass (GLOM sign), indicates that a Bankart lesion is present. Note the Hill Sachs lesion on the posterior humeral head (black arrow), a compression fracture caused by impaction on the anterior glenoid rim during dislocation, resulting in indentation of the round contour of the humeral head with associated high signal intensity marrow contusion.

lesions on the posterior superior humeral head (Figure 2-23B). Hill Sachs lesions represent a compression fracture caused by impaction of the humeral head with the anterior glenoid during anterior dislocation. This results in indentation of the normally round contour of the humeral head.

Neviaser described a variant of the Bankart lesion known as an anterior labroligamentous periosteal sleeve avulsion (ALPSA lesion)(Option A). This lesion is an avulsion of the IGHLLC from the anteroinferior glenoid with an intact scapular periosteum. The avulsed anteroinferior labrum is displaced medially and rotates inferiorly along the anterior scapular neck (Figure 2-4). The lesion eventually heals in this medially displaced position, leading to recurrent anterior instability because of persistent incompetence of the IGHLLC.

The third Bankart variant in this location is known as a Perthes lesion (Option B), named after the German physician who described it in the early 1900s. This lesion is an avulsion of the anteroinferior labrum with an intact scapular periosteum (Figure 2-5). The periosteum is stripped from the anterior glenoid without medial displacement of the labral-periosteal complex. The Perthes lesion is well visualized with abduction and external rotation of the shoulder (Figure 2-6).

The glenoid labrum is a fibrocartilaginous structure that can be triangular or round. There are considerable normal variations of labral attachment and of the morphology in the anterosuperior glenoid region (Table 2-2). Knowledge of the location and appearance of the variants often helps in distinguishing them from tears.

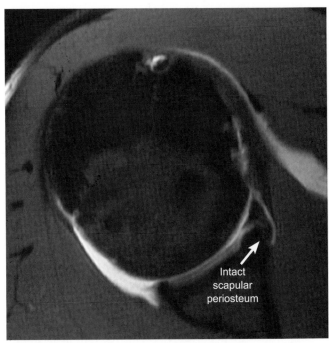

Figure 2-5. Perthes lesion. Shoulder. MR arthrogram. Axial plane. T1-weighted, fat-suppressed. The image shows contrast at the base of the anterior inferior glenoid labrum (arrow) with an intact scapular periosteum, consistent with a Perthes lesion.

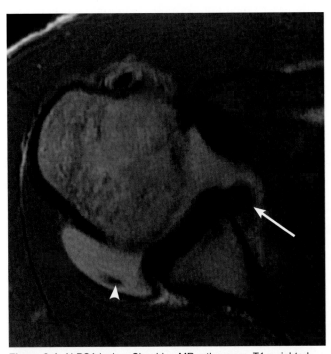

Figure 2-4. ALPSA lesion. Shoulder. MR arthrogram. T1-weighted. Axial plane. Inferior glenohumeral joint. The image shows an anterior labroligamentous periosteal sleeve avulsion (ALPSA lesion) (arrow). Note the inferomedial displacement of the labrum, which is still attached to scapular periosteum. Incidentally noted is a low intensity mass consistent with a cartilaginous body floating in the posterior aspect of the joint (arrowhead).

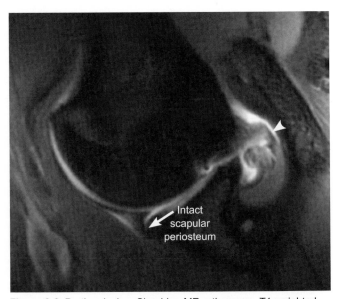

Figure 2-6. Perthes lesion. Shoulder. MR arthrogram. T1-weighted, fat-suppressed. Glenohumeral joint. Abduction and external rotation (ABER) view. This image shows the Perthes lesion with the labrum separated from the glenoid rim at its base (arrow). The labrum is still attached to the scapular periosteum. This patient also has a tear of the infraspinatus tendon (arrowhead).

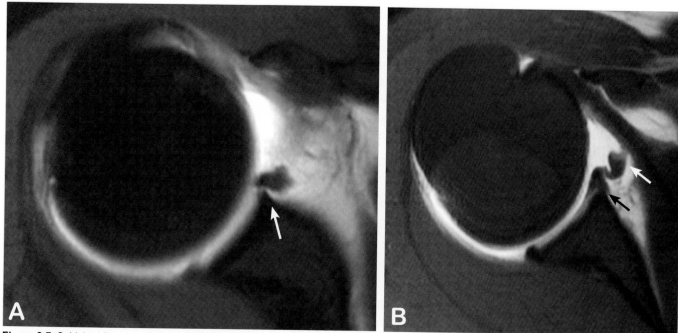

Figure 2-7. Sublabral foramen. Shoulder. MR arthrogram. (A) T1-weighted, fat-suppressed. Axial plane. Superior glenohumeral joint. The image taken in the anterosuperior area demonstrates a sublabral foramen (hole) at the base of the labrum (arrow). (B) An image obtained several sections caudal to the image in panel A at the midportion of the glenoid shows the labrum has reattached to the glenoid (black arrow) and is associated with a cord-like glenohumeral ligament (white arrow).

A sublabral foramen (Option D) is seen in the anterosuperior region of the glenoid labrum in 11% to 15% of cases. This foramen or hole is seen at the base of the anterosuperior labrum and is associated with a cordlike middle glenohumeral ligament (MGHL) in 75% of cases (Figure 2-7B). One should not mistake the cordlike MGHL for a labral detachment.

There may be congenital absence of the anterosuperior labrum. This variant is known as the Buford complex (Figure 2-8) (Option E). It is seen in 1% to 2% of shoulder arthroscopies and is associated with a cord-like MGHL that attaches directly to the superior labrum anterior to the biceps tendon attachment.

The Buford complex and the sublabral foramen sometimes can extend into the anteroinferior portion of the labrum. In addition, a sublabral foramen is usu-

Table 2-2. Normal labral variants

Name	Morphologic Characteristics
Sublabral foramen	Defect at base of anterosuperior labrum
Buford complex	Absence of anterosuperior labrum in association with a cordlike middle glenohumeral ligament
Sublabral recess	Defect at base of superior labrum

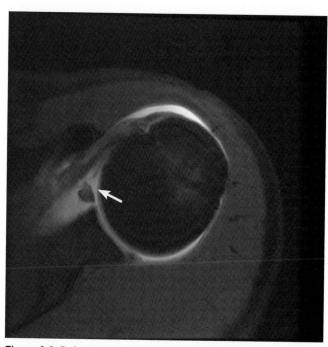

Figure 2-8. Buford complex. Shoulder. MR arthrogram. T1-weighted, fat-suppressed. Axial plane. The image shows congenital absence of labrum anterosuperiorly associated with a cordlike middle glenohumeral ligament (arrow).

ally accompanied by a sublabral recess in the superior labrum.

The sublabral recess is a normal recess that can exist between the superior labrum and the glenoid articular cartilage. This anatomic variant is smooth and 1 mm to 2 mm wide. It does not extend to the top of the labrum (Figure 2-9). It is not associated with a paralabral cyst, as are some superior labral tears. In general, this recess

does not extend posteriorly to the attachment of the long head of the biceps tendon to the superior labrum.

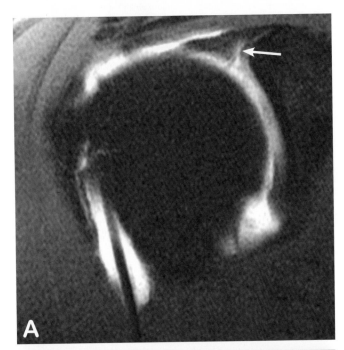

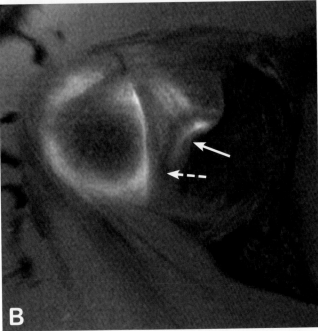

Figure 2-9. Sublabral recess. Shoulder. MR arthrography. T1-weighted, fat-suppressed. (A) Coronal plane. There is a defect at the base of the superior labrum (arrow). (B) Axial plane. An arrow points to the superior labrum defect. It lies anterior to the biceps attachment to the glenoid labrum (anchor) (dashed arrow).

Questions 6 through 9

You are shown MR images of four shoulders with a history of instability and a glenohumeral ligament lesion. For each of the numbered images (Figures 2-10 through 2-13 in the test section), select the one lettered diagnosis (A, B, C, D, or E) that is MOST closely associated with it. Each lettered diagnosis may be used once, more than once, or not at all.

6. Figure 2-10
7. Figure 2-11
8. Figure 2-12
9. Figure 2-13

 (A) HAGL lesion
 (B) BHAGL lesion
 (C) RHAGL lesion
 (D) Superior glenohumeral ligament tear
 (E) Middle glenohumeral ligament tear

Three glenohumeral ligaments provide stability to the glenohumeral joint. The superior glenohumeral ligament (SGHL), MGHL, and IGHL are infoldings of the capsule. The SGHL originates at the superior glenoid tubercle anterior to the insertion of the long head of the biceps tendon and inserts into the fovea capitis line just superior to the lesser tuberosity of the humerus in the region of the bicipital groove. The SGHL is best seen on axial images obtained directly beneath or adjacent to the origin of the long head of the biceps lateral tendon. The SGHL lies lateral and parallel to the coracoid in the rotator interval, just beneath the extraarticular coraco-

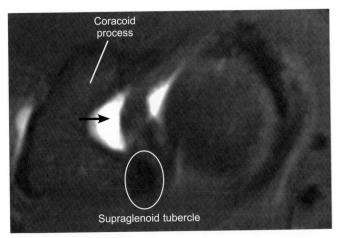

Figure 2-14. MR arthrography. T1-weighted, fat-suppressed. Axial plane. The normal superior glenohumoral ligament (SGHL) is seen extending from the supraglenoid tubercle (circled) anteriorly and parallel to the coracoid process (arrow).

humeral ligament (Figure 2-14). The SGHL varies in size and is present in almost all shoulders. It represents the primary restraint to inferior translation of the unloaded, abducted glenohumeral joint. The SGHL and the extraarticular coracohumeral ligament together form a sling around the intraarticular portion of the biceps tendon in the rotator interval immediately before the entrance of the biceps tendon into the bicipital groove. These two structures prevent posterior and inferior translation of the humeral head. A tear of the SGHL is shown in Figure 2-15 **(Option (D) is the correct answer to Question 6)**.

The MGHL (Figure 2-16) has variable origins from the glenoid, scapula, anterior labrum, biceps tendon, IGHL and SGHL. The MGHL merges with the subscapularis tendon and inserts with it just below the attachment of the SGHL to the lesser tuberosity of the humerus. The MGHL is usually seen en face on axial images as it takes an oblique course from the glenoid to the subscapularis tendon (Figure 2-16A). It is seen as a vertical linear structure in front of the glenoid on oblique sagittal images (Figure 2-16B). Occasionally this ligament can be duplicated, simulating a longitudinal tear. The MGHL can be absent in up to 27% of the population. Absence of this ligament is not associated with an increased incidence of instability, but when it is absent the subscapular recess can be enlarged, and the IGHL will usually originate more superiorly than when an MGHL is present.

MGHL tears occur in a variety of patterns and are best seen on sagittal and axial MR images. The ligament can be proximally detached (Figure 2-17) **(Option (E) is the correct answer to Question 7)**, disrupted along its path, floating in the anterior capsular space, detached from the scapular insertion, foreshortened, thickened, wavy, or a combination of these features.

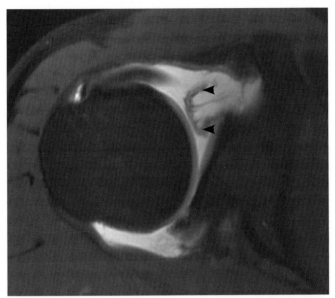

Figure 2-15 (Same as Figure 2-10). MR arthrogram. Shoulder. Axial plane. T1-weighted, fat-suppressed. A disrupted SGHL (arrowheads) can be seen in the rotator interval.

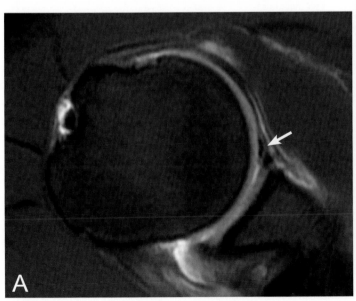

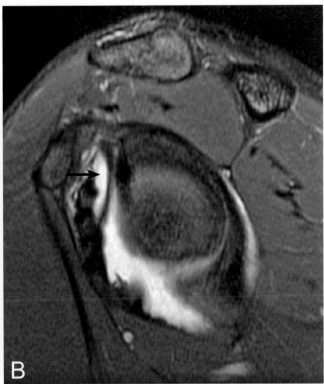

Figure 2-16. Normal middle glenohumeral ligament. MR. Fat-suppressed. (A) Axial plane. T1-weighted. (B) Sagittal plane. T2-weighted. The ligament (arrow) is parallel to the anterior labrum. It has a variable proximal origin, which in this case is the SGHL, and merges with the subscapularis muscle.

Another pattern of rupture is the split longitudinal tear extending along the length of the MGHL without complete disruption of the ligament. When isolated, this injury can simulate the previously mentioned normal bifid variant. MGHL tears are frequently associated with superior labral tears, which are categorized into different types of "SLAP" lesions. SLAP stands for "superor labral anterior to posterior" tears.

The anterior band of the IGHL is the primary restraint to anterior translation of the humeral head when the glenohumeral joint is in 90 degrees of abduction. The IGHL, considered to be the most important stabilizer of the glenohumeral joint, originates at the middle to inferior portion of the anterior glenoid labrum and extends posteriorly. It drapes for a variable distance from an anterior to a posterior direction and inserts into the anatomic neck of the humerus. This ligament originates from the glenoid labrum, forming a labroligamentous complex.

The IGHL has strong collagenous thickenings—the anterior and posterior bands—at its anterior and posterior margins. These are joined by a fibrous thickening of the capsule called the axillary pouch or recess (Figure 2-18). The IGHL functions as a sling to support the humeral head and prevents abnormal anterior and posterior instability. It reinforces the anterior capsule between the subscapularis muscle and the inferior aspect of the glenoid at or near the origin of the long head of the triceps tendon. Various forms of disruption of this important stabilizing ligament are discussed here.

Sagittal (Figure 2-18), axial (Figure 2-19) and coronal (Figure 2-20) T1-weighted, fat-suppressed images from an MR arthrogram demonstrate a normal anterior band of the IGHL. Disruption of the humeral attachment of the anterior band of the IGHL is called a HAGL lesion (Figure 2-21) **(Option (A) is the correct answer to Question 8)**. This lesion results from the forces of anterior instability acting on the anterior band of the IGHL. A HAGL lesion is less common than a Bankart lesion at the glenoid attachment of the IGHL. Approximately 40% of IGHL lesions are seen at the glenoid attachment. Although a HAGL lesion typically results from a first-time dislocation in a patient older than 35 years of age, some patients have not had an earlier dislocation. A HAGL lesion is occasionally associated with a tear of the subscapularis tendon and can cause recurrent anterior instability. Other associations include an anterior labral tear and an osteochondral injury of the humeral head. A history of surgery also leads to a predisposition for HAGL lesions. A HAGL lesion is seen on axial MR images as a thick, wavy and irregular ligament that does not attach to the anatomic neck of the humerus. On coronal MR images, the normal "U" shape of the anterior band of the IGHL looks like a "J" shape when the ligament is disrupted (Fig-

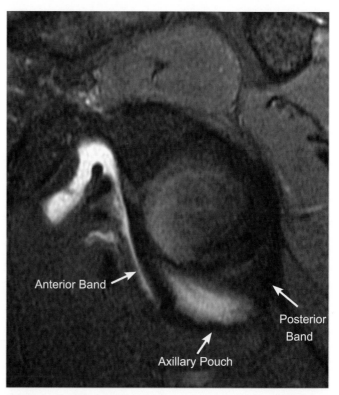

Figure 2-18. MRI. Sagittal view. Fat-suppressed, T1-weighted. The inferior glenohumeral ligament (IGHL) is like a hammock. Its three components are labeled, demonstrating the anterior band, axillary pouch or recess, and posterior band. The axillary pouch forms the inferior aspect of the ligament and the shoulder capsule. The posterior band extends from the posterior labrum and glenoid rim to the posterior humerus and is usually part of the posterior capsule.

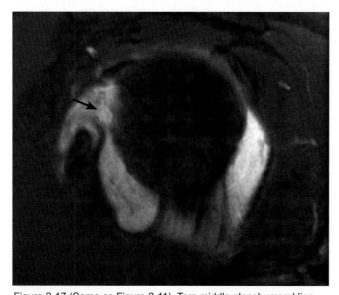

Figure 2-17 (Same as Figure 2-11). Torn middle glenohumeral ligament. MRI. Shoulder. T2-weighted, fat-suppressed. Sagittal plane. The MGHL is torn from its proximal origin (arrow).

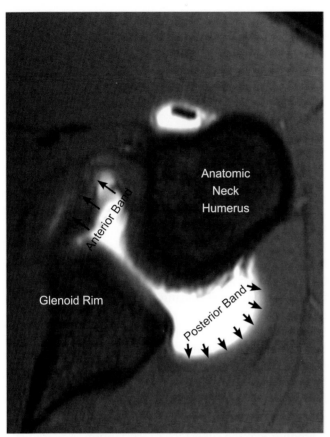

Figure 2-19. Normal anterior band of the IGHL. Shoulder. MR arthrogram. T1-weighted, fat-suppressed. Axial plane. The image shows the anterior band extending from the anterior inferior labrum at the glenoid rim to the anatomic neck of the humerus.

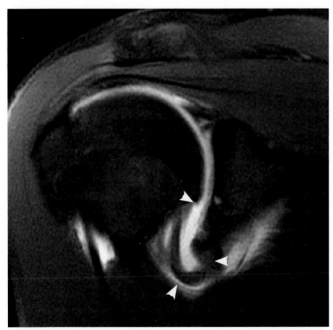

Figure 2-20. Normal anterior band of the IGHL. Shoulder. MR arthrogram. T1-weighted, fat-suppressed. Coronal view. The image shows the anterior band of the IGHL extending from the glenoid rim to the anatomic neck of the humerus. On the coronal image the ligament has a normal "U" shape (arrowheads), as one would expect when a ligament is not disrupted.

ure 2-21). It is important to identify a HAGL lesion. An unrecognized HAGL lesion may be the cause of a failed Bankart lesion repair. Although isolated HAGL lesions can be treated conservatively using immobilization with a sling and physical therapy, arthroscopic or open surgical repair is usually indicated. In up to 20% of cases of HAGL injury, a patient can have an avulsion of a bony fragment along with the IGHL from the humeral attachment. This bony HAGL injury is known as a BHAGL lesion. When the IGHL is avulsed at the humeral and labral attachments, it is called a floating anterior glenohumeral ligament (AIGHL). In 35% of cases, the IGHL can tear in the middle portion and not at either attachment. In 25% of cases, the tear occurs at the humeral attachment. An avulsion of the IGHL at the glenoid attachment can occur without a tear of the anteroinferior labrum. This injury is known as an anterior ligamentous periosteal sleeve avulsion (ALIPSA lesion) or as a glenoid avulsion of the glenohumeral ligament (GAGL lesion).

The posterior band of the IGHL extends from the posteroinferior glenoid to the posterior humeral head

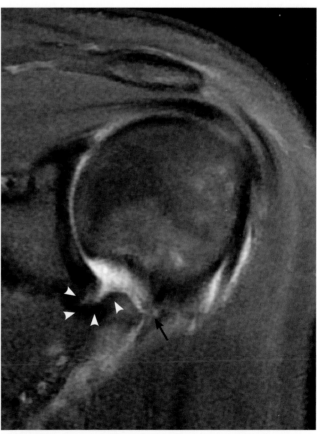

Figure 2-21. (Same as Figure 2-12). HAGL lesion. MRI. Shoulder. Coronal plane. T2-weighted, fat-suppressed. The image of the shoulder shows a disruption of the anterior band of the IGHL at the humeral attachment (black arrow) consistent with a HAGL lesion. This produces a "J"-shaped IGHL (arrowheads).

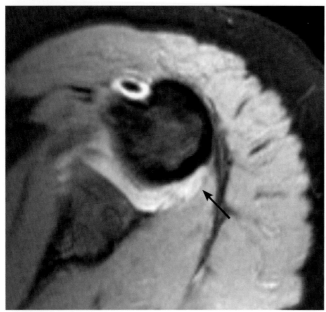

Figure 2-22. (Same as Figure 2-13). Reverse HAGL lesion. Shoulder. MRI. T1-weighted, fat-suppressed. Axial plane. The posterior band of the IGHL (arrow) is disrupted on this arthrographic image, consistent with a reverse HAGL lesion.

(Figure 2-19). A disruption or avulsion of the humeral attachment of the posterior band of the IGHL is known as a reverse HAGL injury (RHAGL lesion) (Figure 2-22) **(Option (C) is the correct answer to Question 9)**. This injury is often caused by a posteriorly directed force on an abducted shoulder and is frequently associated with posterior labral tears and cystic changes in the greater tuberosity. It can also be related to multidirectional instability and microinstability. A RHAGL lesion is characterized by a lack of attachment of the posterior band of the IGHL to the humerus, often with extravasation of fluid or contrast material into the posterior soft tissues. It is important to identify a RHAGL lesion on MRI before surgery, because it can be missed at arthroscopy if no anterior portals are used to search posteriorly. Open repair rather than arthroscopic repair may be used to prevent the leakage of fluid introduced during arthroscopy from the back of the shoulder through the capsular rent. Osseous avulsion of the posterior band of the IGHL from the humeral head can occur but is rare. This injury is known as a reverse or posterior BHAGL lesion. A floating posteroinferior glenohumeral ligament with tears at both ends can also occur.

Question 10

Posterior instability is associated with:

(A) Posterior labrocapsular periosteal sleeve avulsion (POLPSA) lesion
(B) Bennett lesion
(C) Kim lesion
(D) Osseous Bankart lesion
(E) Engagement of the humeral head on the anterior glenoid during internal rotation

Posterior labral and capsular tears are much less common than anterior ones, accounting for up to 5% of all cases of shoulder instability. Posterior instability is usually encountered in association with nontraumatic recurrent posterior multidirectional instability, or repetitive microtrauma; however, it can also be seen with traumatic posterior dislocation, a redundant posterior capsule, osteochondral lesions, or posterior labroligamentous tears, as well as in the setting of injuries due to electric shock or seizures. Subluxations are more common than dislocations.

Like anterior labral tears, posterior tears can be seen with absence of the labrum, with morphologic distortion of the labrum, or with contrast material or fluid extending into the substance of the labrum. A particular type of posterior labral tear is the posterior labrocapsular periosteal sleeve avulsion (POLPSA lesion) **(Option**

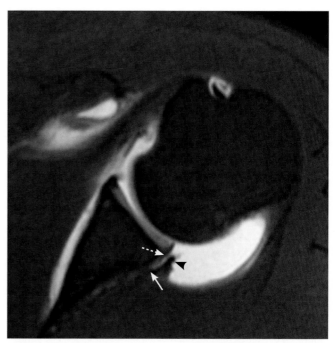

Figure 2-23. POLPSA lesion. MR arthrography. Shoulder. T1-weighted, fat-suppressed. Axial plane. The image shows an avulsion (black arrowhead) of the posterior labrum with a patulous posterior recess (dashed arrow). The labrum is still attached to scapular periosteum (white arrow).

(A) is true). This lesion is an avulsion of the attachment of the posterior capsule and the periosteum, resulting in a patulous recess posteriorly (Figure 2-23). It can represent an acute Bennett lesion.

A Bennett lesion is an extracapsular avulsion injury commonly seen along the posterior glenoid rim in 25% of throwing athletes, such as baseball pitchers. A Bennett lesion is associated with posterior instability **(Option (B) is true)**. This lesion is characterized by heterotopic ossification near the insertion of the posterior band of the IGHL on the glenoid; the ossification is produced by traction of the IGHL during the cocking or follow-through phases of pitching. Although it can be asymptomatic, a Bennett lesion is associated with posterior labral injury and posterior undersurface tears of the rotator cuff. The patient can develop crescentic mineralization adjacent to the posteroinferior osseous glenoid and sclerosis of the posterior glenoid (Figure 2-24). The mineralization can occasionally be identified on MRI but is better seen on axillary radiographs and CT scans. Low signal intensity or fatty marrow signal intensity related to the heterotopic bone is usually present; hyperintensity on T2-weighted MR images in the region of the Bennett lesion can suggest a more acute lesion.

Another posteroinferior labrum lesion that is associated with posterior instability is deep or intrasub-

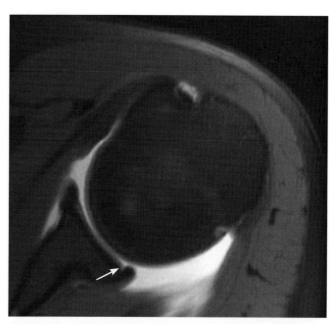

Figure 2-25. Kim lesion of the posterior labrum. MR arthrography. Shoulder. T1-weighted. Fat-suppressed. Axial plane. The image shows a subtle detachment (arrow) at the base of the posterior inferior labrum consistent with a Kim lesion. This patient had posterior instability. There is also extravasation of contrast posteriorly, which was incidental and not related to a posterior capsular tear.

stance incomplete detachment in association with a defect at the chondrolabral junction. This lesion is known as a Kim lesion **(Option (C) is true).** A Kim lesion includes a marginal crack or chondral erosion with incomplete and concealed avulsion of the posteroinferior labrum (Figure 2-25). This lesion is thought to be caused by submaximal posterior force of the labrum at the attachment of the posterior band of the IGHL. With repetitive posterior subluxation of the humeral head, shear force on the chondrolabral junction can cause a marginal crack. With increased force, the tear along the inner portion can propagate to the surface of the chondrolabral junction and become visible at that location on arthroscopy. Arthroscopy can be used to probe for a concealed Kim lesion; if found, such a lesion can be converted to a complete tear and repaired with a suture anchor. This procedure restores the posterior labral height, preventing further posterior instability. A procedure to accomplish a posterior capsular shift toward the superior direction can be performed at the same time. Some patients also undergo a procedure to achieve an inferior capsular shift anterosuperiorly and closure of the rotator interval to address multidirectional instability, if present.

An osseous Bankart lesion is associated with anterior instability, not posterior instability **(Option (D) is false)**. It is the result of impaction of the humeral head

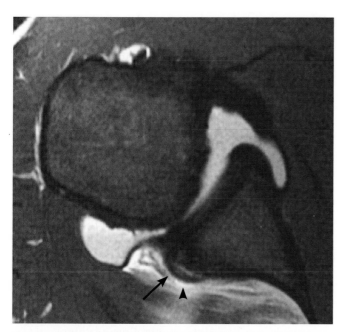

Figure 2-24. Bennett lesion. Shoulder. MR arthrography. Fat-suppressed, T2-weighted. Axial plane. The image demonstrates a crescentic low signal intensity structure adjacent to the posterior scapula near the glenoid rim, consistent with a Bennett lesion (arrow). Extravasation of contrast material into the posterior soft tissues (arrowhead) had no clinical relevance.

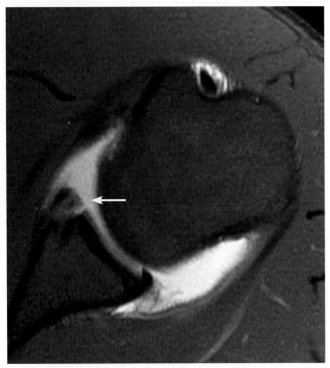

Figure 2-26. Osseous Bankart lesion. MR arthrography. Axial plane. Fat-suppressed, T1-weighted. There is a fracture along the anterior glenoid rim (arrow) related to prior anterior dislocation and consistent with an osseous Bankart lesion.

on the anterior glenoid. An osseous Bankart lesion is well seen on CT as a small fragment of bone associated with irregularity of the adjacent anterior glenoid rim. On MRI, low-signal-intensity cortical fragments or glenoid deficiencies are seen in all planes, but particularly on axial images (Figure 2-26). Very small osseous

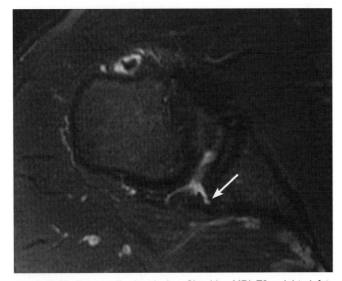

Figure 2-27. Reverse Bankart lesion. Shoulder. MRI. T2-weighted, fat-suppressed. Axial plane. Reverse osseous Bankart lesion represents a fracture of the posterior glenoid rim (arrow) following a posterior glenohumeral joint dislocation.

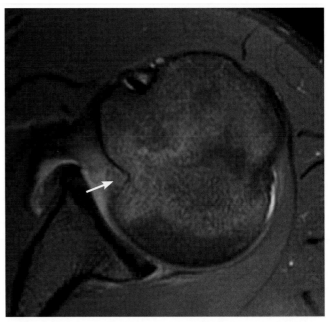

Figure 2-28. Reverse Hill Sachs lesion. MRI. Fat-suppressed, T2-weighted. Axial plane. There is a large compression fracture (arrow) in the anteromedial aspect of the humeral head with overlying large contusion following a posterior dislocation of the glenohumeral joint.

Bankart lesions can be missed on MRI and are better seen on CT.

The osseous lesions associated with posterior instability carry the familiar eponyms associated with anterior instability, except that the word "reverse" is added. A reverse osseous Bankart lesion is an impaction fracture of the posterior glenoid resulting from posterior dislocation of the humerus (Figure 2-27). A reverse Bankart lesion is usually seen after trauma but is occasionally seen with nontraumatic posterior or multidirectional instability. A reverse osseous glenoid rim fracture can be seen in approximately one third of cases of acute traumatic posterior dislocation.

A reverse Hill-Sachs lesion results from an impaction fracture of the anterosuperior humerus on the posterior genoid rim. It involves 10% to 30% of the articular surface of the anterior humeral head. Also referred to as a trough or McLaughlin's fracture, it is seen in up to 86% of cases of acute traumatic posterior dislocation of the shoulder. A reverse Hill-Sachs lesion is diagnosed when there is loss of the normal convexity of the anteromedial aspect of the humeral head. The defect can be classified as small, medium or large. A defect is considered to be small when less than 25% of the articular surface of the humeral head is involved. A medium defect involves between 25% and 50% of the articular surface. A large defect occupies more than 50% of the articular surface (Figure 2-28). A reverse Hill-Sachs defect can engage or lock on the posterior glenoid, not the anterior glenoid **(Option (E) is false)**. Locking of a reverse Hill-Sachs lesion on the posterior glenoid occurs during internal rotation, producing posterior subluxation, attrition of the humerus and a posterior labral tear.

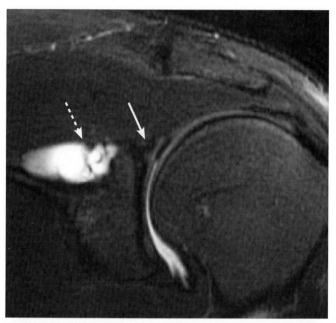

Figure 2-29. SLAP lesion with cyst in the suprascapular notch. MR arthrography. Shoulder. Fat-suppressed, T2-weighted. Coronal plane. MR arthrographic image shows a tear of the superior labrum (SLAP lesion), marked by an arrow and associated with a large paralabral cyst in the suprascapular notch (dotted arrow).

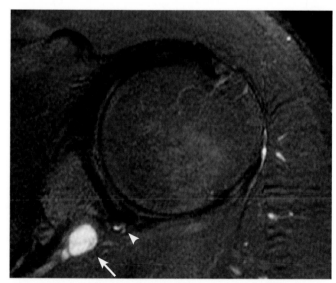

Figure 2-30. Spinoglenoid notch paralabral cyst. MRI. Axial plane. Fat-suppressed, T2-weighted. A cyst (arrow) is seen in the paralabral area associated with a posterior labral tear (arrowhead), but the muscle signal is normal without evidence of muscle denervation on MRI.

Question 11

Concerning paralabral cysts:

(A) They are most commonly associated with anterior labral tears.
(B) Superior labral cysts often extend into the subscapular notch.
(C) Cysts in the spinoglenoid notch can denervate the infraspinatus muscle.
(D) Subacute denervation changes can be seen as both atrophy and fatty infiltration of the muscle.
(E) Inferior cysts can affect the axillary nerve.

A unique subset of shoulder ganglion cysts that arise from glenoid labral tears has been described. The mechanism for the formation of these paralabral cysts is similar to that of meniscal cysts, and is due to extrusion of joint fluid through labrocapsular tears into adjacent tissue planes. The most common locations for a labral cyst-tear complex is posterior (associated with a posterosuperior labral tear) and superior, but not anterior (associated with a SLAP lesion) **(Option (A) is false)**.

Extraarticular extension of a labral cyst into the spinoglenoid notch, the suprascapular notch, or both, is common. Cysts associated with superior labral tears often extend into the suprascapular notch (Figure 2-29), not the subscapular notch **(Option (B) is false)**. Intraosseous extension into the bony glenoid can also occur.

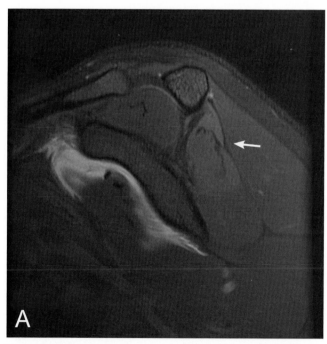

Figure 2-31. Parsonage Turner syndrome. Shoulder. MR arthrography. (A) Fat-suppressed, T2-weighted. Sagittal plane. The muscle is subtly high signal intensity on the T2-weighted image (arrow). Idiopathic neuritis of the suprascapular nerve shows subacute to chronic denervation of the infraspinatus muscle.

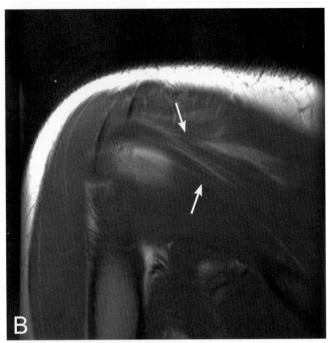

Figure 2-31 (continued). Parsonage Turner syndrome. Shoulder. MR arthrography. (B) T1-weighted. Coronal plane. There is fatty infiltration of the subacute or chronically denervated infraspinatus muscle (arrows) on this T1-weighted image.

When located adjacent to SLAP or posterior labral lesions, these cysts can produce suprascapular nerve entrapment, which is a cause of shoulder pain that can be evaluated on MRI.

The suprascapular nerve is derived from the upper trunk of the brachial plexus. It passes deep relative to the trapezius and omohyoid muscles before entering the supraspinatus fossa through the suprascapular notch. In the supraspinatus fossa, it sends two motor branches to the supraspinatus muscle and receives sensory branches from the capsular and ligamentous structures of the shoulder and acromioclavicular joint. The nerve then runs deep relative to the supraspinatus muscle, entering the infraspinatus fossa through the spinoglenoid notch. In the infraspinatus fossa, the suprascapular nerve sends motor branches to the infraspinatus muscle as well as to the shoulder joint and capsule. Isolated cysts in the spinoglenoid notch are usually caused by posterior labral tears (Figure 2-30), and they occasionally denervate the infraspinatus muscle **(Option (C) is true)** without affecting the supraspinatus muscle.

The suprascapular nerve can become compressed along its path by masses such as paralabral cysts, large vessels and neuromas. These masses are well seen on MRI. Other causes of injury or entrapment of the suprascapular nerve include humeral and scapular fractures, anterior shoulder dislocation, traction or kinking of the nerve and anomalous or thickened transverse scapular ligaments. Idiopathic conditions (neuritis) that cause myopathy from denervation are part of Parsonage-Turner syndrome (Figure 2-31).

Suprascapular nerve entrapment can be diagnosed earlier with MRI, which can localize and characterize the masses causing the syndrome. Denervation appears in the subacute phase as muscle edema with diffuse high T2-weighted signal intensity within the muscle innervated by the affected nerve. Chronic denervation appears as high T1-weighted signal intensity within the muscle (representing fatty infiltration), atrophy of the muscle or both **(Option (D) is false)**. These changes are often seen in the affected supraspinatus muscle, infraspinatus muscle or both. Treatment of a paralabral cyst associated with a labral tear involves arthroscopic debridement of the labrum, removing the frayed edges and any loose parts, as well as possible repair of the labral pathology causing the cyst. If the cyst can be reached with the scope, then it is decompressed. If the cyst cannot be reached and is not surgically removed, then it might spontaneously decompress. If the cyst is still present after surgery, then the radiologist can aspirate the cyst with a large-bore needle guided by sonography or CT.

Cysts associated with inferior labral tears can produce axillary nerve compression in the quadrilateral space (Figure 2-32) **(Option (E) is true)**. Anterior dislocation of the glenohumeral joint or a humeral fracture can also damage the axillary nerve or its branches. In one series, 43% of patients with anterior shoulder dislocation developed axillary nerve damage. The axillary

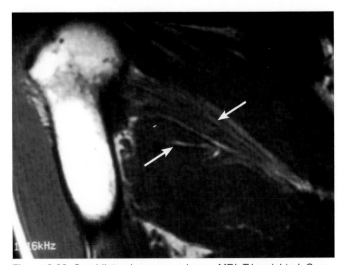

Figure 2-32. Quadrilateral space syndrome. MRI. T1-weighted. Coronal plane. The image shows fatty infiltration in the teres minor muscle (arrows) related to axillary nerve compression in the quadrilateral space.

nerve innervates the teres minor and deltoid muscles; when a nerve injury occurs, these muscles can show the subacute and chronic changes related to denervation. These changes are similar to those seen with suprascapular nerve entrapment.

Another reason for axillary neuropathy is constriction in the quadrilateral space. This feature can produce isolated changes in the teres minor muscle on MRI or can also involve the deltoid muscle. The axillary nerve courses anteriorly to posteriorly through the quadrilateral space, which is defined superiorly by the teres minor muscle, inferiorly by the teres major muscle, medially by the long head of the triceps muscle and laterally by the humeral shaft. The posterior circumflex vessels traverse the quadrilateral space along with the axillary nerve. Therefore, arteriography, either with MRI or with radiography, has been suggested for demonstrating constriction of the vessels when the arm is held in abduction and external rotation. Although masses such as a ganglion or a lipoma can compress the axillary nerve, fibrous bands in the quadrilateral space are often cited in the literature as a common cause of compression of the nerve and vessels. In a recent study, bands were found in this region in 14 of 16 cadaveric specimens. The most common site for such a band was between the teres major muscle and the long head of the triceps muscle. When bands are present, internal and external rotation of the shoulder causes a decrease in the cross-sectional area of the quadrilateral space. These bands are difficult to visualize on MRI. Surgery is indicated when a mass or fibrous bands are suspected.

NOTE: The use of intraarticular gadolinium has not been FDA-approved.

Suggested Readings

ANTERIOR LABRUM

1. Allmann KH, Uhl M, Gufler H, et al. Cine-MR imaging of the shoulder. Acta Radiol. 1997;38:1043–1046.
2. Applegate GR, Hewitt M, Snyder SJ, Watson E, Kwak S, Resnick D. Chronic labral tears: value of magnetic resonance arthrography in evaluating the glenoid labrum and labral-bicipital complex. Arthroscopy. 2004;20:959–963.
3. Beaulieu CF, Hodge DK, Bergman AG, et al. Glenohumeral relationships during physiologic shoulder motion and stress testing: initial experience with open MR imaging and active imaging-plane registration. Radiology. 1999; 212:699–705.
4. Beltran J, Bencardino J, Mellado J, Rosenberg ZS, Irish RD. MR arthrography of the shoulder: variants and pitfalls. RadioGraphics. 1997;17:1403–1412.
5. Beltran J, Rosenberg ZS, Chandnani VP, Cuomo F, Beltran S, Rokito A. Glenohumeral instability: evaluation with MR arthrography. RadioGraphics. 1997;17:657–673.
6. Cardinal E, Buckwalter KA, Braunstein EM. Kinematic magnetic resonance imaging of the normal shoulder: assessment of the labrum and capsule. Can Assoc Radiol J. 1996;47:44–50.
7. Chandnani VP, Yeager TD, DeBerardino T, et al. Glenoid labral tears: prospective evaluation with MR imaging, MR arthrography, and CT arthrography. AJR Am J Roentgenol. 1993;161:1229–1235.
8. Dépelteau H, Bureau NJ, Cardinal E, Aubin B, Brassard P. Arthrography of the shoulder: a simple fluoroscopically guided approach for targeting the rotator cuff interval. AJR Am J Roentgenol. 2004;182:329–332.
9. Detrisac DA, Johnson LL. Arthroscopic Shoulder Anatomy: Pathologic and Surgical Implications. Thorofare, NJ: Slack; 1986.
10. Friedman RJ, Bonutti PM, Genez B. Cine magnetic resonance imaging of the subcoracoid region. Orthopedics. 1998;21:545–548.
11. Gusmer PB, Potter HG, Schatz JA, et al. Labral injuries: accuracy of detection with unenhanced MR imaging of the shoulder. Radiology. 1996;200:519–524.
12. Hall FM, Rosenthal DI, Goldberg RP, Wyshak G. Morbidity from shoulder arthrography: etiology, incidence, and prevention. AJR Am J Roentgenol. 1981;136:59–62.
13. Kwak SM, Brown RR, Trudell D, Resnick D. Glenohumeral joint: comparison of shoulder positions at MR arthrography. Radiology. 1998;208:375–380.
14. Lee SY, Lee JK. Horizontal component of partial-thickness tears of rotator cuff: imaging characteristics and comparison of ABER view with oblique coronal view at MR arthrography—initial results. Radiology. 2002;224:470–476.
15. Magee T, Williams D, Mani N. Shoulder MR arthrography: which patient group benefits most? AJR Am J Roentgenol. 2004;183:969–974.
16. Mäurer J, Rudolph J, Lorenz M, et al. A prospective study on the detection of lesions of the labrum glenoidale by indirect MR arthrography of the shoulder [in German]. Rofo 1999; 171:307–312.
17. Neumann CH, Petersen SA, Jahnke AH. MR imaging of the labral-capsular complex: normal variations. AJR Am J Roentgenol. 1991;157:1015–1021.
18. Newberg AH, Munn CS, Robbins AH. Complications of arthrography. Radiology. 1985;155:605–606.
19. Palmer WE, Brown JH, Rosenthal DI. Labral-ligamentous complex of the shoulder: evaluation with MR arthrography. Radiology. 1994;190:645–651.
20. Pappas AM, Goss TP, Kleinman PK. Symptomatic shoulder instability due to lesions of the glenoid labrum. Am J Sports Med. 1983;11:279–288.
21. Park YH, Lee JY, Moon SH, et al. MR arthrography of the labral capsular ligamentous complex in the shoulder: imaging variations and pitfalls. AJR Am J Roentgenol, 2000;175:667–672.
22. Rockwood CA Jr, Matsen FA III. The Shoulder. Philadelphia: WB Saunders; 1990.

23. Roger B, Skaf A, Hooper AW, Lektrakul N, Yeh L, Resnick D. Imaging findings in the dominant shoulder of throwing athletes: comparison of radiography, arthrography, CT arthrography, and MR arthrography with arthroscopic correlation. AJR Am J Roentgenol 1999; 172:1371–1380.

24. Sans N, Richardi G, Railhac JJ, et al. Kinematic MR imaging of the shoulder: normal patterns. AJR Am J Roentgenol 1996;167:1517–1522.

25. Shankman S, Bencardino J, Beltran J. Glenohumeral instability: evaluation using MR arthrography of the shoulder. Skeletal Radiol. 1999;28:365–382.

26. Smith DK, Chopp TM, Aufdemorte TB, et al. Sublabral recess of the superior glenoid labrum: study of cadavers with conventional nonenhanced MR imaging, MR arthrography, anatomic dissection, and limited histologic examination. Radiology. 1996;201:251–256.

27. Sommer T, Vahlensieck M, Wallny T, et al. Indirect MR arthrography in the diagnosis of lesions of the labrum glenoidale [in German]. Rofo 1997; 67:46–51.

28. Song HT, Huh YM, Kim S, et al. Anterior-inferior labral lesions of recurrent shoulder dislocation evaluated by MR arthrography in an adduction internal rotation (ADIR) position. J Magn Reson Imaging. 2006;23:29–35.

29. Steinbach LS, Palmer WE, Schweitzer ME. Special focus session: MR arthrography. RadioGraphics. 2002;22:1223–1246.

30. Tirman PF, Bost FW, Steinbach LS, et al. MR arthrographic depiction of tears of the rotator cuff: benefit of abduction and external rotation of the arm. Radiology. 1994;192:851–856.

31. Tirman PF, Feller JF, Palmer WE, Carroll KW, Steinbach LS, Cox I. The Buford complex—a variation of normal shoulder anatomy: MR arthrographic imaging features. AJR. 1996;166:869–873.

32. Tuite MJ, Blankenbaker DG, Seifert M, Ziegert AJ, Orwin JF. Sublabral foramen and Buford complex: inferior extent of the unattached or absent labrum in 50 patients. Radiology. 2002;223:137–142.

33. Tuite MJ, Orwin JF. Anterosuperior labral variants of the shoulder: appearance on gradient-recalled-echo and fast spin-echo MR images. Radiology. 1996;199:537–540.

34. Tuite MJ, Rutkowski A, Enright T, Kaplan L, Fine JP, Orwin J. Width of high signal and extension posterior to biceps tendon as signs of superior labrum anterior to posterior tears on MRI and MR arthrography. AJR Am J Roentgenol. 2005;185:1422–1428.

35. Williams MM, Snyder SJ, Buford D Jr. The Buford complex—the "cord-like" middle glenohumeral ligament and absent anterosuperior labrum complex: a normal anatomic capsulolabral variant. Arthroscopy. 1994;10:241–247.

36. Yeh L, Kwak S, Kim YS, et al. Anterior labroligamentous structures of the glenohumeral joint: correlation of MR arthrography and anatomic dissection in cadavers. AJR Am J Roentgenol. 1998;171:1229–1236.

GLENOHUMERAL LIGAMENTS

37. Beltran J, Bencardino J, Padron M, Shankman S, Beltran L, Ozkarahan G. The middle glenohumeral ligament: normal anatomy, variants and pathology. Skeletal Radiol. 2002;31:253–262.

38. Flannigan B, Kursunoglu-Brahme S, Snyder S, et al. MR arthrography of the shoulder: comparison with conventional MR imaging. AJR Am J Roentgenol.1990;155:829–832.

39. Loredo R, Longo C, Salonen D, et al. Glenoid labrum: MR imaging with histologic correlation. Radiology. 1995;196:33–41.

40. Neviaser RJ, Neviaser TJ, Neviaser JS. Anterior dislocation of the shoulder and rotator cuff rupture. Clin Orthop Relat Res. 1993;(291):103–106.

41. Neviaser RJ, Neviaser TJ, Neviaser JS. Concurrent rupture of the rotator cuff and anterior dislocation of the shoulder in the older patient. J Bone Joint Surg Am. 1988;70:1308–1311.

42. Neviaser TJ. The anterior labroligamentous periosteal sleeve avulsion lesion: a cause of anterior instability of the shoulder. Arthroscopy. 1993;9:17–21.

43. Neviaser TJ. The GLAD lesion: another cause of anterior shoulder pain. Arthroscopy. 1993;9:22–23.

44. Oberlander MA, Morgan BE, Visotsky JL. The BHAGL lesion: a new variant of anterior shoulder instability. Arthroscopy 1996;12:627–633.

45. Sanders TG, Tirman PF, Linares R, Feller JF, Richardson R. The glenolabral articular disruption lesion: MR arthrography with arthroscopic correlation. AJR Am J Roentgenol. 1999;172:171–175.

46. Tirman PF, Steinbach LS, Feller JF, Stauffer AE. Humeral avulsion of the anterior shoulder stabilizing structures after anterior shoulder dislocation: demonstration by MRI and MR arthrography. Skeletal Radiol. 1996;25:743–748.

47. Warner JJ, Beim GM. Combined Bankart and HAGL lesion associated with anterior shoulder instability. Arthroscopy. 1997; 13:749–752.

POSTERIOR INSTABILITY

48. Chung CB, Sorenson S, Dwek JR, Resnick D. Humeral avulsion of the posterior band of the inferior glenohumeral ligament: MR arthrography and clinical correlation in 17 patients. AJR Am J Roentgenol. 2004;183:355–359.

49. De Maeseneer M, Jaovisidha S, Jacobson JA, et al. The Bennett lesion of the shoulder. J Comput Assist Tomogr. 1998;22:31–34.

50. Hottya GA, Tirman PF, Bost FW, Montgomery WH, Wolf EM, Genant HK. Tear of the posterior shoulder stabilizers after posterior dislocation: MR imaging and MR arthrographic findings with arthroscopic correlation. AJR Am J Roentgenol. 1998;171:763–768.

51. Jin W, Ryu KN, Park YK, Lee WK, Ko SH, Yang DM. Cystic lesions in the posterosuperior portion of the humeral head on MR arthrography: correlations with gross and histologic findings in cadavers. AJR Am J Roentgenol. 2005;184:1211–1215.

52. Jobe CM. Posterior superior glenoid impingement: expanded spectrum. Arthroscopy. 1995;11:530–536.

53. Liu SH, Boynton E. Posterior superior impingement of the rotator cuff on the glenoid rim as a cause of shoulder pain in the overhead athlete. Arthroscopy. 1993;9:697–699.

54. Richards RD, Sartoris DJ, Pathria MN, Resnick D. Hill-Sachs lesion and normal humeral groove: MR imaging features allowing their differentiation. Radiology. 1994;190:665–668.

55. Simons P, Joekes E, Nelissen RG, Bloem JL. Posterior labrocapsular periosteal sleeve avulsion complicating locked posterior shoulder dislocation. Skeletal Radiol. 1998;27:588–590.

56. Steinbach LS, Tirman PFJ, Peterfy CA, Feller J. eds. Shoulder Magnetic Resonance Imaging. Philadelphia: Lippincott-Raven; 1998.

57. Tirman PF, Bost FW, Garvin GJ, et al. Posterosuperior glenoid

impingement of the shoulder: findings at MR imaging and MR arthrography with arthroscopic correlation. Radiology. 1994;193:431–436

58. Weishaupt D, Zanetti M, Nyffeler RW,Gerber C, Hodler J. Posterior glenoid rim deficiency in recurrent (atraumatic) posterior shoulder instability. Skeletal Radiol 2000;29:204–210.

59. Workman TL, Burkhard TK, Resnick D, et al. Hill-Sachs lesion: comparison of detection with MR imaging, radiography, and arthroscopy. Radiology. 1992;185:847–852.

60. Yu JS, Ashman CJ, Jones G. The POLPSA lesion: MR imaging findings with arthroscopic correlation in patients with posterior instability. Skeletal Radiol. 2002;31:396–399.

PARALABRAL CYSTS

61. Fritz RC, Helms CA, Steinbach LS,Genant HK. Suprascapular nerve entrapment: evaluation with MR imaging. Radiology. 1992;182:437–444.

62. Nobuhara K, Ikeda H. Rotator interval lesion. Clin Orthop Relat Res. 1987;223:44–50.

63. Sanders TG, Tirman PF. Paralabral cyst: an unusual cause of quadrilateral space syndrome. Arthroscopy. 1999;15:632–637.

64. Tirman PF, Feller JF, Janzen DL, Peterfy CG, Bergman AG. Association of glenoid labral cysts with labral tears and glenohumeral instability: radiologic findings and clinical significance. Radiology. 1994;190:653–658.

65. Visser CP, Coene LN, Brand R, Tavy DL. The incidence of nerve injury in anterior dislocation of the shoulder and its influence on functional recovery: a prospective clinical and EMG study. J Bone Joint Surg Br. 1999;81:679–685.

Case 3

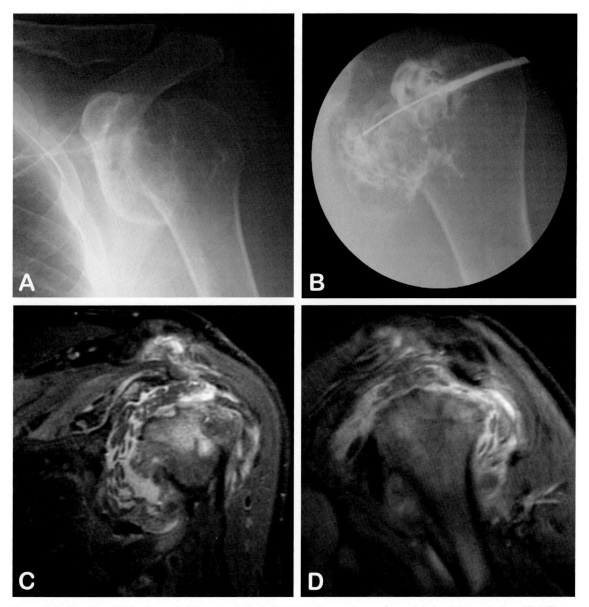

Figure 3-1. Shoulder. (A) Radiograph (internal rotation). (B) MR arthrography, performed during joint aspiration. (C) MRI. Proton-density, fat-saturated. Coronal oblique view. (D) MRI. Proton-density, fat-saturated. Sagittal oblique view.

Question 12

You are shown four images (Figure 3-1) from the shoulder MRI examination of a 36-year-old man who presents with shoulder pain. Which *one* of the following is the MOST likely diagnosis?

(A)   Rheumatoid arthritis
(B)   Synovial osteochondromatosis
(C)   Pigmented villonodular synovitis
(D)   Lipoma arborescens

David P. Fessell, M.D.

Synovial Osteochondromatosis

Question 12

Which *one* of the following is the MOST likely diagnosis?

(A) Rheumatoid arthritis
(B) Synovial osteochondromatosis
(C) Pigmented villonodular synovitis
(D) Lipoma arborescens

The shoulder radiograph demonstrates remodeling of the glenoid, a large cyst in the humeral head, and an absence of ossified intraarticular bodies. The arthrogram shows multiple small filling defects. The proton-density, fat-saturated coronal and sagittal oblique MR images demonstrate multiple, small rice bodies, with signal intensity that is isointense to muscle. No foci of signal void or foci with fat signal are noted to suggest calcification or ossification within the bodies. Small, erosive changes of the humeral head are also noted. These findings are consistent with a chronic synovial process, and of the choices in Question 12, most consistent with rheumatoid arthritis **(Option (A) is correct).**

Rice bodies within a joint were initially described in the setting of tuberculosis. Nowadays they are most commonly seen in patients with rheumatoid arthritis or, less commonly, in the setting of seronegative arthropathies or chronic joint or bursal inflammation. Macroscopically they resemble grains of polished rice, with 90% percent being less than 7 mm in length. Rice bodies comprise fibrin and fibronectin, and may also contain collagen, reticulin, and elastin. They appear isointense to muscle on both T1- and T2-weighted sequences, consistent with a fibrous composition. They are seen best on T2-weighted sequences as small, low-signal, discrete nodules outlined by fluid. The absence of prominent regions of high signal on T2- or proton-density-weighted

sequences helps distinguish rice bodies from the cartilaginous bodies of synovial chondromatosis (chondroid bodies). Because of their intermediate to high signal on proton-density or T2 sequences, the cartilaginous bodies of synovial chondromatosis may not be distinguishable from the underlying high intensity signal of joint fluid on these sequences. On MRI, the intraarticular bodies seen with synovial osteochondromatosis (also known as the ossified form of synovial chondromatosis) demonstrate a signal void due to calcification or fat signal due to ossification. Mineralized bodies may also be noted on radiographs. The absence of these findings helps distinguish rice bodies from synovial osteochondromatosis. In addition to large joints like the knee and shoulder, rice bodies have also been reported in bursa, secondary to rheumatoid arthritis or chronic inflammation.

Rice bodies are thought to evolve from one of two processes: synovial microinfarction with subsequent sloughing of synovial fragments into the joint and their encasement by fibrin from the synovial fluid; or de novo formation of fibrin/fibronectin aggregates in the synovial fluid that progressively enlarge over time. If saline lavage of the joint is done with a large bore (8-14G) needle, rice bodies can be found in the knee joint aspirate of approximately 70% of rheumatoid arthritis patients, versus only about 15% if aspiration is performed without lavage.

With the recent advent of new and highly effective therapies, the treatment of rheumatoid arthritis has undergone a revolution. Such therapies include very costly drugs such as anti-tumor necrosis factor agents. The availability of such effective therapies has created an urgent need for early diagnosis as well as better ways of monitoring the disease during the course of treatment. The hands, wrists, and feet are most frequently affected by rheumatoid arthritis and are thus the most frequently evaluated joints. Larger joints such as the shoulder can also be affected, especially with more advanced or long-standing disease.

Radiographs are widely used for the diagnosis and followup of rheumatoid arthritis. They are relatively insensitive, however, and can only detect more advanced disease. The classic radiographic findings of rheumatoid arthritis are osteopenia, erosions, and joint space narrowing. Radiographs do not visualize synovial inflammation, and are also insensitive to such bone changes as bone marrow edema and early erosions, thereby limiting the usefulness of this modality for early detection of rheumatoid arthritis.

Arthrography, while not typically used for the diagnosis of rheumatoid arthritis, can suggest a synovial process when filling defects are noted, as in Figure 3-2B. Intraarticular bodies may also be seen as filling defects on arthrograms, with the bodies often noted on the pre-arthrogram "scout" radiographs. For arthrography, iodinated contrast is injected into a joint, usually as part of a fluoroscopically guided joint aspiration or joint

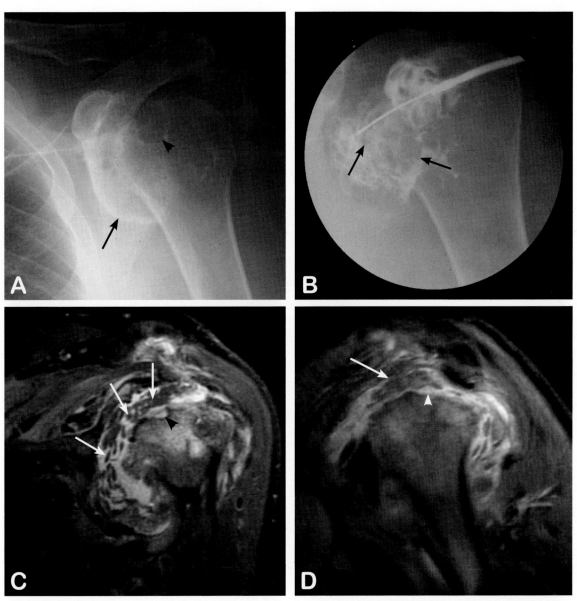

Figure 3-2 (same as Figure 3-1). Rice bodies in the shoulder joint. Shoulder. (A) Radiograph (internal rotation). Remodeling of the glenoid is noted (arrow). There is a large cyst in the humeral head (arrowhead). (B) Arthrogram (performed during joint aspiration). Contrast is noted in the glenohumeral joint containing multiple small filling defects (arrows). (C) MRI. Proton-density, fat-saturated. Coronal plane. (D) MRI. Proton-density, fat-saturated. Sagittal plane. The images demonstrate multiple small low-signal rice bodies (arrows in panels C and D) with small erosive changes of the humeral head (arrowheads in panels C and D). Findings are consistent with a chronic synovial process such as rheumatoid arthritis.

injection. When used in this way, the iodinated contrast assures proper needle placement within the joint. Joint aspiration is typically performed to assess for infection or crystal deposition disease. Joint injection can also be performed for an MR arthrogram. A combined steroid and anesthetic injection can be performed for symptomatic relief in the setting of degenerative joint disease or rotator cuff disease. Since it is an invasive and relatively insensitive procedure for the detection of synovitis, ar-

thrography is not used in the diagnosis or for monitoring of rheumatoid arthritis.

MR imaging provides global imaging of a joint, including the osseous and soft tissue structures. On MR imaging, synovitis, bone edema and erosions are the hallmarks of rheumatoid arthritis (Figure 3-3). Tenosynovitis and bursitis may also be present. Synovitis is noted as thickening of the synovial membrane and usually shows rapid enhancement after intravenous gado-

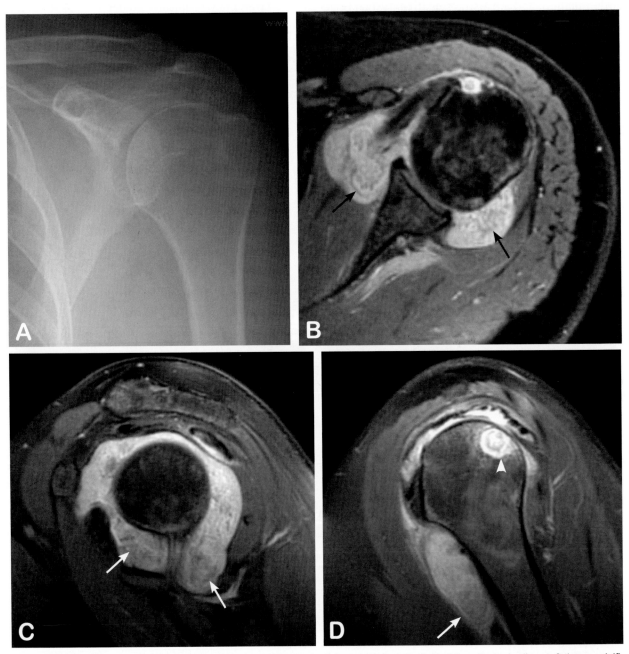

Figure 3-3. Synovitis of rheumatoid arthritis. Shoulder. (A) Radiograph (in external rotation). No intraarticular bodies, soft tissue calcifications or definite erosions are demonstrated. (B, C, D) MRI. Proton-density, fat-saturated. (B) Axial plane. Vague regions of low signal visible in the glenohumeral joint are consistant with synovitis. (C) Sagittal plane. Vague regions of low signal (arrows in panels C and D) can be seen in the glenohumeral joint, consistent with synovitis. (D) Sagittal oblique plane. The arrowhead denotes a subchondral cyst at the posterior aspect of the humeral head in panel D, with surrounding bone edema.

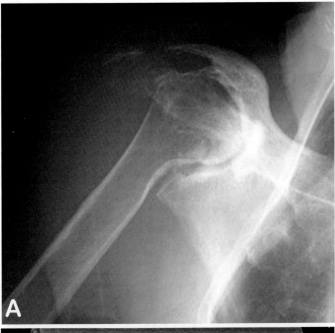

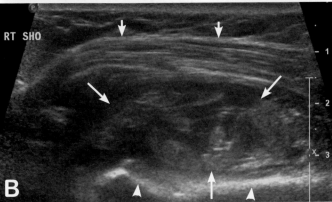

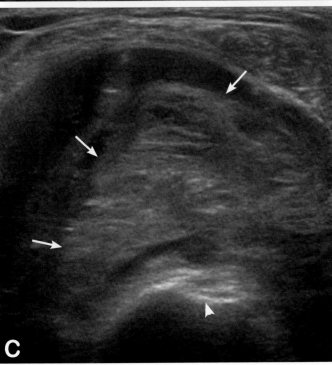

linium administration. Bone edema, noted as ill-defined high signal on T2-weighted, fat-saturated, or short tau inversion recovery (STIR) sequences, may be seen before erosions. Erosions are noted as a cortical defect, which may also show trabecular bone loss, often with associated synovial proliferation and bone edema.

Ultrasound can also be used to assess a joint for changes of rheumatoid arthritis (Figure 3-4). On ultrasound examination, synovial proliferation is noted as a hypoechoic or isoechoic mass, relative to subcutaneous fat. Synovial proliferation may distend joint recesses, tendon sheaths, and bursae. Increased Doppler signal is noted on color or power Doppler evaluation. Erosions are noted as discontinuities of the cortical bone adjacent to or involving the joint surface. Such discontinuities should be visible on images obtained in perpendicular planes, e.g. longitudinal and transverse planes relative to the long axis of the extremity. Ultrasound can also detect tenosynovitis, seen as anechoic or hypoechoic thickening of the synovial sheath of the tendon. Bursitis is noted as heterogeneous (hypoechoic and hyperechoic) regions in the expected location of a bursa, often with hyperemia on Doppler imaging. Ultrasound cannot detect bone edema but can detect enthesitis, such as that at the Achilles insertion. Thickening and hypoechogenicity of the entheses can be noted, along with hyperemia, during color Doppler evaluation.

Synovial osteochondromatosis, also known as the mineralized form of synovial chondromatosis or synovial (osteo) chondromatosis, is typically seen as multiple osseous joint bodies (Figure 3-5). At histology, synovial chondromatosis is classically termed a "synovial metaplasia." Its etiology is uncertain but is commonly thought to be secondary to transformation of pluripotent mesenchymal cells (located at the junction of the synovium) and cartilage into nests of chondrocytes, which eventually pedunculate and slough into the joint space as intraarticular bodies. If the bodies mineralize, they may be termed synovial osteochondromatosis. The terminology in the literature is inconsistent, with some authors lumping both mineralized and unmineralized

Figure 3-4. Bursitis and erosions of rheumatoid arthritis. Shoulder. (A) Radiograph. The radiograph demonstrates extensive erosive changes of the glenoid, humeral head, and proximal humerus. (B) Ultrasound (along the long axis of the proximal humerus). Extensive synovial proliferation in the subacromial-subdeltoid bursa (long arrows) is demonstrated. Arrowheads denote the cortex of the neck and diaphysis of the proximal humerus. Short arrows point to the proximal deltoid muscle. (C) Ultrasound (along the short axis of the proximal humerus). Synovial proliferation can be seen in the bursa (long arrows). The arrowheads denote the cortex of the proximal humerus with erosive changes. RT SHO = right shoulder.

forms into the heading of "synovial chondromatosis," and other authors placing both forms under the heading of "synovial osteochondromatosis." Primary (de novo) and secondary forms of synovial osteochondromatosis have been described, though the secondary form is something of a misnomer and is simply the name given

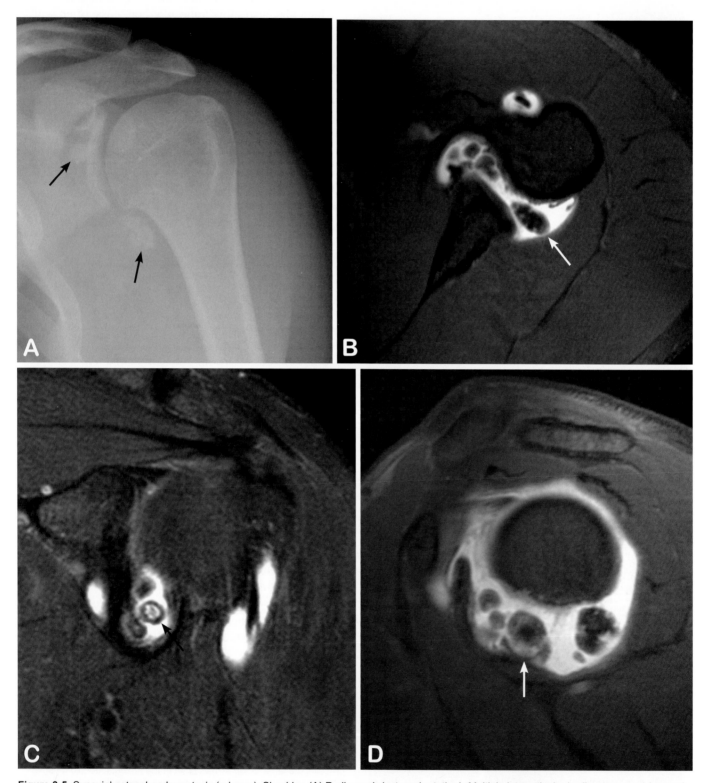

Figure 3-5. Synovial osteochondromatosis (primary). Shoulder. (A) Radiograph (external rotation). Multiple intraarticular bodies are noted (arrows) with absence of marked degenerative disease. (B, C, D) MR arthrography. T1-weighted, fat-saturated. (B) Axial plane. (C) Coronal plane. (D) Sagittal oblique plane. Multiple small low-signal intraarticular bodies are marked with arrows in panels B, C, and D. Findings are consistent with primary synovial osteochondromatosis. The signal intensity of these bodies can vary depending on the relative amounts of ossification.

by some to describe multiple intraarticular bodies secondary to osteoarthrosis. While the MR appearance in Figure 3-2 shows multiple bodies, they are not ossified and thus not visible on the radiograph **(Option (B) is false)**. They also do not have high internal signal on proton density images to suggest that they are cartilaginous in origin.

Pigmented villonodular synovitis (PVNS) of the shoulder is a proliferative synovial process of unknown etiology. It can cause osseous erosions and can occur in the glenohumeral joint as in Figure 3-2. PVNS has a variable appearance and signal intensity on MR imaging, depending on the relative proportions of hemosiderin, lipid, fibrous elements, fluid, cystic components, and cellular aggregates. Its presence can be strongly suggested when low signal foci are noted on all MR sequences. "Blooming" artifact at the site of PVNS can also occur on gradient echo sequences, which are extremely sensitive to magnetic field inhomogenity. The low signal hemosiderin deposition deposits appear to enlarge or "bloom" due to magnetic field inhomogenity induced by the hemosiderin in the tissue adjacent to the a blood clot. The "bloom" increases in size as TE increases. PVNS also demonstrates strong enhancement after intravenous gadolinium administration. While PVNS can range from small foci of low signal to larger masslike regions, it does not have the appearance of multiple discrete, small, rice bodies **(Option (C) is false)**.

Lipoma arborescens of the shoulder is a synovial abnormality with villous, lipomatous proliferation of the synovium. It is noted as frond- or tree-like ("arbor" is Latin for "tree"), lipomatous hypertrophy within a joint or bursa, most commonly involving the knee joint, glenohumeral joint, or the subacromial-subdeltoid bursa. It is typically seen in association with a joint effusion and may be seen with synovial cysts and erosions. In Figure 3-2, no frond-like fat signal is noted **(Option (D) is false)**.

Question 13

Regarding synovial chondromatosis of the shoulder:

(A) Treatment may include removal of bodies, synovectomy, or arthroplasty.
(B) It is the same as "rice bodies" in the shoulder.
(C) The shoulder is the most commonly involved joint.
(D) Malignant transformation into chondrosarcoma is uncommon.

The typical treatment of synovial chondromatosis usually involves at least removal of the joint bodies and partial synovectomy. Depending on the degree of erosions or associated joint pathology, arthroplasty may also be performed **(Option (A) is true)**.

Rice bodies are composed predominantly of fibrin/fibronectin and are seen in patients with rheumatoid arthritis, or less commonly in patients with other arthritides or chronic infection. Synovial chondromatosis is composed of cartilage rests, which, if ossified or calcified, may be referred to as synovial osteochondromatosis. Rice bodies are low in signal on all MR sequences, due to their fibrous composition **(Option (B) is false)**. Cartilaginous bodies have intermediate to high signal on proton-density and T2-weighted sequences.

While synovial chondromatosis can be seen in the shoulder, the knee is by far the most commonly involved joint **(Option (C) is false)**. At least 80% to 95% of cases occur in the knee, hip, and elbow. Synovial chondromatosis has also been reported in the ankle, wrist, spine, and smaller joints such as the acromioclavicular joint, temperomandibular joint and sternoclavicular joint.

Though it is a very rare event, synovial chondromatosis can undergo malignant transformation to chondrosarcoma **(Option (D) is true)**. At least 33 cases of histologically confirmed malignant transformation of synovial chondromatosis have been reported. Typically this occurs in the setting of a protracted clinical course, with rapid, frequent, or multiple recurrences of synovial chondromatosis prior to the malignant transformation.

Question 14

Which *one* of the following is the MOST sensitive modality for detecting early erosions in rheumatoid arthritis of the shoulder?

(A) Radiography
(B) Ultrasound
(C) MR imaging

While all of the above modalities can detect findings of rheumatoid arthritis, MR imaging has been shown to be the most sensitive for detecting early erosions **(Option (C) is correct)**. Ultrasound is less sensitive than MR imaging for detecting erosions (Figure 3-2) **(Option (B) is incorrect)** but it is more sensitive than radiography. Radiographs are thus the least sensitive of these three modalities **(Option (A) is incorrect)**. The differences in sensitivity between MR and radiography and between MRI and ultrasound are statistically significant.

MR is also superior to ultrasound for detecting synovitis, tenosynovitis, and bursitis. The expense and availability of MR limits its application. Ultrasound is widely available and relatively inexpensive. Radiographs are clearly useful for monitoring known joint destruction in the setting of established rheumatoid arthritis.

Question 15

Regarding pigmented villonodular synovitis of the shoulder,

(A) Radiographs can provide definitive diagnosis.
(B) Erosions are not always present.
(C) MR imaging is the modality of choice for diagnosis and pre-operative planning.
(D) Malignant degeneration is rarely associated with this entity.
(E) Recurrence is more common in the shoulder than in the knee.

Radiographs can show soft tissue swelling and erosions, but are not definitive for PVNS **(Option (A) is false).** The radiographic findings of PVNS can be seen with many other entities including rheumatoid arthritis and other arthritides, infection, and lipoma arborescens. Secondary changes of osteoarthrosis can be seen in chronic cases of PVNS. Radiographs can be helpful to exclude mineralized bodies, such as those seen in synovial osteochondromatosis, and to assess for erosions or degenerative joint disease.

Erosions are not always present **(Option (B) is true)** and are not necessary to make the diagnosis of PVNS. They have been reported in approximately 25% to 60% of cases. MR imaging is more sensitive and can detect the erosive changes earlier than radiographs or sonography.

MR imaging provides global imaging with excellent soft tissue resolution and is therefore the most optimal modality for imaging suspected PVNS **(Option (C) is true)** and monitoring its treatment. PVNS can involve synovial spaces about the shoulder, including the glenohumeral joint and subacromial-subdeltoid bursa (Figure 3-6). Though not always definitive, MR imaging can in some cases provide the diagnosis if the classic findings are noted. These include heterogeneous synovial thickening with areas of low signal on all sequences, "blooming" on gradient echo sequences, and rapid enhancement with contrast. Even when not definitive for the diagnosis, MR is the optimal modality for determining the extent of disease. MR imaging aids preoperative planning and can monitor for

recurrence after treatment. Intravenous gadolinium should always be used, if the patient's condition permits. PVNS strongly enhances with gadolinium, which helps detection and diagnosis. Gradient echo

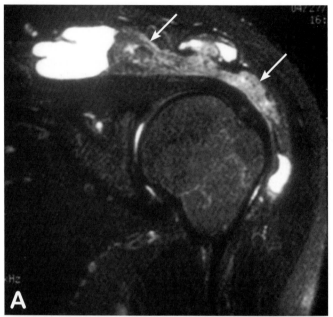

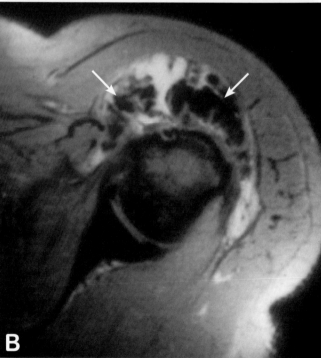

Figure 3-6. Pigmented villonodular synovitis. MRI. Shoulder. (A) T2-weighted. Coronal oblique view. The image demonstrates fluid as well as nodular tissue of intermediate signal in the subacromial/subdeltoid bursa (arrows). (B) Gradient echo. Axial plane. Low-signal hemosiderin (arrows) can be seen within the nodular bursal tissue. In combination with the clinical history of pain and swelling, findings are consistent with pigmented villonodular synovitis. *Case courtesy of Jon A. Jacobson, University of Michigan.*

sequences have increased sensitivity to local magnetic susceptibility from hemosiderin and are thus useful for detecting hemorrhagic processes. Other causes of joint hemorrhage such as trauma, surgery, hemophilia, and synovial hemangioma can also demonstrate "blooming" on gradient echo sequences. Clinical history as well as absence of the serpentine vascular mass seen with synovial hemangioma, can thus aid in the diagnosis of PVNS.

PVNS can be found diffusely within a joint, or be seen as a more focal mass of variable size. Treatment of PVNS is typically undertaken to relieve pain, restore joint motion, and prevent joint destruction. It can include synovectomy, radiation therapy, and arthroplasty. Malignant degeneration of PVNS, while rare, has been reported and can occur in association with recurrent PVNS, or de novo **(Option (D) is true)**. Given its rare occurrence, the imaging features of malignant PVNS have not been well described Murphey and colleagues note that extensive bone marrow involvement should raise concern for malignancy. With malignant PVNS, lymph node involvement, pulmonary metastases and multiple local recurrences are not uncommon.

PVNS of the shoulder is a relatively rare condition; it occurs much less commonly than in the knee where approximately 80% of cases are noted. Recurrence in the shoulder is also very uncommon **(Option (E) is false)**, in contrast to recurrence at the knee. This may be due to the ease of performing a synovectomy at the shoulder compared to the knee. The knee joint has multiple recesses and internal structures including the cruciate ligaments and menisci, making a "curative" synovectomy more difficult.

Question 16

Regarding lipoma arborescens of the shoulder:

(A) The diagnosis can be made with radiographs.
(B) T1-weighted MR imaging is helpful in making the diagnosis.
(C) It only occurs in joints.
(D) It is caused by prior hemarthrosis.
(E) It only occurs in patients over 40.

Lipoma arborescens has no specific radiographic findings **(Option (A) is false)**. Soft tissue swelling may be seen, but the villous, lipomatous synovial hypertrophy that characterizes lipoma arborescens is not seen with radiographs. Erosions have been reported with lipoma arborescens, but erosions are not specific for this diagno-

sis. Radiographs are helpful to exclude other joint processes such as synovial osteochondromatosis.

T1-weighted imaging aids detection of the high (fat) signal in the villous, hypetrophic synovium of patients with lipoma arborescens (Figure 3-7 and Figure 3-8) **(Option (B) is true)**. Fat-suppressed or T2-weighted MR sequences will demonstrate low signal in the frondlike fat, which is usually outlined by high signal joint fluid. STIR sequences will show a similar appearance.

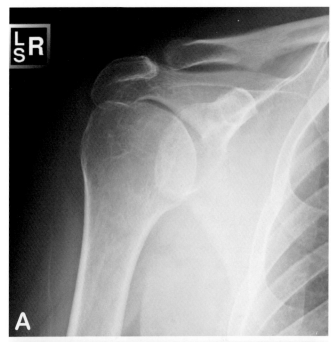

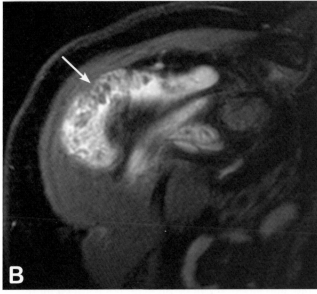

Figure 3-7. Lipoma arborescens of the subacromial-subdeltoid bursa. Shoulder. (A) Radiograph (slight external rotation). No intraarticular bodies or soft tissue calcifications are seen. (B) MRI. Proton-density, fat-saturated. Coronal plane.

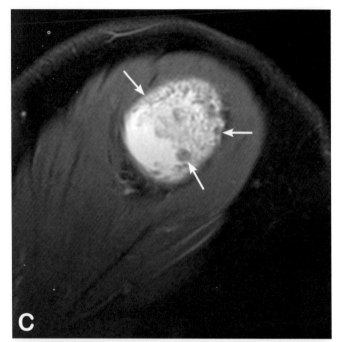

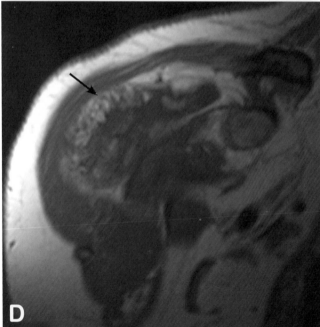

Figure 3-7 (continued). (C) MRI. Proton-density, fat-saturated. Sagittal oblique plane. Panels B and C both demonstrate foci of low signal (arrows) in the subacromial-subdeltoid bursa. (D) MRI. T1-weighted. Coronal plane. These foci (arrow) have fat signal on T1, consistent with lipoma arborescens.

Lipoma arborescens most commonly occurs in the knee joint. It can also occur in the shoulder joint and subdeltoid-subacromial bursa **(Option (C) is false)** (Figure 3-7). It has been reported in the hip, elbow, hand, and ankle. It can be bilateral but is much more commonly monoarticular.

While the etiology of lipoma arborescens is not well understood, it is not thought to be due to prior

hemarthrosis **(Option (D) is false).** Primary and secondary forms have been postulated, with the secondary form associated with a chronic joint process such as degenerative disease, meniscal pathology in the knee, or rotator cuff tear in the shoulder (Figure 3-8). The primary form has no underlying joint pathology. Lipomatous hypertrophy of the synovium is the predominant feature. The secondary form is thus thought to be a re-

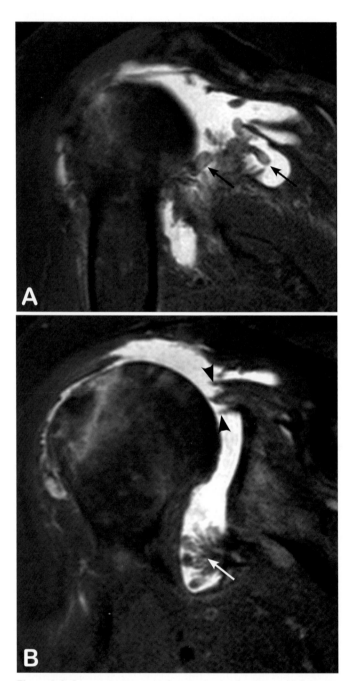

Figure 3-8. Supraspinatus and infraspinatus tendon tears with lipoma arborescens of the glenohumeral joint. (A, B, C) MRI. Shoulder. Proton-density, fat-saturated. (A) Coronal plane. Black arrows point to frond-like foci of low signal. (B) Coronal plane. Arrowheads denote the ends of the torn tendon. A white arrow points to frond-like foci of low signal.

active process due to prior trauma and/or arthritis, and is much more common than the primary form.

Lipoma arborescens typically occurs in patients in their fifth to seventh decades of life, but it has been reported in younger patients **(Option (E) is false).** The more common secondary form of lipoma arborescens is typically seen in older patients, whose age makes them more likely to have a chronic joint process.

Note: The use of intraarticular gadolinium has not been FDA-approved.

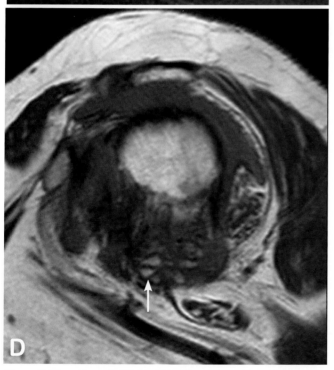

Figure 3-8 (continued). (C) Sagittal oblique plane. Frond-like foci of low signal (arrow) are also seen in this plane at the inferior aspect of the glenohumeral joint. (D) T1-weighted. Sagittal plane. The frond-like foci (arrow) have fat signal similar to subcutaneous fat on T1, consistent with a diagnosis of lipoma arborescens.

Suggested Readings

RHEUMATOID ARTHRITIS AND RICE BODIES

1. Boutry N, Morel M, Flipo RM, Demondion X, Cotten A. Early rheumatoid arthritis: a review of MRI and sonographic findings. AJR Am J Roentgenol. 2007;189:1502–1509.

2. Chen A, Wong LY, Sheu CY, Chen BF. Distinguishing multiple rice body formation in chronic subacromial-subdeltoid bursitis from synovial chondromatosis. Skeletal Radiol. 2002;31:119–121.

3. Griffith JF, Peh WC, Evans NS, Smallman LA, Wong RW, Thomas AM. Multiple rice body formation in chronic subacromial/subdeltoid bursitis: MR appearances. Clin Radiol 1996; 51:511–514.

4. Hermann KG, Backhaus M, Schneider U, et al. Rheumatoid arthritis of the shoulder joint: comparison of conventional radiography, ultrasound, and dynamic contrast-enhanced magnetic resonance imaging. Arthritis Rheum 2003;48:3338–3349.

5. Popert AJ, Scott DL, Wainwright AC, Walton KW, Williamson N, Chapman JH. Frequency of occurrence, mode of development, and significance or rice bodies in rheumatoid joints. Ann Rheum Dis. 1982;41:109–117.

6. Sheldon PJ, Forrester DM, Learch TJ. Imaging of intraarticular masses. RadioGraphics 2005;25:105–119.

7. Spence LD, Adams J, Gibbons D, Mason MD, Eustace S. Rice body formation in bicipito-radial bursitis: ultrasound, CT, and MRI findings. Skeletal Radiol. 1998;27:30–32.

PVNS

8. Cotten A, Flipo RM, Mestdahg H, Chastanet P. Diffuse pigmented villonodular synovitis of the shoulder. Skeletal Radiol. 1995;24:311–313.

9. Hughes TH, Sartoris DJ, Schweitzer ME, Resnick DL. Pigmented villonodular synovitis: MRI characteristics. Skeletal Radiol. 1995;24:7–12.

10. Mulier T, Victor J, Van Den Bergh J, Fabry G. Diffuse pigmented villonodular synovitis of the shoulder. A case report & review of literature. Acta Orthop Belg. 1992;58:93–96.

11. Murphey MD, Rhee JH, Lewis RB, Fanburg-Smith JC, Flemming DJ, Walker EA. Pigmented villonodular synovitis: Radiologic-pathologic correlation. RadioGraphics. 2008;28:1493–1518.

12. Wirbel RJ, Braun C, Blandfort R, Pahl S, Mutschler WE. Villon-odular synovitis of the shoulder. Orthopedics. 2000;23:731–733.

SYNOVIAL CHONDROMATOSIS AND OSTEOCHONDROMATOSIS

13. Milgram JW. Synovial osteochondromatosis: a histopathological study of thirty cases. J Bone Joint Surg Am .1977;59:792–80.

14. Sah AP, Geller DS, Mankin HJ, et al. Malignant transformation of synovial chondromatosis of the shoulder to chondrosarcoma. A case report. J Bone Joint Surg Am. 2007;89:1321–1328.

15. Wirbel RJ, Braun C, Blandfort R, Pahl S, Mutschler WE. Vil-lonodular synovitis of the shoulder. Orthopedics. 2000;23:731–733.

LIPOMA ARBORESCENS

16. Nisolle JF, Blouard E, Baudrez V, Boutsen Y, De Cloedt P, Es-selinckx W. Subacromial-subdeltoid lipoma Arborescens as-sociated with a rotator cuff tear. Skeletal Radiol. 1999;28:283–285.

17. Pandey T, Alkhulaifi Y. Bilateral lipoma arborescens of the subdeltoid bursa. Australasian Radiol. 2006;50:487–489.

18. Vilanova JC, Barcelo J, Villalon M, Aldoma J, Delgado E, Za-pater I. MR imaging of lipoma arborescens and the associated lesions. Skeletal Radiol. 2003;32:504–509.

Case 4

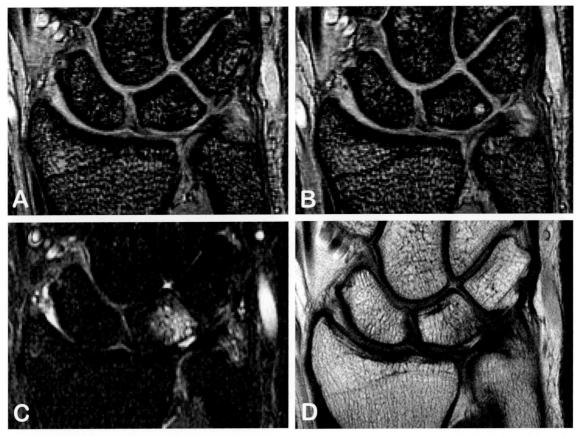

Figure 4-1. Wrist. MRI. Coronal plane. (A) T2*-weighted, three-dimensional (3-D) gradient echo. (B) T2*-weighted, 3-D gradient echo. (C) Fast inversion recovery (FIR). (D) Proton-density-weighted, moderate echo time, fast spin-echo.

Question 17

You are shown four MR images (Figure 4-1) from the right wrist of a right-hand-dominant 36-year-old man. The patient presented with ulnar-sided wrist pain. Which *one* of the following is the MOST likely diagnosis?

(A)   Kienböck's disease
(B)   Giant cell tumor of the lunate
(C)   Ulnar impaction syndrome
(D)   Ulnar styloid abutment syndrome

Triangular Fibrocartilage Complex

Question 17

Which *one* of the following is the MOST likely diagnosis?

(A) Kienböck's disease
(B) Giant cell tumor of the lunate
(C) Ulnar impaction syndrome
(D) Ulnar styloid abutment syndrome

The coronal fast spin-echo (FSE) image demonstrates full-thickness cartilage loss (Figure 4-2D) over the ulnar margin of the proximal lunate, adjacent to the prominent cysts and edema pattern noted on the inversion recovery image (Figure 4-2C). The superior (1mm) slice resolution of the three-dimensional gradient echo images demonstrates central thinning (Figure 4-2A) but

no defect of the triangular fibrocartilage (TFC) adjacent to the cyst. In addition, there is a focal full-thickness tear of the lunotriquetral ligament (Figure 4-2B). These findings are indicative of ulnar impaction syndrome **(Option (C) is correct).**

Ulnar impaction syndrome represents a constellation of findings, including central TFC lesions, cartilage loss over the ulnar proximal pole of the lunate and lunotriquetral instability. Cartilage loss is occasionally seen over the proximal aspect of the triquetrum.

Ulnar impaction is commonly seen in the setting of pronounced ulnar positive variance (Figure 4-3). Ulnar variance is generally described on a posteroanterior (PA) radiograph view of the wrist obtained with neutral rotation. Most MR imaging of the wrist is performed with the wrist in full pronation, a position

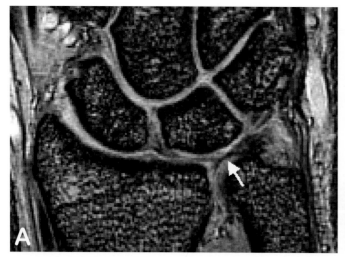 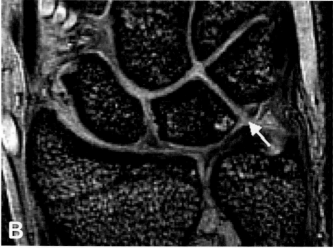

Figure 4-2 (same as 4-1). Ulnar impaction syndrome. Wrist. MRI. Coronal plane. (A) T2*weighted, 3-D gradient echo. The image shows contral thinning (arrow) of the central triangular fibrocartilage (TFC) but no defect. (B) T2*-weighted, 3-D gradient echo. The image shows a focal full-thickness tear of the lunotriquetral ligament (arrow). A subchondral cyst is also present in the proximal lunate.

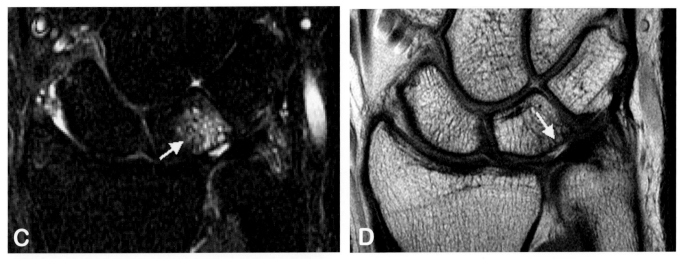

Figure 4-2 (continued). Ulnar impaction syndrome. (C) Fast inversion recovery. An edema pattern is revealed in the lunate (arrow). (D) Moderate echo time, proton-density-weighted, fast spin-echo. There is full-thickness cartilage loss (arrow) over the ulnar margin of the proximal lunate.

which acts to physiologically shorten the radius. Previous studies have correlated the relative thickness of the TFC with ulnar variance, where the TFC or articular disc tends to be thinner in the presence of positive variance and thicker in the presence of ulnar negative variance.

The differential diagnosis for ulnar impaction includes Kienböck's disease; however, Kienböck's disease typically generates a more global bone marrow edema pattern throughout the lunate or preferential involvement of the radial margin of the lunate. Kienböck's disease is not typically associated with full-thickness cartilage loss in the absence of collapse **(Option (A) is incorrect).**

Giant cell tumors of bone may be found in the carpal bones but are typically associated with large cystic expansion and are not associated with cartilage loss **(Option (B) is incorrect).** Ulnar styloid abutment is typically associated with ulnar styloid non-union (not demonstrated in this case), or in the setting of a prominent ulnar styloid process that abuts or impinges against the cartilage of the triquetrum **(Option (D) is incorrect).**

Treatment for ulnar impaction generally involves ulnar osteotomy and triangular fibrocartilage debridement. Ulnar impingement may occur secondary to shortening of the ulna proximal to the sigmoid notch and loss of cartilage over the distal radius at the distal

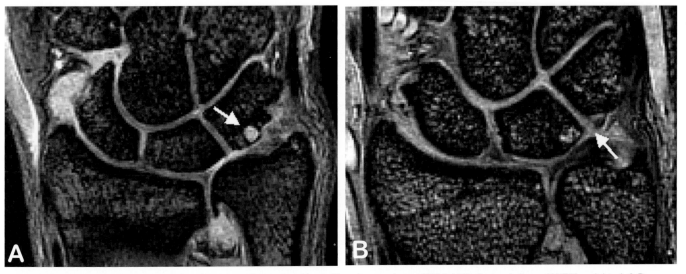

Figure 4-3. Ulnar impaction syndrome in a 65-year-old woman with positive ulnar variance. Wrist. MRI. Coronal plane. (A) T2*-weighted, 3-D, gradient-echo. The image shows a cyst (arrow) in the proximal triquetrum. (B) Moderate-echo-time, proton-density-weighted, fast spin-echo. An associated central perforation (arrow) of the TFC is seen.

radioulnar joint, with reactive cystic change or scalloping of the cortex proximal to the level of the joint (Figure 4-4).

Ulnar impingement may also be seen in the absence of previous ulnar osteotomy due to prior growth disturbance with premature closure of the physis. When this occurs in young individuals, it characteristically creates pronounced ulnar minus variance with compensatory thickening of the TFC (Figure 4-5). This results in abnormal mechanical stresses upon the distal radioulnar joint as well as the proximal carpal row.

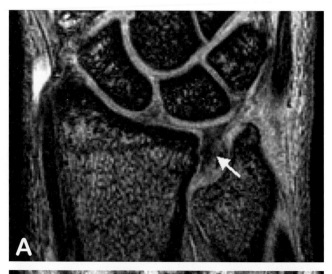

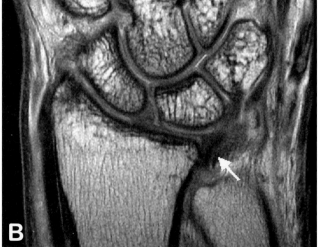

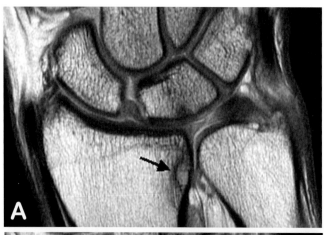

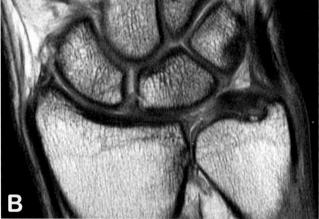

Figure 4-4. Ulnar impingement in a 59-year-old woman 18 months after ulnar osteotomy and TFC debridement for ulnar impaction syndrome. Wrist. MRI. Coronal plane. (A & B) Moderate echo time, proton-density-weighted, fast spin-echo. There is prominent cystic change (arrow) as well as bony sclerosis of the distal radius just below the joint, where there is a full-thickness cartilage loss.

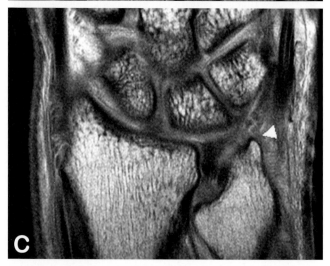

Figure 4-5. Ulnar impingement in a 40-year-old woman who was a long-standing competitive gymnast. Wrist. MRI. Coronal plane. (A) T2*-weighted, 3-D gradient echo. The image shows pronounced ulnar minus variance with secondary deformity of the distal radioulnar joint, irregular contour of the TFC and marked degeneration of the TFC remnant (arrows). (B & C) Moderate echo time, proton-density-weighted, fast spin-echo images demonstrate marked degeneration of the TFC remnant (arrow) as well as the elongated ulnar styloid (arrowhead) abutting the synovium in the prestyloid recess.

Question 18

You are shown three MR images (Figure 4-6 in the Test section) of the right wrist in an 18-year-old, right-hand-dominant female gymnast, who presents with ulnar-sided wrist pain.

This case illustrates which *one* of the following?

(A) Peripheral detachment of the triangular fibrocartilage
(B) Tear of the extensor carpi ulnaris tendon sheath
(C) Lunotriquetral ligament tear
(D) Central defect of the triangular fibrocartilage

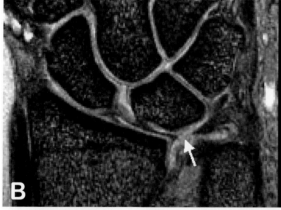

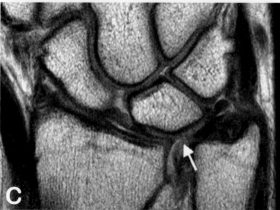

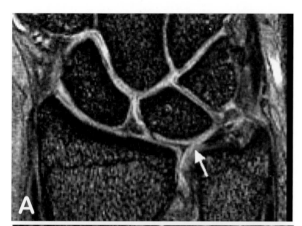

Figure 4-7. (same as Figure 4-6) Wrist. MRI. Coronal plane. (A & B) T2*-weighted, 3-D gradient echo. The images show a central defect of the TFC (arrows). (C) Moderate echo time, proton-density-weighted, FSE. A defect (arrow) in the central portion of the TFC is seen. The peripheral attachment of the TFC is intact.

This case illustrates a central defect of the TFC **(Option (D) is correct)**. The peripheral or ulnar attachment is intact, as is the lunotriquetral ligament **(Options (A) and (C) are incorrect)**. The extensor carpi ulnaris tendon and its sheath are best evaluated on axial acquisitions and appear intact in this case **(Option (B) is incorrect)**.

Question 19

Which *one* of the following is NOT a component of the triangular fibrocartilage complex?

(A) Ulnolunate ligament
(B) Ulnotriquetral ligament
(C) Lunotriquetral ligament
(D) Meniscal homologue

The triangular fibrocartilage complex (TFCC) is a major stabilizer of the distal radioulnar joint. The complex is composed of the triangular fibrocartilage (or articular disc), the dorsal and volar distal radioulnar ligaments, meniscal homologue (ulnar carpal meniscus), the ulnolunate and ulnotriquetral ligaments, and the ulnar collateral ligament/sheath of the extensor carpi ulnaris tendon. There is a surgical classification for lesions of the TFCC (Table 4-1) **(Option (C) is correct; Options (A), (B) and (D) are incorrect)**.

Table 4-1. Palmer Classification of Triangular Fibrocartilage Complex Injuries	
Class I : Traumatic	*Class II : Degenerative*
A. Central perforation	A. TFCC wear
B. Ulnar avulsion with or without distal ulnar fracture	B. TFCC wear, lunate and/or ulnar chondromalacia
C. Distal avulsion	C. TFCC perforation, lunate and/or ulnar chondromalacia
D. Radial avulsion with or without sigmoid notch fracture	D. TFC perforation, lunate and/or ulnar chondromalacia, and lunotriquetral ligament perforation
	E. TFC perforation, lunate and/or ulnar chondromalacia, lunotriquetral ligament perforation, and ulnocarpal arthritis

Question 20

Regarding lesions of the triangular fibrocartilage, which *one* of the following statements is true?

(A) Only central lesions of the triangular fibrocartilage can be successfully repaired.
(B) Peripheral tears are associated with ulnar positive variance.
(C) Tears are characteristically associated with lesions of the extensor carpi ulnaris tendon.
(D) Diagnosis requires the presence of disproportionate. amount of fluid in the distal radioulnar joint.
(E) None of the above is correct.

Similar to meniscus surgery of the knee, surgical intervention of TFC lesions is strongly influenced by the distribution of vascular supply of the disc. Small vessels perforate the peripheral 10% to 40%, leaving the inner margin and radial attachment of the TFC relatively avascular. Central lesions of the TFC are generally considered not repairable **(Option (A) is incorrect).** Central, rather than peripheral, tears of the TFC are often associated with ulnar positive variance **(Option (B) is incorrect).**

As the vascular portion of the TFC is in the peripheral or ulnar margin, primary repairs of the TFC are generally confined to the ulnar attachment, which is typically bifurcate in appearance (Figure 4-8). Note should be made that peripheral detachments of the TFC may be associated with disruption of the distal radioulnar ligaments, thus rendering the distal radioulnar joint grossly unstable (Figure 4-9).

Differential diagnoses for TFC lesions include traumatic cartilage injury of the distal radioulnar joint and distal radioulnar joint degenerative arthritis, as well as tendinosis or tears of the sixth dorsal compartment/extensor carpi ulnaris tendon. The latter may be associated

but is often seen in isolation **(Option (C) is incorrect).** The diagnosis of TFC tears on MRI is made by recognition of either a central defect or peripheral detachment

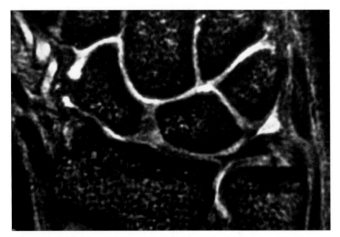

Figure 4-8. Wrist. MRI. Coronal plane. This inversion recovery image shows normal bifurcate appearance of the TFC ulnar (peripheral) attachment.

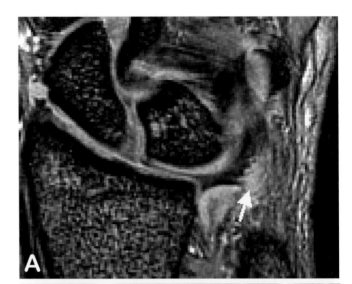

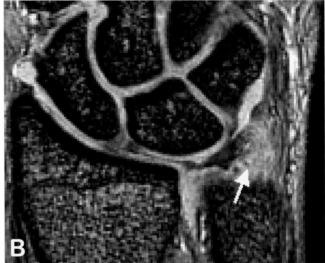

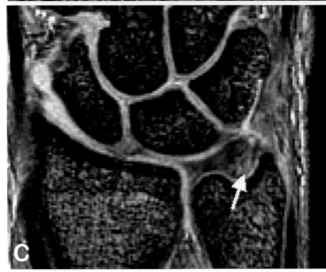

of the disc. This may or may not be associated with the presence of fluid in the distal radioulnar joint **(Option (D) is incorrect), (Option (E) is correct).** In patients with ulnar-sided wrist pain, however, careful scrutiny of the TFC, distal radioulnar joint, and extensor carpi ulnaris tendon is necessary to provide a more definitive and accurate diagnosis, particularly as clinical diagnosis may often be confounded in this region.

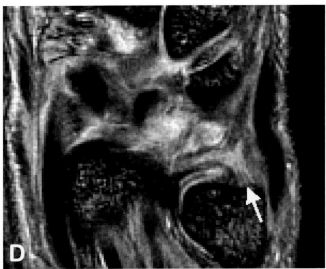

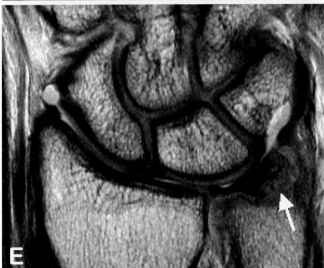

Figure 4-9. Triangular fibrocartilage tear in a 44-year-old woman presenting with ulnar-sided wrist pain. Wrist. MRI. Coronal plane. (Panels A to D) T2*-weighted, 3-D gradient-echo. In panels A and B, peripheral detachment of the ulnar margin of the volar distal radioulnar ligament can be seen, extending to the peripheral margin of the TFC (arrows). Panel C shows the peripheral attachment to be more dorsally intact (arrow), indicating that the tear is focal. Panel D shows fraying of the ulnar attachment of the dorsal distal radioulnar ligament (arrow). (E) Moderate echo time, proton-density-weighted, fast spin-echo. This image shows scarring of the synovium in the prestyloid recess (arrow).

Question 21

Which *one* of the following is true regarding imaging of the triangular fibrocartilage?

(A) Fast spin-echo imaging is useful for assessment of cartilage loss adjacent to the TFC.

(B) Accurate diagnosis requires the use of MR arthrography.

(C) Optimal positioning is at the isocenter of the magnet in the "Superman" position.

(D) Slice resolution should be 3 mm.

The addition of cartilage-sensitive, fast spin-echo images will further increase diagnostic accuracy and also assess for associated cartilage loss adjacent to the TFC **(Option (A) is correct).** With appropriate pulse sequences, high accuracy in the detection of TFC lesions is possible, with reported accuracies as high as 97% for noncontrast MRI and 95% for MR arthrography **(Option (B) is incorrect).** The "Superman" position should be avoided when possible, as this may place traction on the brachial plexus and lead to excessive motion **(Option (C) is incorrect).** Three-dimensional gradient echo imaging obtained with a small field of view (8 cm) and superior slice resolution (1 mm), performed using a dedicated wrist coil, is recommended **(Option (D) is incorrect).** Optional positioning is with the hand at the side, using standardized neutral positioning with regard to radial or ulnar deviation.

Suggested Readings

1. Bednar MS, Arnoczky SP, Weiland AJ. The microvasculature of the triangular fibrocartilage complex: its clinical significance. J Hand Surg [Am]. 1991;16:1101-1105.

2. Bell MJ, Hill RJ, McMurtry RY. Ulnar impingement syndrome. J Bone Joint Surg [Br]. 1985;67:126-129.

3. Berná-Serna JD, Martinez F, Reus M, et al. Evaluation of the triangular fibrocartilage in cadaveric wrists by means of arthrography, magnetic resonance (MR) imaging, and MR arthrography. Acta Radiol. 2007;48: 96-103.

4. Cerezal L, del Pinal F, Abascal F, et al. Imaging findings in ulnar-sided wrist impaction syndromes. RadioGraphics 2002; 22:105-121.

5. Escobedo EM, Bergman AG, Hunter JC. MR imaging of ulnar impaction. Skeletal Radiol. 1995;24:85-90.

6. Imaeda T, Nakamura R, Shionoya K, et al. Ulnar impaction syndrome: MR imaging findings. Radiology. 1996; 201:495-500.

8. Palmer AK. Triangular fibrocartilage complex lesions: a classification. J Hand Surg [Am] 1989;14:594-606.

9. Potter HG, Asnis-Ernberg L, Weiland AJ, et al. The utility of high-resolution magnetic resonance imaging in the evaluation of the triangular fibrocartilage complex of the wrist. J Bone Joint Surg [Am]. 1997; 79:1675-1684.

10. Yoshioka H, Tanaka T, Ueno T, et al. Study of ulnar variance with high-resolution MRI: correlation with triangular fibrocartilage complex and cartilage of ulnar side of wrist. J Magn Reson Imaging. 2007;26:714-719.

11. Zlatkin MB, Rosner J. MR imaging of ligaments and triangular fibrocartilage complex of the wrist. Radiol Clin North Am. 2006;44:595-623.

Case 5

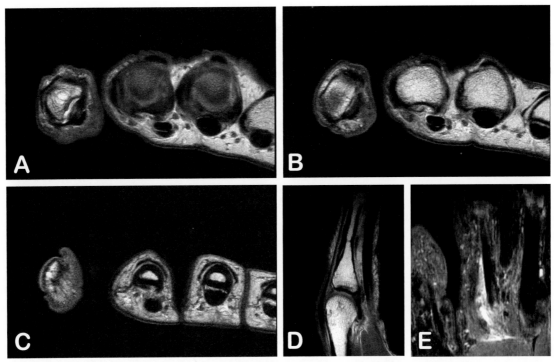

Figure 5-1. Index finger. MRI. (A to C) Proton-density-weighted, fast spin-echo (FSE). Axial plane. (D) Moderate-echo-time, proton-density-weighted, FSE. Sagittal plane. (E) Fast inversion recovery (FIR). Coronal plane.

Question 22

You are shown axial, sagittal, and coronal MR images through the right index finger of a 33-year-old woman with a recent history of trauma. Which *one* of the following is the MOST likely diagnosis?

(A)   Flexor tendon laceration
(B)   Metacarpophalangeal joint subluxation
(C)   Pulley disruption
(D)   Vincula disruption

Hollis G. Potter, M.D.

Finger Pulley Injuries

Question 22

Which *one* of the following is the MOST likely diagnosis?

(A) Flexor tendon laceration
(B) Metacarpophalangeal joint subluxation
(C) Pulley disruption
(D) Vincula disruption

The three axial fast spin-echo images of the index finger are obtained at the level of the metacarpophalangeal joint (Panel 5-2A), base of the proximal phalanx (Panel 5-2B), and midportion of the proximal phalanx (Panel 5-2C), respectively. Figure 5-2A demonstrates a tear of the distal A1 pulley **(Option (C) is correct).** Panels 5-2B and 5-2C show a tear of the A2 pulley. For

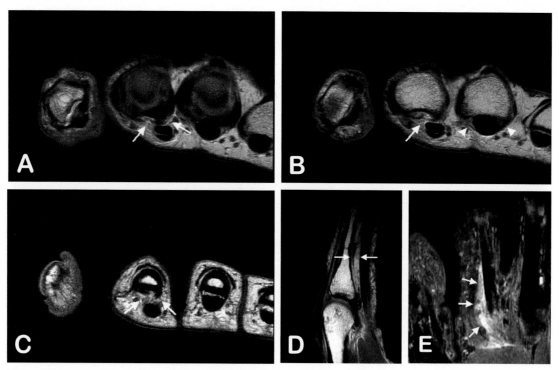

Figure 5-2 (same as Figure 5-1). Disruption of the pulley system. MRI. Index finger. (A) Proton-density-weighted, FSE. Axial plane at the level of the metacarpophalangeal joint. There is a tear of the A1 pulley (arrows). (B) Proton-density-weighted, FSE. Axial plane at the level of the base of the proximal phalanx. A tear of the A2 pulley (arrows) can be seen. Note the intact A2 pulley of the long finger (arrowheads) (C) Proton-density-weighted, FSE. Axial plane at the level of the mid portion of the proximal phalanx. Disruption of the A2 pulley (arrows) is shown. (D) Moderate-echo- time, proton-density-weighted, FSE. Sagittal plane. The image reveals palmar displacement of the flexor tendon from the proximal phalanx (arrows) with the characteristic "bow-string" sign. (E) Fast inversion recovery (FIR). Coronal plane. Palmar extracapsular soft-tissue edema (arrows) is seen.

comparison, note the intact A2 pulley of the long finger (Panel 5-2B).

Disruption of the A2 pulleys is not typically associated with concomitant flexor tendon damage, and careful scrutiny of the tendon in the case provided shows that the tendon signal is preserved **(Option (A) is incorrect).** The joint alignment of the index finger is maintained on the sagittal image, indicating that there is no metacarpophalangeal joint subluxation. Note the intact normal volar plate at the palmar margin of the metacarpophalangeal joint (Panel 5-2D) **(Option (B) is incorrect).**

The pulley system is an important stabilizer of the finger flexor system, representing focal thickenings of the flexor tendon sheaths. The system acts to provide a smooth gliding motion for the flexor tendons, and thereby maintains a more normal range of motion throughout flexion and extension. Tears of the major flexor pulleys, most commonly encountered at the level of the A2 pulley, result in a characteristic "bow-string sign," reflecting the palmar displacement of the flexor tendon from the proximal phalanx. This may be seen on MR imaging (Figure 5-2D), and in the acute

setting, extracapsular palmar soft tissue edema is typically noted on fat-suppressed images (Panel 5-2E).

The major components of the pulley system include the annular or "A" pulleys. The first annular pulley (A1) begins at the region of the volar plate of the metatarsophalangeal joint and extends to the base of the proximal phalanx, the second arises from the proximal aspect of the proximal phalanx and extends to the junction between the distal two-thirds of the proximal phalanx, the third extends over the proximal interphalangeal joint, the fourth over the middle portion of the middle phalanx, and the fifth at the distal interphalangeal joint (Figure 5-3). Whereas the annular pulleys are considered of vital importance, the cruciate or "C" pulleys provide for a degree of flexibility.

Differential diagnostic consideration includes that of vincula disruption. Vincula are specialized mesotenon-containing arteries derived from the four digital volar arterial arches. These small vessels provide the vast majority of blood supply to the superficial flexor tendons. Damage to the vincula results in soft tissue swelling surrounding the flexor sheath, simulating a pulley rupture (Figure 5-4). However, careful scrutiny of the axial images will demonstrate intact A2 pulley arms (Panel 5-4D) **(Option (D) is incorrect).**

Figure 5-3. Sagittal (left) and coronal (right) depictions of the pulley system of a typical flexor tendon (black areas) of the finger. Fibro-osseous annular pulleys (A2, A4), palmar plate annular pulleys (A1, A3, A5), and cruciate pulleys (C1, C2, C3). Dotted lines represent the division of the flexor digitorum superficialis into two bands at this level. [Reprinted with permission Hauger O, Chung CB, LektraKul N et al. Pully system in the fingers: normal anatomy and simulated lesions in cadavers at MR imaging, CT and US with and without contrast material extension of the tendon sheath. Radiology 2000;217:201-212].

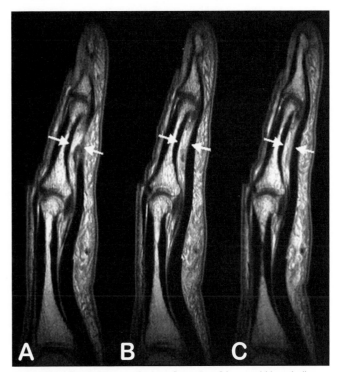

Figure 5-4. Vincula injury to the long finger in a 24-year-old baseball player. MRI. (A to C) Moderate-echo-time, proton-density-weighted, FSE. Sagittal plane. Note the increased signal intensity between the flexor tendon and the proximal phalanx (arrows).

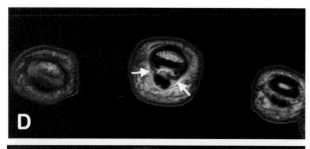

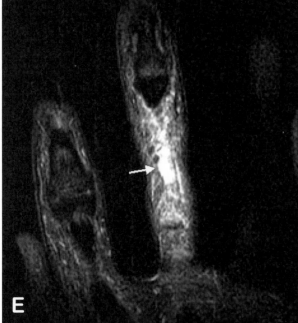

Figure 5-4 (continued). Vincula injury to the long finger in a 24-year-old baseball player. (D) Proton-density-weighted, fast spin-echo. Axial plane. There is increased signal intensity between the flexor tendon and underlying phalanx with intact arms of the A2 pulley (arrows). (E) Fast inversion recovery. Coronal plane. The image demonstrates associated extracapsular palmar soft tissue edema (arrow).

Question 23

Which *one* of the following sports is most commonly associated with pulley injuries?

(A) Basketball
(B) Football
(C) Rock climbing
(D) Squash

Pulley injures are most common among rock climbers, whose climbing techniques often involve the entire body weight being placed on fingers that are gripping small ledges or wedged into small holes. Pulley rupture can cause subsequent loss of strength and significant disability **(Option (C) is correct).** Professional baseball players may also sustain pulley injuries; these are more

clinically severe injuries than those associated with vincula disruption, the latter being an important differential diagnosis in the setting of palmar flexor tendon injuries in a throwing athlete.

Flexor tendons injuries among basketball players are not uncommon. More characteristic in basketball players, however, are deformities due to traumatic impaction-of the lateral bands of the extensor tendons, or subluxations at the metacarpophalangeal joints. While these are typically associated with flexion deformities, the primary pathology is on the extensor tendon side, rather than the flexor side (Figure 5-5) **(Option (A) is incorrect).** Injuries to the upper extremity sustained in squash are much more common at the wrist due to the high rotation forces necessary for playing **(Option (D) is incorrect).**

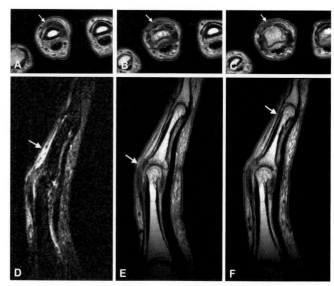

Figure 5-5. Extensor tendon injury to the long finger in a professional basketball player. MRI. Finger. (A to C) Proton-density-weighted, FSE. Axial plane. All three images show a tear of the extensor tendon of the middle phalanx (arrows). (D) Fast inversion recovery. Sagittal plane. The image reveals associated soft tissue edema (arrow). (E) Moderate echo time, proton-density-weighted, FSE. Sagittal plane. The image demonstrates the traumatic boutonniere deformity as a result of the injury to the dorsal capsule of the proximal interphalangeal joint (arrow). (F) Proton-density-weighted. Moderate echo time, FSE. Sagittal plane. A thin remnant of the extensor tendon can be seen reaching the distal interphalangeal joint and distal phalanx (arrow).

Question 24

Surgical management of pulley disruption typically involves which one of the following:

(A) Flexor tendon transfer
(B) Primary repair
(C) Allograft reconstruction
(D) Autograft reconstruction

Whereas vincula disruption is treated conservatively, pulley disruption may require surgical repair, which is characteristically performed with a palmaris longus tendon graft (Figure 5-6) **(Option D is correct; Options A, B and C are incorrect).**

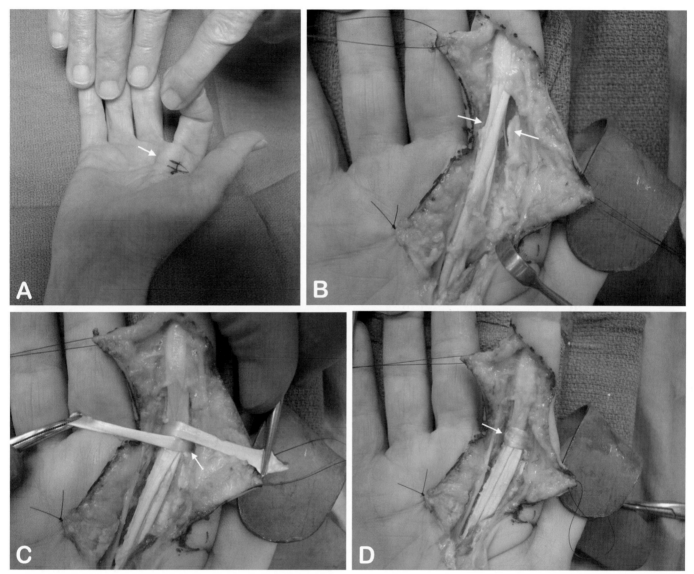

Figure 5-6. (A) Clinical examination demonstrates characteristic bowstringing of the flexor tendon (arrow) of the right index finger in a patient similar to that shown in Figure 5-1. (B) Intraoperative exposure demonstrates complete disruption of the pulleys with bowstringing of the tendon (arrow). (C & D) Preparation and placement of the palmaris longus tendon graft to surgically reconstruct the A2 pulley mechanism (arrows).

Suggested Readings

1. Armenta E, Lehrman A. The vincula to the flexor tendons of the hand. J Hand Surg [Am]. 1980;5:127–134.
2. Guntern D, Goncalves-Matoso V, Gray A, et al. Finger A2 pulley lesions in rock climbers: detection and characterization with magnetic resonance imaging at 3 Tesla--initial results. Invest Radiol. 2007;42:435–441.
3. Hauger O, Chung CB, Lektrakul N, et al. Pulley system in the fingers: normal anatomy and simulated lesions in cadavers at MR imaging, CT, and US with and without contrast material distention of the tendon sheath. Radiology. 2000;217:201–212.
4. Klauser A, Frauscher F, Bodner G, et al. Finger pulley injuries in extreme rock climbers: depiction with dynamic US. Radiology. 2002;222:755–761.
5. Martinoli C, Bianchi S, Cotten A. Imaging of rock climbing injuries. Semin Musculoskelet Radiol. 2005;9:334–345.
6. Schoffl VR, Schoffl I. Injuries to the finger flexor pulley system in rock climbers: current concepts. J Hand Surg [Am] 2006;31:647–654.
7. Schoffl VR, Schoffl I. Finger pain in rock climbers: reaching the right differential diagnosis and therapy. J Sports Med Phys Fitness 2007;47:70–78.

Case 6

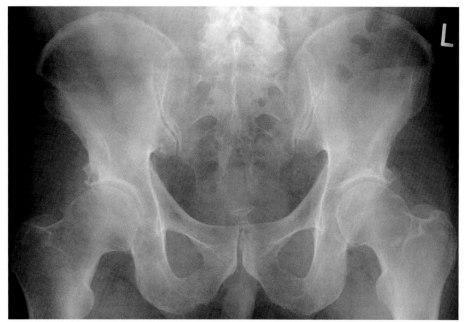

Figure 6-1. (A) Pelvis. Radiograph. Anteroposterior view.

Question 25

This 56-year-old man presented with right hip pain. You are shown a radiograph of his pelvis (Figure 6-1). Which *one* of the following is the MOST likely underlying cause of this patient's advanced degenerative joint disease involving both hips?

(A)   Ankylosing spondylitis
(B)   Cam femoroacetabular impingement
(C)   Pincer femoroacetabular impingement
(D)   Osteonecrosis
(E)   Rheumatoid arthritis

Kirkland W. Davis, M.D.

Femoroacetabular Impingement

Question 25

Which *one* of the following is the MOST likely underlying cause of the advanced degenerative joint disease involving both hips?

(A) Ankylosing spondylitis
(B) Cam femoroacetabular impingement
(C) Pincer femoroacetabular impingement
(D) Osteonecrosis
(E) Rheumatoid arthritis

The key finding for diagnosing this case is the morphology of the proximal femurs shown in the test image. On both sides, there are convex bumps (arrows) at the anterolateral junction of the femoral head and neck (Figure 6-2). This differs from the expected normal anatomy (Figure 6-3), in which there is a "waist" at this junction causing the lateral femoral neck to be concave. The normal morphology, with the waist at the femoral head-neck junction, causes the normal femoral head to have a spherical shape on all projections; however, if there is a bump at the anterior lateral head-neck junction, the femoral head is no longer spherical.

Cam femoroacetabular impingement (FAI) is a condition in which an aspherical femoral head, with a bump or lack of a waist at the head-neck junction, abnormally abuts the anterior acetabulum during extremes of hip flexion (**Option (B) is correct**). For decades, surgeons have known that prominent deformities of the femoral head-neck junction from various childhood conditions or as a result of prior fracture could be the cause of accelerated degenerative arthrosis. However, the term

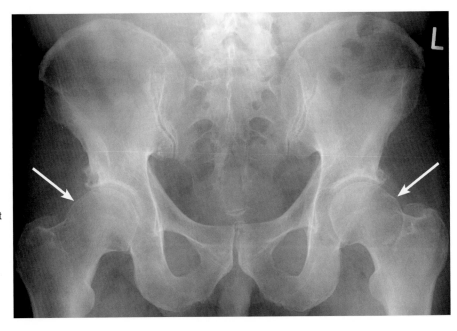

Figure 6-2 (same as Figure 6-1). Pelvis. Radiograph. Anteroposterior view. The image demonstrates degenerative changes bilaterally. The joint spaces narrow superiorly and laterally, and there are subchondral cysts. A mild degree of sclerosis may be present, but it is not a dominant feature in this case. As is typically the case, it is difficult to determine whether or not there are acetabular osteophytes. The arrows denote convex bumps at the junctions of the femoral heads and necks laterally.

femoroacetabular impingement has only been in use for about a decade. In the last few years, the concept of FAI causing hip osteoarthrosis has become widely accepted, though a true causal relationship remains to be established. Certainly, not all patients with cam FAI develop advanced hip degenerative joint disease (DJD) at an early age. With the popularization of the concept of cam FAI has come the realization that many patients have that morphology but do not develop significant DJD any earlier than patients without cam FAI. Presumably, patients with cam FAI who are more active and routinely subject their hips to greater ranges of motion are more likely to develop early DJD. With the development of various surgical options to treat FAI and possibly ward off DJD, determining which patients with cam FAI are prone to early DJD is paramount. When and in whom to intervene remain poorly answered questions.

The man in this case has moderate DJD. At the age of 56, he may have developed DJD regardless of whether his head-neck junctions were abnormal. However, the large femoral neck bumps could have contributed substantially to the degeneration.

The best method to diagnose cam FAI before surgery remains elusive. Physical diagnosis, including the internal impingement test, is purported to be as reliable as any test. Radiographic assessment can demonstrate bumps at the junction of the femoral head and neck, but correlation with surgical findings has not proved reliable. In 2002, a new measurement, the alpha angle, was described on MR arthrograms. Initial results were promising that this would be an accurate method for diagnosing cam FAI. The alpha angle is measured on

an oblique axial series from an MR arthrogram (Figure 6-4). Choosing the center slice extending along the

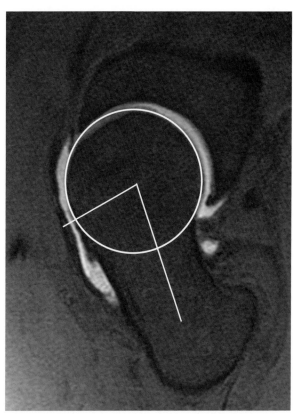

Figure 6-4. Measurement of the alpha angle. MR arthrogram. Oblique view. A best-fit circle is placed around the femoral head. One limb of the alpha angle is a line drawn up the femoral neck to the center of the head. The other limb is drawn to the point at which the femoral head extends beyond the circle anteriorly (to the left of the image). Less than 55 degrees is considered normal.

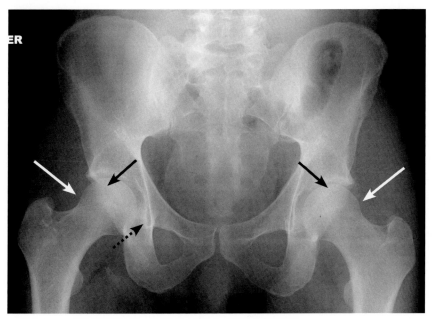

Figure 6-3. Morphologically normal pelvis. Pelvis. Radiograph. Anteroposterior view. The femoral heads are spherical; the white arrows denote the normal waists at the junction of each femoral head and neck. Black arrows demonstrate the anterior walls of the acetabula, which remain medial to the posterior walls throughout their courses. The dotted arrow shows the right teardrop (indicating the medial wall of the acetabulum), which normally remains lateral to the ilioischial line. The patient is a 30-year-old man.

femoral neck and head, a circle is drawn around the femoral head. A line is then drawn up the femoral neck to the center of the head. From this point, an angle is made by drawing a line to the point at which the anterior head/neck exits the circle. Most authors use a cutoff of 55 degrees for this alpha angle: below 55 degrees is normal and above 55 indicates cam FAI. Despite initial widespread enthusiasm for this measurement, several investigators subsequently have shown that the alpha angle has poor sensitivity and specificity for cam FAI; in addition, the alpha angle is not easily reproduced, with considerable interobserver and intraobserver variability. Furthermore, several investigators have noted that the bump is not always most prominent anteriorly, and may be underestimated on oblique axial images. Some have suggested radial imaging and other techniques to overcome this limitation. Ultimately, while there are some cases in which the radiologic and/or clinical findings indicate a straightforward diagnosis of cam FAI, we await more accurate methods of noninvasively diagnosing cam FAI.

Ankylosing spondylitis (AS), one of the seronegative spondyloarthropathies, is a relatively uncommon condition. Cases of significant hip involvement by AS are few and far between. Typical cases of AS affecting the hip demonstrate more axial (toward the center of the pelvis) joint space narrowing than superolateral joint space narrowing. At the age of 56, almost all patients with AS have severe involvement of the sacroiliac joints; the SI joints are normal in this case **(Option (A) is incorrect).**

There is a second type of FAI, known as pincer type, which also leads to advanced DJD. Pincer FAI is discussed in more detail below. In this type of FAI, abnormal contact between the acetabulum and femur is a result of acetabular abnormalities that cause overcoverage of the femoral head. Several different conditions can lead to this overcoverage of the femoral head, including acetabular retroversion, coxa profunda, and protrusio acetabuli. None of these conditions is present in this case **(Option (C) is incorrect).**

End-stage osteonecrosis of the femoral head causes degeneration of the hip joint. Osteonecrosis affects the hips more commonly than AS or rheumatoid arthritis (RA). However, this case does not demonstrate any expected findings of osteonecrosis. Radiographic early stage osteonecrosis (ON) presents as patchy sclerosis within the femoral head, sometimes with intervening lucencies (Figure 6-6). In the next radiographic stage, a curvilinear lucency referred to as the "subchondral crescent sign" underlies the femoral articular cortex. The subchondral crescent precedes overt collapse of the

femoral head, which in turn causes joint degeneration, the final stage. The patient in Figure 6-1 does not demonstrate sclerosis of the femoral head or collapse of the articular surface **(Option (D) is incorrect).**

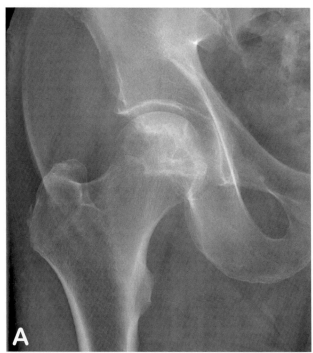

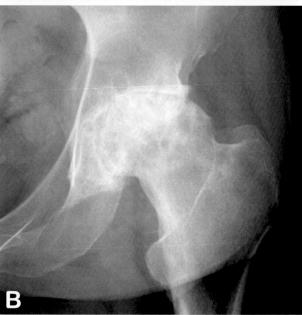

Figure 6-5. Osteonecrosis. Radiograph. Anteroposterior view. (A) Right hip. The image demonstrates early-stage osteonecrosis. The findings include patchy sclerosis and lucency in the femoral head, but there is no collapse of the articular surface, and the joint space is preserved. The patient is a 66-year-old man being treated with corticosteroids. (B) Left hip. The image depicts advanced osteonecrosis. Not only are there extensive areas of sclerosis and lucency, but also the head is collapsed, and there is obliteration of the joint space with severe secondary degenerative changes. The patient is a 57-year-old woman transplant recipient on corticosteroids.

Like AS, RA causes axial joint space narrowing (JSN), rather than superolateral JSN **(Option (E) is incorrect)**. Rheumatoid arthritis occasionally involves the hips; when it does, it usually causes widespread erosions or global erosion of the femoral head, similar to erosion of the humeral head when the shoulder is involved. The femoral head is not eroded in this case.

Question 26

All of the following statements are true EXCEPT:

(A) Cam femoroacetabular impingement primarily leads to damage of the acetabular articular cartilage.

(B) Femoroacetabular impingement does not lead to accelerated degeneration of the hip joint.

(C) Pincer femoroacetabular impingement first leads to damage of the acetabular labrum.

(D) Patients with surgically proven femoroacetabular impingement most commonly have a combination of cam and pincer types.

(E) Patients suffering from slipped capital femoral epiphysis may develop cam morphology as adults.

During the last decade, the field of hip surgery has expanded considerably. That has been due largely to an explosion in the number of arthroscopies performed for tears of the acetabular labrum and, to a lesser degree, treatment of articular cartilage damage. Increasing frequency of hip surgery for femoroacetabular impingement has lagged the expansion of hip surgery in general, but the last few years have brought a noticeable increase in the number of procedures performed specifically or in part to address FAI. At the time of arthroscopic or open hip surgery, the surgeon can evaluate more accurately for FAI because the hip can be manipulated through full ranges of motion with direct visualization of any impingement that may occur.

Surgeons are particularly interested in treating patients who are prone to but have not yet developed significant arthrosis. Readily available arthroscopic techniques now allow debridement or reattachment of labral tears and various treatments for articular cartilage defects. As surgeons have become more aggressive in treating these abnormalities, they have increasingly recognized the tie between FAI and early joint degeneration. It is now generally accepted that FAI can contribute to advanced degenerative changes of the hip at a younger age than otherwise expected **(Option (B) is false and therefore correct)**.

With the increasing frequency of these surgeries, we now have a better picture of the demographics of these patients and the pattern of injuries they sustain. Patients with cam FAI first develop acetabular hyaline cartilage damage where the femoral bump impacts the acetabulum. This cartilage injury often presents as a delaminated flap tear. **(Option (A) is true and therefore incorrect).** If the condition progresses, the adjacent labrum often tears also. For patients with pincer FAI, labral tears often precede articular cartilage defects, **(Option (C) is true and therefore incorrect)**, but both will likely be present if the injury is advanced. These patients also frequently develop a contre-coup injury to the cartilage on the opposite (typically posterior) side of the acetabulum.

Several authors note a typical demographic pattern for patients that present with symptoms from femoroacetabular impingement. Patients presenting with cam FAI typically are athletic males in their 30s. The typical patient with pincer FAI is a woman in her 40s. However, recent surgical series make the point that most patients treated for FAI have a combination of both types, rather than one or the other. **(Option (D) is true and therefore incorrect).**

The etiology of the femoral head asphericity in cam FAI is unknown. Some authors consider it a devel-

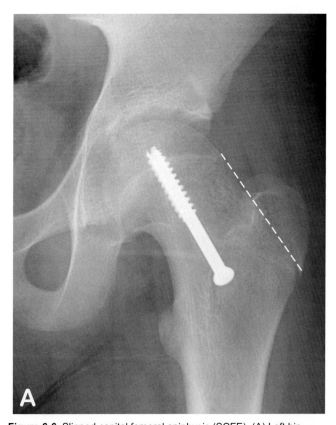

Figure 6-6. Slipped capital femoral epiphysis (SCFE). (A) Left hip. Radiograph. Anteroposterior view. Klein's line along the lateral femoral neck (dashed white line) is abnormal, in that it does not intersect the epiphysis, consistent with the diagnosis of SCFE. This morphology eliminates the expected "waist" at the femoral neck. The patient is an 11-year-old girl who recently had her hip pinned to stabilize a SCFE.

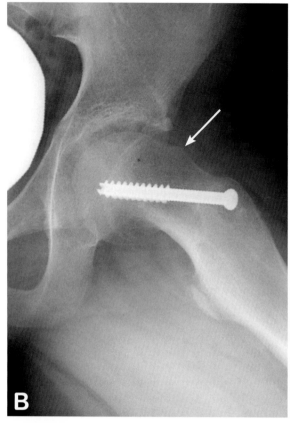

Figure 6-6 (continued). Slipped capital femoral epiphysis. (B) Left hip. Radiograph. Frogleg view. A bump can be seen on the anterolateral femoral neck (arrow).

opmental anomaly. Others suggest FAI is the result of subclinical cases of slipped capital femoral epiphysis (SCFE), which did not come to medical attention at the time of the injury but caused residual deformity of the head-neck junction in adulthood. This theory stems from the longstanding knowledge that significantly displaced cases of SCFE often cause early and advanced hip DJD in adults **(Option (E) is true and therefore incorrect).** Figure 6-6 demonstrates a recently pinned case of SCFE in which one can recognize an anterolateral bump at the head-neck junction. It is easy to imagine this morphology leading to accelerated arthrosis. Other injuries to the hip that leave residual deformity, such as Legg-Calvé-Perthes disease and fractures of the proximal femur, are also suspected of causing accelerated DJD.

Question 27

Regarding Figure 6-7 (in the Test section), what condition does the patient have that may cause accelerated degenerative joint disease involving the right hip?

(A) Ankylosing spondylitis
(B) Cam femoroacetabular impingement
(C) Pincer femoroacetabular impingement
(D) Osteonecrosis
(E) Rheumatoid arthritis

The crossover sign is evidence of acetabular retroversion, which causes overcoverage of the femoral head anteriorly by the anterior wall of the acetabulum. This is the most common form of pincer FAI, which can lead to accelerated hip DJD **(Option (C) is correct).** This figure-8 morphology of the crossover sign is often easy to recognize; however, appropriate radiographic positioning must be present to confidently make this diagnosis. First, the pelvis must be straight. If there is any obliquity, the anterior wall could artifactually extend beyond the posterior wall. Likewise, one must ensure there is not too much pelvic tilt. When the pelvis is posteriorly tilted, the anterior walls of the acetabula

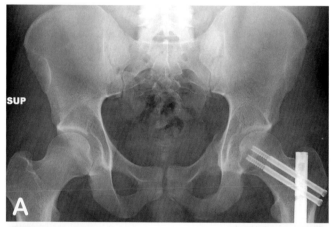

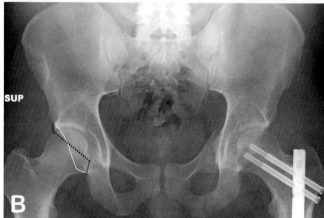

Figure 6-8 (same as Figure 6-7). Pincer femoroacetabular impingement. Pelvis. Radiograph. Anteroposterior view. (A) The anterior wall of the right acetabulum is lateral to the posterior wall along the more superolateral aspect of the acetabulum. (B) The anterior wall is traced as a dashed line, and the posterior wall is the solid line. This is termed the "crossover sign." The fractures and trochanteric fixation nail on the patient's left side are not related to this case.

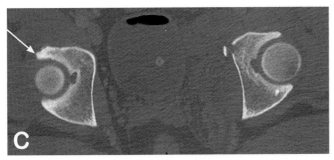

Figure 6-8 (continued). Pincer acetabular impingement. (C) CT. Axial plane at the level of the superior hip joints. The CT image from the same patient demonstrates the anterior wall (arrow) of the right acetabulum extending lateral to the posterior wall. The patient is an 18-year-old man.

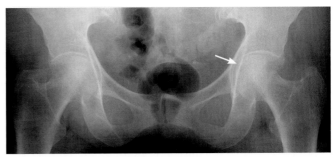

Figure 6-10. Protrusio acetabuli. Pelvis. Radiograph. Coned-down anteroposterior view. The image demonstrates the findings of mild protrusio. The femoral heads overlap the ilioischial lines bilaterally, especially on the left (arrow). The patient is a 57-year-old woman.

drop down on an AP radiograph and appear to declare overcoverage; instead there is just excessive tilt. When assessing the AP radiograph, there is excessive tilt if the sacrococcygeal junction is more than 4.7 cm above the pubic symphysis in women and more than 3.2 cm above the symphysis in men. In normal patients without retroversion, the anterior wall of the acetabulum projects medial to the posterior wall at all points (Figure 6-3).

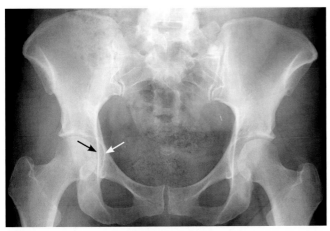

Figure 6-9. Coxa profunda. Pelvis. Radiograph. Anteroposterior view The image demonstrates the medial walls of both acetabula (white arrow) to extend medial to the ilioischial lines (black arrow). The patient is a 48-year-old woman.

Acetabular retroversion may also be visible on computed tomography (CT) or magnetic resonance (MR) scans (Figure 6-8). On the more cranial axial images through the hip, the anterior acetabular wall extends lateral to the posterior wall.

Acetabular retroversion is not the only cause of overcoverage of the femoral head. Other recognized causes include coxa profunda and acetabular protrusio. On a well positioned radiograph, coxa profunda is determined when the medial wall of the acetabulum (lat-

eral teardrop line) projects medial to the ilioischial line (Figure 6-9). Protrusio acetabuli is defined when the head of the femur crosses medial to the ilioischial line (Figure 6-10). Any of these causes of pincer FAI may result in abnormal contact of the femur with the excessively prominent acetabular rim, leading to labral tears and cartilage damage.

The young patient in Figure 6-8 has no stigmata of hip arthritis on the image. This patient has none of the signs of ankylosing spondylitis **(Option (A) is incorrect)**, osteonecrosis **(Option (D) is incorrect),** or rheumatoid arthritis **(Option (E) is incorrect)**, all described in the discussion of Question 25. While this patient does have pincer FAI, there is normal morphology of the femoral head and neck, arguing against cam FAI **(Option (B) is incorrect).**

Question 28

For the patient with a combination of a focal acetabular labral tear, localized articular cartilage defects, and femoroacetabular impingement, surgical options include all of the following EXCEPT:

    (A) Cartilage treatment techniques, such as microfracture, chondroplasty, and mosaicplasty
    (B) Labral debridement or repair
    (C) Hip resurfacing
    (D) Femoroplasty
    (E) Resection of the acetabular rim

The patient described in this question presents a common scenario encountered by hip surgeons today. A focal labral tear and localized articular cartilage damage, in association with cam or pincer FAI, may predict early advanced DJD in this patient's future. However, with the damage relatively mild at this point, the surgeon will take steps to relieve pain and attempt to forestall the development of more severe joint degeneration. Depending on their training and expertise, some surgeons will undertake attempts to regenerate functional articular cartilage using such techniques as microfracture and mosaicplasty **(Option (A) is true and therefore incorrect).** Likewise, debridement of labral tears and cartilage damage often relieves pain for months or years **(Option (B) is true and therefore incorrect).** Recently, more surgeons have begun to repair the labrum when appropriate, hoping to restore more normal joint function. Similarly, correction of impingement morphology may reduce the likelihood of accelerated arthrosis. Patients with cam FAI now may undergo resection of the femoral neck bump via a shaving procedure best termed "femoroplasty" **(Option (D) is true and therefore incorrect).** When pincer morphology is present, exuberant portions of the acetabular rim may be resected **(Option (E) is true and therefore incorrect).** During these procedures, the surgeon can repeatedly evaluate the patient's full range of motion, determining when the resection is sufficient to relieve impingement.

Once a patient's cartilage damage has progressed to the point of marked DJD, labral and cartilage debridement may provide temporary relief of pain but are not expected to be a long-term solution. By the time the degenerative change is widespread, relieving impingement morphology has little purpose. At this point, if activity modification and other conservative measures fail, the remaining options are various forms of joint replacement and resurfacing.

The patient with advanced DJD often must resort to total hip replacement to improve symptoms and function. In younger patients, some of whom have FAI as a cause of their accelerated DJD, the prospects of total joint replacement are not inviting. Because the life expectancy of these patients far exceeds the expected life of a total hip prosthesis, they may be faced with two or more revisions of a total hip replacement as time passes. Some patients choose to delay total joint replacement by undergoing resurfacing of the femoral head and acetabulum, or the femoral head alone (Figure 6-11). When these resurfacing devices eventually fail, they can be replaced by a standard total hip prosthesis, rather than a revision, long-stemmed prosthesis. The patient described in question 27 does not have widespread joint deterioration, and would not warrant resurfacing **(Option (C) is false and therefore correct).**

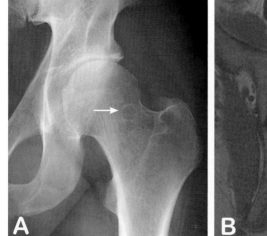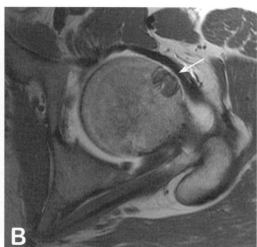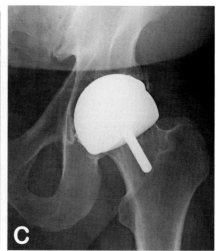

Figure 6-11. Hip resurfacing. Pelvis. (A) Radiograph. Coned down anteroposterior view. The image demonstrates a small bump at the lateral head/neck junction and fibrocystic change of the anterior femoral neck (arrow pointing at lucencies). There is moderate to severe joint space loss, mild sclerosis, and subchondral cyst formation in the acetabulum. (B) Left hip. MR arthrogram. T1-weighted. Axial plane. The femoral head is seen to be aspherical, and the fibrocystic change is evident (arrow). (C) Radiograph. Anteroposterior view. This radiograph demonstrates the femoral head and acetabulum to have been resurfaced. When these devices need to be revised, they often can be converted to a standard hip prosthesis, because the surgeon is able to leave sufficient native femoral bone in place.

Suggested Readings

ARTHRITIDES AND OSTEONECROSIS OF THE HIP

1. Boutry N, Khalil C, Jaspart M, et al. Imaging of the hip in patients with rheumatic disorders. Eur J Radiol. 2007;63:49–58.
2. Jacobson JA, Girish G, Jiang Y, Resnick D. Radiographic evaluation of arthritis: inflammatory conditions. Radiology. 2008; 248:378–389.
3. Joshi AB, Markovic L, Hardinge K, Murphy JCM. Total hip arthroplasty in ankylosing spondylitis. J Arthroplasty. 2002;17:427–433.
4. Lang P, Genant HR, Jergesen HE, Murray WR. Imaging of the hip joint: computed tomography versus magnetic resonance imaging. Clin Orthop Relat Res. 1992;274:135–153.
5. Malizos KN, Karantanas AJ, Varitimidis SE, et al. Osteonecrosis of the femoral fead: Etiology, imaging and treatment. Eur J Radiology. 2007; 3:16–28.
6. Troum OM, Crues JV. The young adult with hip pain: diagnosis and medical treatment, circa 2004. Clin Orthop Relat Res. 2004;418:9–17.

FEMOROACETABULAR IMPINGEMENT: CLINICAL EVALUATION AND SURGICAL MANAGEMENT

7. Beck M, Kalhor M, Leunig M, Ganz R. Hip Morphology influences the pattern of damage to the acetabular cartilage: femoroacetabular impingement as a cause of early osteoarthritis of the hip. J Bone Joint Surg (Br). 2005;87-B:1012-1018.
8. Beck M, Leunig M, Parvizi J, et al. Anterior femoroacetabular impingement: Part II. midterm results of surgical treatment. Clin Orthop Relat Res. 2004;418:67–73.
9. Bedi A, Chen N, Robertson W, Kelly BT. The management of labral tears and femoroacetabular impingement of the hip in the young, active patient. Arthroscopy. 2008;24:1135–1145.
10. Bharam S. Labral tears, extra-articular injuries, and hip arthroscopy in the athlete. Clin Sports Med. 2006;25:279–292.
11. Byrd JW, Jones KS. Arthroscopic femoroplasty in the management of cam-type femoroacetabular impingement. Clin Orthop Relat Res. 2009;467:739–746.
12. Ganz R, Parvizi J, Beck M, et al. Femoroacetabular impingement: a cause of osteoarthritis of the hip. Clin Orthop Relat Res. 2003;417:112–120.
13. Ilizaliturri VM. Complications of arthroscopic femoroacetabular impingement treatment. Clin Orthop Relat Res. 2009;467:760–768.
14. Keogh MJ, Batt ME. A review of femoroacetabular impingement in athletes. Sports Med. 2008;38:863–878.
15. Laude F, Sariali E, Nogier A. Femoroacetabular impingement treatment using arthroscopy and anterior approach. Clin Orthop Relat Res. 2009;467:747–752.
16. Leunig M, Beaulé PE, Ganz R. The concept of femoroacetabular impingement: current status and future perspectives. Clin Orthop Relat Res. 2009;467:616–622.
17. Murphy S, Tannast M, Kim Y, et al. Debridement of the adult hip for femoroacetabular impingement. Clin Orthop Relat Res 2004; 429:178–181.
18. Philippon MJ, Stubbs AJ, Schenker ML, et al. Arthroscopic management of femoroacetabular impingement: osteoplasty technique and literature review. Am J Sports Med. 2007;35:1571–1580.
19. Standaert CJ, Manner PA, Herring SA. Expert opinion and controversies in musculoskeletal and sports medicine: femoroacetabular impingement. Arch Phys Med Rehabil. 2008;89:890–893.

FEMOROACETABULAR IMPINGEMENT AND LABRAL AND CARTILAGE TEARS: IMAGING

20. Armfield DR, Towers JD, Robertson DD. Radiographic and MR imaging of the athletic hip. Clin Sports Med. 2006;25:211–239.
21. Beall DP, Sweet CF, Martin HD, et al. Imaging findings of femoroacetabular impingement syndrome. Skelet Radiol. 2005;34:691–701.
22. Blankenbaker DG, Tuite MJ. The painful hip: new concepts. Skelet Radiol 2006; 35:352–370.*
23. MR imaging of femoroacetabular impingement. Bredella MA, Stoller DW. Magn Reson Imaging Clin N Am. 2005;13:653–664.
24. Dudda M, Albers C, Mamisch TC, et al. Do normal radiographs exclude asphericity of the femoral head-neck junction? Clin Orthop Relat Res. 2009;467:651–659.
25. James SLJ, Ali K, Malara F, et al. MRI Findings of femoroacetabular impingement. AJR Am J Roentgenol. 2006;187:1412–1419.
26. Kassarjian A, Brisson M, Palmer WE. Femoroacetabular impingement. Europ J Radiol. 2007;63:29–35.
27. Kassarjian A, Yoon LS, Belzile E, et al. Triad of MR arthrographic findings in patients with cam-type femoroacetabular impingement. Radiology. 2005;236:588–592.
28. Leunig M, Beck M, Kalhor M, et al. Fibrocystic changes at anterosuperior femoral neck: prevalence in hips with femoroacetabular impingement. Radiology. 2005;236:237–246.
29. Notzli HP, Wyss TF, Stoecklin CH. The contour of the femoral head-neck junction as a predictor for the risk of anterior impingement. J Bone Joint Surg (Br). 2002;64-B:556–560.
30. Nouh MR, Schweitzer ME, Rybak L, Cohen J. Femoroacetabular impingement: can the alpha angle be estimated? AJR Am J Roentgenol. 2008;190:1260–1262.
31. Rakhra KS, Sheikh AM, Allen D, Beaulé PE. Comparison of MRI alpha angle measurement planes in femoroacetabular impingement. Clin Orthop Relat Res. 2009;467:660–665.
32. Pfirrmann CWA, Duc SR, Zanetti M, et al. MR arthrography of acetabular cartilage delamination in femoroacetabular cam impingement. Radiology. 2008;249:235–241.
33. Pfirrmann CWA, Mengiardi B, Dora C, et al. Cam and pincer femoroacetabular impingement: characteristic mr arthrographic findings in 50 patients. Radiology. 2006;240:778–785.
34. Pulido L, Parvizi J. Femoroacetabular impingement. Sem Musculoskel Radiol. 2007;11:66–72.
35. Tannast M, Siebenrock KA, Anderson SE. Femoroacetabular Iimpingement: radiographic diagnosis—what the radiologist should know. AJR Am J Roentgenol. 2007;188:1540–1552.

Case 7

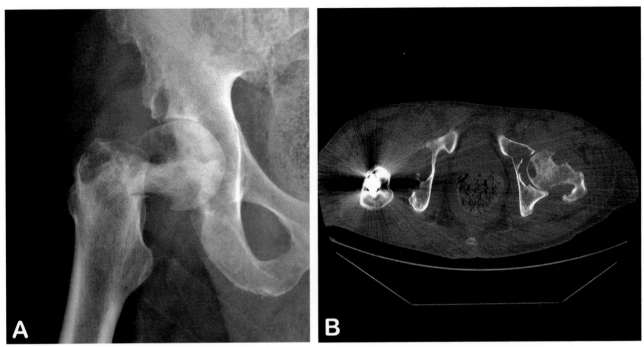

Figure 7-1. (A) Right hip. Radiograph. Anteroposterior view. (B) Pelvis. Thin-section CT. Axial plane.

Question 29

A 78-year-old African-American man presents after falling at his home. You are shown an initial radiograph (Figure 7-1A) and a CT image (Figure 7-1B) obtained later in the workup. The patient has a past medical history of end-stage renal disease secondary to hypertensive nephrosclerosis and is maintained on hemodialysis. His medical history also includes hypertension for more than 15 years, diabetes for more than 30 years, and bowel issues for a few years. What is the *one* MOST likely underlying cause of the patient's pathologic fracture?

(A)   Metastases
(B)   Multiple myeloma
(C)   Pigmented villonodular synovitis
(D)   Amyloidosis
(E)   Rheumatoid arthritis

Osteoarticular Amyloidosis

Question 29

What is the MOST likely underlying cause of the patient's pathologic fracture?

(A) Metastases
(B) Multiple myeloma
(C) Pigmented villonodular synovitis
(D) Amyloidosis
(E) Rheumatoid arthritis

An anteroposterior radiograph of the right hip (Figure 7-2A) demonstrates a pathologic femoral neck fracture secondary to a large osteolytic lesion involving the femoral neck. There are multiple osteolytic lesions on both sides of the hip joint.

A skeletal survey (not shown) was obtained. It showed another lesion involving the left tibial intercondylar eminence and left acetabulum, evoking suspicion for either multiple myeloma or metastatic disease. A nuclear three-phase bone scan (Figure 7-3) was obtained for whole-body evaluation for metastatic disease. It did not reveal additional osseous-based lesions. Instead, the bone scan showed circumferential increased radiotracer activity at the right hip, with a central area of photopenia of the right femoral head suggesting avascularity.

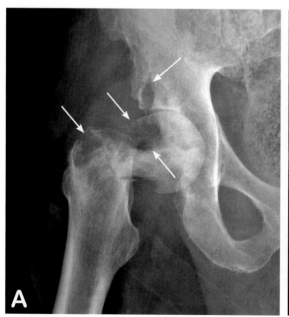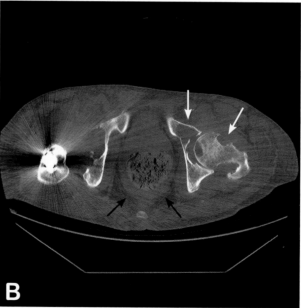

Figure 7-2 (same as Figure 7-1). (A) Right hip. Radiograph. Anteroposterior view. A pathological femoral neck fracture can be seen, with multiple osteolytic lesions (arrows) about the joint. (B) Pelvis. Thin-section CT. Axial plane. This scan of the bony pelvis shows multiple osteolytic lesions (white arrows) involving both hip joints, including the left femur and both actabuli. The patient is status post right hip hemiarthroplasty. There was superior and lateral dislocation of the right hip. Incidentally noted is rectal wall thickening (black arrows), presumably from amyloid infiltration.

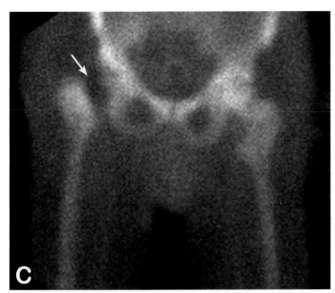

Figure 7-3. Pelvis. Nuclear medicine bone scan. Anteroposterior view. A photopenic area (arrow) can be seen in the vicinity of the expected femoral head. The finding suggests avascularity of the right femoral head.

The patient underwent surgical excision and right hip hemiarthroplasty. At histologic examination, thin sections of the femoral head were obtained for ultrastructural examination. The Congo Red stain (Figure 7-4A) showed a focal area of green birefringence. Similarly, there was thioflavin T staining for beta-2-microglobulin (beta-2-MG) (Figure 7-4B). Ultrastructural examination with electron microscopy (not shown) revealed nonbranching fibrils, 7.7 to 11.5 nm in width, arranged in a haphazard fashion, which were in keeping with amyloidosis **(Option (D) is correct).**

Subsequently, a thin section computed tomography (CT) scan of the pelvis was obtained using a high frequency filter (Figure 7-2B). Osteolytic erosions in a juxtaarticular distribution of the contralateral hip joint and associated capsular thickening were verified. Incidentally, there was also marked rectal wall thickening, presumably from amyloid infiltration.

Amyloidosis related to dialysis is a well-known complication affecting many organ systems, in particular the musculoskeletal system. In 1985, Shirahama et al identified the beta-2 microglobulin as the offending constituent by using protein purification techniques. Amyloidosis has been increasing in prevalence due to longer life spans and a corresponding increase in chronic medical conditions such as end-stage renal disease.

Amyloidosis, the abnormal deposition of extracellular proteins in tissues, can affect many organ systems. It is classically divided into primary and secondary forms. The primary form of amyloidosis is defined by a unique fibrillar protein, 7-10 micrometer thick. However, secondary amyloidosis is associated with more ubiquitous components called serum amyloid P and charged glycosaminoglycans. Amyloid, Greek for "starch," was derived from the tendency of glycosaminoglycan to stain blue with iodine. This extracellular protein is always a byproduct of the acute phase reactant protein serum amyloid A, which is secreted by the liver in chronic disease conditions. Definitive diagnosis is made histologically by showing apple-green birefringence when stained with Congo red and viewed under polarized light microscopy.

Beta-2 microglobulin amyloidosis associated with chronic hemodialysis invariably affects the musculo-

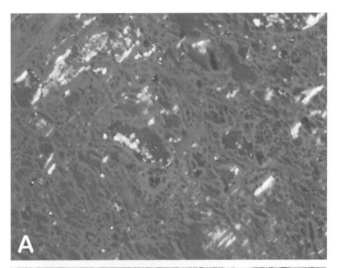

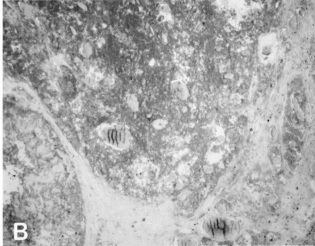

Figure 7-4. Thin sections of the femoral head obtained during surgical excision and right hip hemiarthroplasty. (A) Polarized Congo Red stain demonstrates apple-green birefringence, characteristic of amyloid. (B) T staining for B2-microglobulin. *[Lee KS, van Holsbeeck MT, Abbud A. Skeletal Radiol. Atypical rapid progression of osteoarticular amyloidosis involving the hip in a patient on hemodialysis using polyacrylonitrile membranes. 2009 Aug (Epub ahead of print) with kind permission of Springer Science and Business Media]*

skeletal system. Osseous and articular abnormalities can occur as a result of amyloid deposition in periarticular tissue, synovium, and bone. In the musculoskeletal system, amyloid deposition was first described in the wrist, where it often leads to carpal tunnel syndrome. Other osteoarticular manifestations include osteoporosis, lytic lesions, pathologic fractures, osteonecrosis, periarticular soft tissue masses, subchondral cysts and erosions, contractures, and joint subluxations. Clinical manifestations of osteoarticular amyloidosis are dependent on the duration of hemodialysis, typically 6 to 8 years from onset. However, recent improvements in hemofiltration technology have delayed the onset of dialysis-related amyloid.

Although metastatic disease to bone may present as osteolytic lesions, the juxtaarticular distribution of the lesions in this case make it unlikely **(Option (A) is incorrect).** A key feature of this case is the distribution of these osteolytic lesions affecting both the femoral head and the acetabulum suggesting a joint centered process.

Metastatic lesions to bone account for 700,000 new cases of cancer annually. Common primary tumors that metastasize to bone are prostate, breast, lung, renal, thyroid, and endometrial cancers. However, osteolytic metastases are usually seen in lung, renal, and thyroid carcinomas. Breast metastases may be entirely lytic or mixed lytic-blastic. Patients will present with bone pain and have significant morbidity.

Osteolytic metastases are often multifocal. However, renal and thyroid carcinomas may present as a solitary osteolytic lesion. At presentation, the most common site of bone metastasis is the axial skeleton, followed by the proximal femora, and then the proximal humeri. About one third of all patients will have metastatic involvement of the spine at autopsy (see Suggested Reading #28).

Clinical presentation of a patient with bone metastatic disease can vary from having pain to having no symptoms at all. A fracture after an insignificant injury or out of proportion to its causative mechanism should alert the clinician to a possible underlying lesion. Initial workup usually consists of radiographs, but significant bone loss must occur before the osteolytic metastasis becomes evident on radiographs. Often, advanced cross sectional imaging is required for further workup. CT provides excellent bone detail for fracture or cortical destruction (Figure 7-5). MR imaging is well-suited for assessing bone marrow involvement, especially for early metastatic lesions that may not be detected with CT.

The goals of treatment after a pathologic fracture are stabilization and pain relief. However, these cases

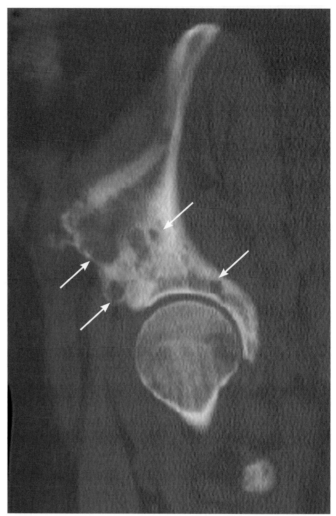

Figure 7-5. Hip. Bone CT. Reformatted in sagittal plane. There are multiple lytic metastases of the pelvis (arrows) in a nonarticular distribution (lesions seen on only one side of the joint). The patient had lung carcinoma.

can be difficult for the clinician when patients present with significant bone destruction, osteopenia of the elderly, and inadequate healing response at the pathologic fracture site from underlying disease. A difficult area for clinicians is deciding when to treat an impending fracture. To facilitate clinical decision making, Mirels et al in 1989 designed a scoring system that helped to predict the risk of pathologic fracture in the extremities. The scoring system (Table 7-1) is based on pain, lesion size, lesion type (lytic or blastic), and lesion location (weight-bearing or non–weight-bearing). Painful lytic lesions in weight-bearing joints are at greatest risk for fracture. According to Mirels criteria, a score of 9 or more carries a 33% probability of fracture and suggests the need for prophylactic fixation. Some authors cite limitations to Mirels scoring system and argue instead that the most reliable marker for impending fracture is mechanical pain—that is, a mechanical pain is a strong indication that the diseased bone cannot withstand the

Table 7-1. Mirels scoring system			
Variable score	*1*	*2*	*3*
Site	Upper limb	Lower limb	Peritrochanteric
Pain	Mild	Moderate	Mechanical pain
Lesion	Blastic	Lytic	
Size	< 1/3 diameter	1/3 to 2/3 diameter	> 2/3 diameter

physical stresses placed upon it and therefore should be prophylactically fixated. Others claim that Mirels criteria may overestimate the risk of fracture. Alternatively, their research showed that simple objective measures of cortical involvement in the axial plane of greater than 30mm and circumferential cortical involvement of greater than 50% were the most reliable risk factors predicting fracture. Nevertheless, outcomes are generally poor for pathologic fractures in cases of metastatic disease, especially with aggressive lytic-type lesions. The main goal for internal fixation is to provide pain relief and long-term durability of the fixation in treated patients.

Regarding the diagnostic choices in the test case, multiple myeloma is a well-known disease that causes osteolytic lesions. It is usually considered in patients over the age of 50. However, the distribution of myeloma is not characteristically articular-based as is the distribution seen in this case. **(Option (B) is incorrect).**

Multiple myeloma is a common hematopoietic neoplastic process that has been extensively studied since its first report in 1845. It is characterized by the uncontrolled monoclonal proliferation of plasma cells within the bone marrow. According to the National Institutes of Health 2004 statistic, there are approximately 63,000 people living with multiple myeloma in the United States. The annual incidence of a multiple myeloma diagnosis is slightly more than 14,000 people diagnosed each year, according to the American Cancer Society. The median prognosis is about three years. Multiple myeloma accounts for 1% of all malignancies and 10% of all blood malignancies, making it the second most common such disease after non-Hodgkin's lymphoma. The peak age of onset for multiple myeloma is 65 to 70 years of age, but recent data have shown a trend towards an earlier age of onset. Men are slightly more likely than women to be diagnosed with multiple myeloma. African Americans and Native Pacific Islanders are twice as likely to be diagnosed as are Caucasian Americans or Europeans. Asians have the lowest risk. It is worth noting that amyloidosis can complicate multiple myeloma at a frequency up to 15%.

The majority of patients who present with multiple myeloma demonstrate plasma cell proliferation in the bone marrow, osteolytic lesions, and positive serum or urine analysis for monoclonal proteins. Unlike the articular pattern of this osteoarticular amyloid case, multiple myeloma has varied patterns of imaging presentation: solitary plasmacytoma, diffuse myelomatosis, diffuse osteopenia, or a sclerosing type known as POEMS syndrome.

The bone involvement of multiple myeloma is characteristically medullary-based with sharply defined lytic lesions and no reactive associated bone formation. Multiple myeloma classically inhibits osteoblastic activity, and there are often false-negative bone scans. Although it primarily starts in the medullary cavity, multiple myeloma often causes endosteal scalloping when it involves the cortex. It can also extend through the cortex to involve the periosteum, with or without soft tissue involvement. Multiple myeloma most commonly affects the spine (66%), ribs (45%), skull (40%), and the pelvis (30%) (Winterbottom, 2009). The rare sclerotic form of myeloma known as POEMS syndrome is characterized by *p*olyneuropathy, *o*rganomegaly, *e*ndocrinopathy, *m*onoclonal gammopathy, and *s*kin changes.

Imaging plays an important role in the initial diagnosis of multiple myeloma, as well as staging and followup after treatment. Initial workup is performed with a radiographic skeletal survey of the axial skeleton, skull, ribs, and proximal extremities. Multiple myeloma rarely involves the distal appendicular skeleton. The sensitivity of the skeletal survey is low; some authors report a sensitivity of 47.4%. The low sensitivity is due to the inability of radiographs to detect bone loss until at least 30% of cancellous bone is gone. Bone scintigraphy also has low sensitivity (40% to 60%) due to lack of bone turnover and osteoblastic activity. Some regions of myeloma involvement may be photopenic. Our case demonstrated a relative photopenic area involving the femoral head, which was proven to be due to avascular necrosis rather than myeloma involvement. Although skeletal surveys have a reported low sensitivity for detection of myeloma, it is the most commonly accepted initial workup with an average radiation dose of 2.5mSv. However, more recent research investigating cost-effective approaches to the diagnosis and follow-up treatment of myeloma notes that utilizing MRI (Figure 7-6) and PET-CT is a promising approach.

Pigmented villonodular synovitis (PVNS) is a rare but benign proliferative disorder of the synovium with pigmentation from hemosiderin. It can affect the synovium of joints, bursae, and tendon sheaths. PVNS was first described as a distinct disorder by Jaffe in 1941 (Murphey, 2008). It may present in one of two forms: a focal form or, more often, a diffuse form. Focal PVNS usually occurs in females, affecting smaller joints such as the finger tendon sheaths, also referred to as giant cell tumor of the tendon sheath.

Incidence of intraarticular PVNS is estimated at 1.8 cases per 1 million people. The most common joints affected are the large joints, such as the knees (70% to

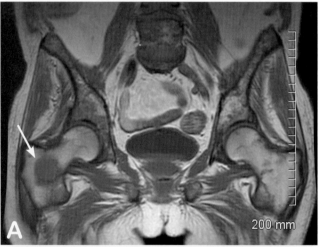

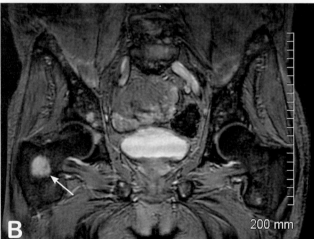

Figure 7-6. Multiple myeloma. Pelvis. MRI. Coronal plane. (A) T1-weighted. There are numerous low intensity T1 lesions thoroughout the pelvis and a large lesion in the right intertrochanteric region (arrow), consistent with multiple myeloma. (B) T2-weighted, fat-saturated. The lesions are high intensity on T2. An arrow points to a high-intensity right intertrochanteric lesion.

80%) and hips (5% to 15%). When PVNS affects the joint, a patient may present with a large joint effusion with osseous erosions that affect both sides of the joint, as seen in the test case. Similar to amyloidosis, articular PVNS is a joint-centered process with relatively good preservation of the joint space until its later stages. Radiographic features include extrinsic erosions with well-defined sclerotic margins in up to 25% of cases. MRI features of the synovial masses seen in PVNS will demonstrate low T1- and T2-weighted signal abnormality due to hemosiderin deposition (Figure 7-7). Gradient echo imaging will cause blooming artifact from the hemosiderin deposition seen in PVNS. Sonographic appearance of intraarticular PVNS is nonspecific. It includes joint effusion synovial thickening, and complex heterogenously hyperechoic masses. However, PVNS is a monoarticular process, whereas amyloidosis tends to be polyarticular **(Option (C) is incorrect).** Polyarticular PVNS is rare but has been reported in children. Synovial masses from PVNS or amyloidosis tend not to ossify, a differentiating feature from synovial osteochondromatosis.

PVNS is usually treated by synovectomy, but there is a recurrence rate of approximately 45%, especially for the diffuse form. Some authors advocate a combined treatment approach for diffuse PVNS with both synovectomy and low dose radiation, which has been shown to reduce pain, edema, and recurrence. Advanced stages of PVNS accompanied by joint destruction may need to be treated with total joint arthroplasty.

Rheumatoid arthritis (RA) is a chronic inflammatory arthritis due to synovitis. Radiographically it is characterized by marginal osseous erosions, bone resorption, and symmetric joint space loss from articular cartilage destruction. Clinically, rheumatoid arthritis presents as a polyarthritis that affects the proximal small joints of the hands, the feet, and spine. Larger joints such as the shoulder and knee may also be affected. Although there are cases in which large lytic erosions involve the hip joint (in an articular distribution in this case), the hip joint space is maintained, which is typical for osteoarticular amyloidosis **(Option (E) is incorrect).**

Rheumatoid arthritis afflicts approximately 1% of the world's population and is three times more prevalent in women. It is a chronic, systemic inflammatory disorder of the synovium that characteristically affects small joints, but can also involve the lung, heart, pleura, and skin. Rheumatoid arthritis usually affects joints in a symmetric distribution but can sometimes demonstrate an asymmetric distribution in its early presentation.

Differential considerations of RA include crystal-induced arthropathy, osteoarthritis, systemic lupus erythematosus, reactive arthritis and psoriasis. There have been reports of amyloidosis presenting as a polyarticular arthritis mimicking rheumatoid arthritis.

Radiographs of the hand and feet are used as the initial imaging workup of rheumatoid arthritis. Radiographs classically show a proximal distribution of RA with marginal erosions, osteopenia, and joint space loss, most often in a symmetric distribution (Figure 7-8). Involvement most typically favors the carpus, distal radio-ulnar joint and ulnar styloid. High resolution ultrasound has been increasingly used to look for synovitis involving the small joints of the hands. Power Doppler (Figure 7-9) allows for sensitive detection of synovial inflammation centered at the joint. Ultrasound may show small osseous erosions. Some research has shown that quantitative analysis by summation of color pixels in a defined region of interest may help to predict development of bone erosions and assess the effect of treatment. MRI is also sensitive for detecting synovitis and joint erosions. Unlike amyloidosis, which demonstrates low T1- and T2-weighted signal intensities in cases of synovial hypertrophy, rheumatoid arthritis will show low T1- and high T2-weighted signal abnormalities.

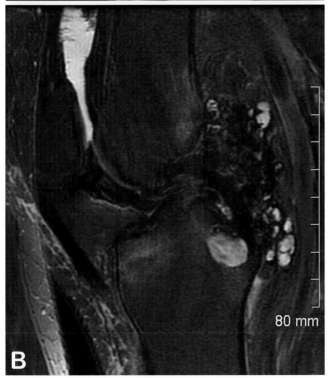

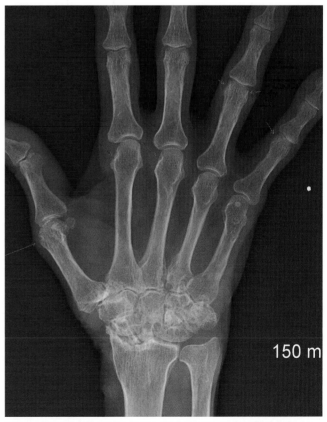

Figure 7-7. Pigmented villonodular synovitis (PVNS). Knee. MRI. Sagittal plane. Fast spin-echo. (A) Proton-density-weighted. The image demonstrates low proton density lesions, diffusely involving the knee joint, consistent with PVNS. There were multiple osseous erosions, the largest one depicted here, involving the posterior tibial plateau (arrow). (B) T-2 weighted, fat-saturated. The posterior tibial plateau mass is high-intensity under T2 weighting as are densities within the knee joint.

Figure 7-8. Rheumatoid arthritis. Radiograph. Hand. Posterior-anterior view. Multiple erosions can be seen involving the carpus. There is joint space loss and osteopenia. The contralateral hand (not shown) showed symmetric involvement.

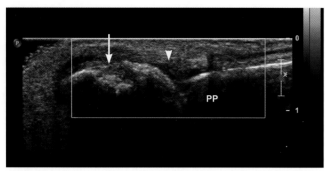

Figure 7-9. Rheumatoid arthritis. Metacarpophalangeal joint. Power Doppler ultrasound. Longitudinal plane. The image shows synovitis (arrowhead) involving the joint and osseous erosion (arrow) of the metacarpal head. PP = proximal phalanx.

Question 30

Musculoskeletal manifestations of dialysis-related amyloidosis include all of the following EXCEPT?

(A) Shoulder pad sign
(B) Osteolytic lesions
(C) Carpal tunnel syndrome
(D) Pathologic fractures
(E) Rheumatoid arthritis

When dialysis-related amyloidosis involves the musculoskeletal system, it affects the shoulder girdle, wrist, hip, knee, and spine. It occurs as a result of amyloid deposition in peri-articular tissue, synovium, and bone. When it affects the bone, it may manifest as osteolytic erosions **(Option (B) is true and therefore incorrect)**, sometimes large, as seen in the test case images. Large osteolytic lesions, especially in the weight-bearing portions, may predispose patients to pathologic fractures **(Option (D) is true and therefore incorrect)**, such as in our case.

It has been well documented that the prevalence of amyloid is dependent on the duration of hemodialysis. There is a reported incidence of greater than 90% in patients dialyzed over 7 years. However, a recent change to high flux membranes used in hemofiltration has been reported to delay the onset of amyloidosis .

The association of osteoarticular amyloidosis deposition in hemodialysis patients was first reported in the wrist, where it often manifested as carpal tunnel syndrome **(Option (C) is true and therefore incorrect)** and small lytic lesions involving the carpal bones. Osteolytic involvement of bone is known to increase in size and number with duration of hemodialysis. Osteoarticular amyloidosis commonly involves

the shoulder girdle. Patients will often present with muscle enlargement from amyloid infiltration, yet have muscle weakness and pain. Affected patients appear to have well-developed shoulder musculature, the so-called "shoulder pad sign" **(Option (A) is true and therefore incorrect)**. Men and women are equally affected. Other areas of involvement include the knees and the small joints of the hand. Less commonly, patients may develop destructive spondyloarthropathy.

Rheumatoid arthritis is not a musculoskeletal manifestation of osteoarticular amyloidosis **(Option (E) is not true and therefore correct)**. However, the polyarticular involvement and stiffness seen in osteoarticular amyloidosis have been confused with rheumatoid arthritis (Katoh, 2008). Helpful differentiating features are clinical labs. Patients with amyloidosis will lack autoantibodies and have negative results for inflammatory markers.

Question 31

True or False? Amyloidosis usually presents as a focal disease.

Osteoarticular amyloidosis is a polyarticular process. It is a systemic disease and should be regarded as a diffuse process affecting major organ systems such as in the cardiopulmonary, gastrointestinal, and genitourinary systems. **The answer to Question 31 is "False."**

Amyloid cardiomyopathy can lead to arrhythmias, diastolic dysfunction, and heart failure, which may complicate treatment regimens. Pulmonary involvement is relatively rare. When it does occur, amyloid may present as recurrent pneumonia from bronchial obstruction, or more rarely as focal amyloidoma. Amyloid involvement of the gastrointestinal system can lead to bowel wall thickening as well as abnormal resorption, and eventual malnutrition. The most common finding in amyloid involvement of the GI tract is colonic dilatation. Liver involvement is often nonspecific, and splenic involvement usually is seen as splenomegaly. Renal involvement in primary systemic amyloidosis is quite common. Amyloid can infiltrate the skin and resemble scleroderma. Other known soft tissue involvement of amyloid includes macroglossia, submandibular swelling, lymphadenopathy, and muscle hypertrophy.

Question 32

What factor(s) affect quality of hemofiltration in preventing or delaying onset of osteoarticular dialysis-related amyloidosis?

    (A)   Porosity
    (B)   Membrane thickness
    (C)   Material composition
    (D)   All of the above

Osteoarticular amyloidosis is a well-known dialysis-related complication in which a protein, beta-2-microglobulin (beta-2-MG), that is normally soluble deposits extracellularly in tissue as insoluble fibrils. It is deposited at 40 to 50 times higher levels in chronic hemodialysis patients. Clinical manifestations usually develop about 5 to 8 years after beginning hemodialysis. Risk factors for this complication include duration of dialysis, age of patient at start of dialysis, and type of hemodialysis membrane used. However, recent advances in hemodialysis filtrate technology have improved hemofiltration quality leading to less long-term morbidity.

Hemofiltration quality is determined by the porosity, thickness, and material composition of the membrane **(Option (D) is correct)**. Recent developments in new membrane technology have included high flux membranes made of polymethylmethacrylate (PMMA), polyacrylonitrile (AN-69), and polysulfone. PMMA membranes were the first commercially available noncellulose high flux membranes. Unlike the older cellulose or cuprophane membranes, these new high flux membranes have the ability to filter larger molecules, such as beta-2 microglobulin, thereby increasing their clearance by both filtration and adsorption. Prospective randomized studies have shown the use of high flux membranes to delay the clinical onset of osteoarticular amyloidosis. It is important to note, however, that higher filtration techniques still fail to return serum concentration levels of beta-2-MG to normal.

Clinical manifestations of osteoarticular amyloidosis commonly involve the shoulder, wrist, hip, and knee, most often in a polyarticular distribution. Involvement is a result of amyloid deposition in periarticular tissue, synovium, and bone. Onset may be delayed or even prevented with continued advances in hemofiltration technology.

Question 33

The imaging characteristics of osteoarticular amyloidosis include all of the following EXCEPT:

    (A)   Erosions or osteolytic lesions with preservation of the joint space
    (B)   Decreased signal intensity on T1-weighted MR images
    (C)   Nondistended joint capsule on sonographic evaluation
    (D)   Moderate enhancement of bone lesions after gadolinium-based contrast injection
    (E)   Variable signal intensity on T2-weighted MR images

Osteoarticular amyloid is characterized by bulky soft tissue masses, well-defined osteolytic, or erosive lesions, and preservation of the joint space of the involved bone **(Option (A) is true and therefore incorrect)**. Clinical manifestations of osteoarticular amyloidosis are typically not seen before 5 years from the onset of hemodialysis. When patients undergo imaging, findings are often nonspecific and may be misdiagnosed, or even unrecognized. Radiographic findings of osteolytic change, or osseous erosions are often seen in later stages, usually in a juxtaarticular distribution. MRI imaging usually reveals more extensive disease than first indicated by radiographs. MRI features of osteoarticular amyloidosis include decreased signal intensity on T1-weighted images **(Option (B) is true and therefore incorrect)**, and variable intensity on T2-weighted images **(Option (E) is true and therefore incorrect)** with approximately 50% demonstrating increased signal intensity. All bone lesions showed moderate enhancement after gadolinium-based contrast injection **(Option (D) is true and therefore incorrect)**. Postcontrast MR imaging can also help to differentiate synovial infiltration from joint fluid.

Ultrasonography can demonstrate the typical distention in the affected joint capsule **(Option (C) is false and therefore correct)**. Distention may be due to synovial infiltration or fluid accumulation. Ultrasonography can also be useful for guiding biopsy.

The radiographic features in the test case suggested the pathologically proven diagnosis of osteoarticular amyloidosis. Radiologic exam of the pathologic fracture through the right femoral neck showed large lytic lesions involving the femoral neck and superior femoral head initially suggesting an underlying malignant process. In addition, an osteolytic lesion was seen in the superior acetabulum and greater trochanter. Bone scan (Figure 9-2) did not show additional lesions, but did demonstrate relative photopenia of the right femoral head suggestive of avascularity.

Differential considerations include multiple myeloma, metastatic disease, and Waldenstrom's macroglobulinemia. Other diagnostic considerations include cystic change from brown tumors of hyperparathyroidism, subchondral degenerative cysts, or infection. Distinguishing multiple myeloma from osteoarticular amyloidosis is difficult because both can demonstrate subcortical radiolucent lesions with scalloping of the adjacent cortex. Compounding this problem is that myeloma can be complicated by osteoarticular amyloidosis in 15% of cases. However, a juxtaarticular distribution of lesions favors osteoarticular amyloidosis. Osteolysis in Waldenström's macroglobulinemia is practically identical to that found in osteoarticular amyloidosis. Metastatic lesions also appear destructive, but tend to be located in the spine or the metaphyseal/diaphyseal regions of tubular bones, such as the femur. They are not typically seen on both sides of a joint space.

Articular processes such as rheumatoid arthritis, gout, xanthomatosis, and pigmented villonodular synovitis (PVNS) may also mimic osteoarticular amyloidosis. Unlike osteoarticular amyloidosis, however, rheumatoid arthritis causes early joint space loss, marginal erosions of bone, and symmetric soft tissue masses. Gout and xanthomatosis can appear like amyloid, but is easily excluded by laboratory and clinical findings. PVNS can be difficult to distinguish from osteoarticular amyloidosis. Both are associated with osteolytic lesions with soft tissue masses and preserved joint space. However, lack of MRI features of chronic hemorrhage with hemosiderin deposition may help to distinguish osteoarticular amyloidosis from PVNS.

Histologically, osteoarticular amyloidosis secondary to hemodialysis is associated with beta-2 MG, an amyloid variant. The diagnosis is classically made by demonstration of apple-green birefringence on Congo Red staining when viewed under polarized light scanning (Figure 7-4A). Immunostaining for beta-2-MG also aids in making the diagnosis (Figure 7-4B). Ultrastructural examination of amyloid with electron microscopy reveals nonbranching fibrils, 7 to 10 nm thick that are usually arranged in a beta-pleated sheet secondary structure. On a macroscopic level, amyloid infiltration has been known to cut off the vascular supply to the femoral head and neck causing avascular necrosis, femoral head subchondral fractures, and subsequent pathologic neck fractures, as in the test case.

Question 34

Which *one* of the following is the BEST method for the treatment of osteoarticular amyloidosis?

(A) Prevention by use of high flux hemodialysis membranes
(B) Surgery involving curettage and bone grafting of bone lesions
(C) Percutaneous cementoplasty of bone lesions to prevent pathologic fracture
(D) Proper insulin therapy to maintain target Hemoglobin A1C levels
(E) None of the above

The goals for treatment of osteoarticular amyloidosis include preventative and palliative measures. Preventing the development of the many systemic manifestations of dialysis-related amyloidosis depends on the improved filtration of the beta-2-MG molecules by high flux hemodialysis membranes. Continuous improvement in membrane technology will help to further delay onset, or perhaps even completely eliminate the soft tissue deposition of amyloid in the future, but the technology is still evolving **(Option (A) is incorrect).** Palliative measures include surgery, which involves curettage and bone grafting, but this carries with it a high risk of infection and failed graft incorporation **(Option (B) is incorrect).** Percutaneous cementoplasty, a less invasive alternative in preventing pathologic fractures, has been performed with some reported success, but is limited in practice. **(Option (C) is incorrect).** Insulin therapy alone, in the setting of hemodialysis, will not treat or delay onset of osteoarticular amyloidosis **(Option (D) is incorrect).** Kidney transplantation, and with it the avoidance of hemodialysis, is the only ideal preventative measure **(Option (E) is correct),** but it would not affect the osteolytic lesions that had already formed.

Suggested Readings

SYSTEMIC AMYLOIDOSIS

1. Aoike I, Geyjo F, Arakawa M and Niigata Research Programme for Beta-2-microglobulin Removal Membrane: Learning from the Japanese Registry: How will we prevent long-term complications? Nephrol Dial Transplant. 1995;10:7–15.
2. Arakawa M and Niigata Research Programme for Beta-2-microglobulin Removal Membrane: Long-term multicentre study

on beta-2-microglobulin removal by PMMA-BK membrane. Nephrol Dial Transplant. 1991;2:69–74.

3. Beirao I, Lobato L, Guimaraes SM, et al. Early destructive spondyloarthropathy from combined beta2-microglobulin and transthyretin Met30 amyloidosis in a dialysed patient. Nephrol Dial Transplant. 1998;13:3223–3225.

4. Bely M, Kapp P, Szabo TS, Lakatos T, Apathy A. Electron microscopic characteristics of beta2-microglobulin amyloid deposits in long-term haemodialysis. Ultrastruct Pathol. 2005;29:483–491.

5. Campistol JM, Torregrosa JV, Ponz E, Fenollosa B. Beta-2-microglobulin removal by hemodialysis with polymethylmethacrylate membranes. Contrib Nephrol. 1999;125:76–85.

6. Chang SW, Murphy KP. Percutaneous CT-guided cementoplasty for stabilization of a femoral neck lesion. JVIR. 2005;16:889–890.

7. Chow KM, Griffith JF, Fung KY, Szeto CC. Rapid progression of destructive spondyloarthropathy. Spine. 2005;30:E31–33.

8. Danesh F, Ho LT. Dialysis-related amyloidosis: History and clinical manifestations. Semin Dial. 2001;14:80–85.

9. Dember LM, Jaber BL. Dialysis-related amyloidosis: Late finding or hidden epidemic? Semin Dial. 2006;19:105–109.

10. Escobedo EM, Hunter JC, Zink-Brody GC, Andress DL. Magnetic resonance imaging of dialysis-related amyloidosis of the shoulder and hip. Skeletal Radiol. 1996;25:41–48.

11. Gejyo F, Kawaguchi Y, Hara S, et al. Arresting dialysis-related amyloidosis: A prospective multicenter controlled trial of direct hemoperfusion with a beta2-microglobulin adsorption column. Artif Organs. 2004;28:371–380.

12. Gejyo F, Narita I. Current clinical and pathogenetic understanding of beta2-m amyloidosis in long-term haemodialysis patients. Nephrology [Carlton]. 2003;8(Suppl):S45–S49.

13. Georgiades CS, Neyman EG, Barish MA, Fishman EK. Amyloidosis. Review and CT manifestations. RadioGraphics. 2004;24:405–416.

14. Gielen JL, van Holsbeeck MT, Hauglustaine D, et al. Growing bone cysts in long-term hemodialysis. Skeletal Radiol. 1990;19:43–49.

15. Isaacs M, Bansal M, Flombaum CD, Lane J, Smith J. Case report 772. Stress fracture of the hip secondary to renal osteodystrophy and erosion of ischium due to amyloid deposition. Skeletal Radiol.1993;22:129–133.

16. Jadoul M. Dialysis-related amyloidosis: importance of biocompatibility and age. Nephrol Dial Transplant. 1998; 3:61–64.

17. Kunitomo T, Takeyama T, Kataoka H. Development of PMMA membrane which can remove beta-2-microglobulin and its clinical significance. Contrib Nephrol. 1995;112:145–155.

18. Little MA, Cafferky M, Menon S, Farrington K. Dialysis amyloid: The bottom line. Nephrol Dial Transplant. 2005;20:462–463.

19. Mahmood A, Sodano D, Dash A, Weinstein R. Therapeutic plasma exchange performed in tandem with hemodialysis for patients with M-protein disorders. J Clin Apher 2006; 21:100–104

20. Nangaku M, Miyata T, Kurokawa K. Pathogenesis and management of dialysis-related amyloid bone disease. Am J Med Sci. 1999;317:410–415.

21. Otake S, Tsuruta Y, Yamana D, Mizutani H, Ohba S. Amyloid arthropathy of the hip joint: MR demonstration of presumed amyloid lesions in 152 patients with long-term hemodialysis. Eur Radiol. 1998;8:1352–1356.

22. Prokaeva T, Spencer B, Kaut M, et al. Soft tissue, joint, and bone manifestations of AL amyloidosis. Arthritis & Rheum. 2007;56:3858–3868.

23. Resnick D. Diagnosis of Bone and Joint Disorders, 4th Ed. Philadelphia, PA: WB Saunders;2002: pp 2054-2058 and 2176–2183.

24. Shirahama T, Skinner M, Cohen AS, et al. Histochemical and immunohistochemical characterization of amyloid associated with chronic hemodialysis as beta-2-microglobulin. Biochem Biophys Res Commun. 1985;53:705–709.

METASTATIC DISEASE

25. Miric A, Banks M, Allen D, et al. Cortical metastatic lesions of the appendicular skeleton from tumors of known primary origin. J Surg Oncol. 1998:67:255–260.

26. Soderlund V. Radiological diagnosis of skeletal metastases. EurRadiol. 1996;6:587–595.

27. Van der Linden YM, Dijkstra PDS, Kroon HM, et al. Comparative analysis of risk factors for pathological fracture with femoral metastases: results based on a randomized trial of radiotherapy. J Bone Joint Surg Br. 2004;86:566–573.

28. Wong DA, Fornasier VL, MacNab I. Spinal metastases: the obvious, the occult, and the imposters. Spine. 1990;15:1–4.

MULTIPLE MYELOMA

29. Baur-Melnyk A, Buhmann S, Durr HR, Reiser M. Role of MRI for the diagnosis and prognosis of multiple myeloma. Eur J Radiol. 2005;55:56–63.

30. International Myeloma Working Group. Criteria for the classification of monoclonal gammopathies, multiple myeloma and related disorders: a report of the International Myeloma Working Group. Br J Haematol. 2003;121:749–757.

31. Larson RS, Sukpanichnant S, Greer JP, Cousar JB, Collins RD. The spectrum of multiple myeloma: diagnostic and biologic implications. Hum Pathol. 1997;28:1336–1347.

32. Winterbottom AP, Shaw AS. Imaging patients with myeloma. Clinical Rad. 2009;64:1–11.

PIGMENTED VILLONODULAR SYNOVITIS

33. Al-Nakshabandi NA, Ryan AG, Choudur H, et al. Pigmented villonodular synovitis. Clinical Radiol. 2004;59:414–420.

34. Blanco CE, Leon HO, Guthrie TB. Combined partial arthroscopic synovectomy and radiation therapy for diffuse pigmented villonodular synovitis of the knee. Arthroscopy. 2001;17:527–531.

35. Hughes TH, Sartoris DJ, Schweitzer ME, Resnick DL. Pigmented villonodular synovitis: MRI characteristics. Skeletal Radiol. 1995;24:7–12.

36. Murphey MD, Rhee JH, Lewis RB, Fanburg-Smith JC, Flemming DF, Walker EA. From the Archives of the AFIP: Pigmented villonodular synovitis: radiologic-pathologic correlation. RadioGraphics. 2008;28:1493–1518.

37. Vastel L, Lambert P, De Pinieux G, Charrois O, Kerboull M, Courpied JP. Surgical treatment of pigmented villonodular synovitis of the hip. JBJS Am. 2005;87:1019–1024.

RHEUMATOID ARTHRITIS

38. de Ruiter EA, Ronday HK, Markusse HM. Amyloidosis mimicking rheumatoid arthritis. Clinical Rheumatol. 1998;17:409–411.

39. Kamishima T, Tanimura K, Henmi M, et al. Power Doppler ultrasound of rheumatoid synovitis: quantification of vascular signal and analysis of interobserver variability. Skeletal Radiol. 2009:38:467–472.

40. Katoh, N, Tazawa K, Matsuda M, Ikeda S. Systemic AL amyloidosis mimicking rheumatoid arthritis. Intern Med. 2008;47:1133–1138.

41. Yamane T, Hashiramoto A, Tanaka Y, et al. Easy and accurate diagnosis of rheumatoid arthritis using anti-cyclic citrullinated peptide 2 antibody, swollen joint count, and C-reactive proteína/rheumatoid factor. J Rheumatol. 2008;35:414–420.

42. Yao L, Magalnick M, Wilson M, Lipsky P, Goldnbach-Mansky R. Periarticular bone findings in rheumatoid arthritis: T2-weighted versus contrast-enhanced T1-weighted MRI. AJR Am J Roentgenol. 2006;187:358–363.

Case 8

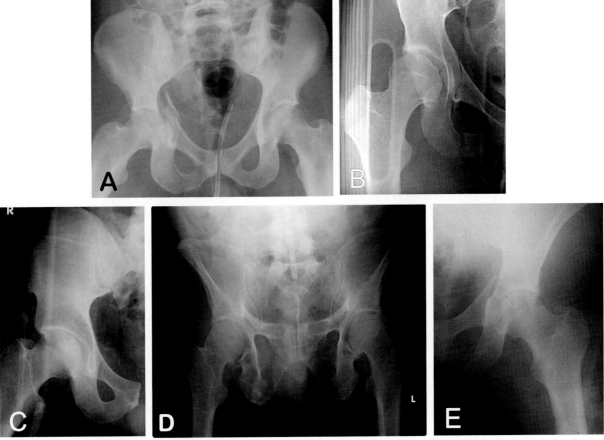

Figure 8-1. Radiographs. (A) Pelvis. Anteroposterior view. (B) Right hip. Anteroposterior view. (C) Right hip. Anteroposterior view. (D) Pelvis. Outlet view. (E) Left hip. Anteroposterior view.

Questions 35 through 39

You are shown five radiographs of the pelvis or hip from *five different patients* (Figures 8-1A through 8-1E) each of whom presented with pain after significant trauma. Select the one lettered diagnosis (A, B, C, D, or E) for each figure. Each lettered diagnosis should be used once.

35. Figure 8-1A
36. Figure 8-1B
37. Figure 8-1C
38. Figure 8-1D
39. Figure 8-1E

     (A) Transverse acetabular fracture
     (B) Posterior wall acetabular fracture
     (C) Both-column acetabular fracture
     (D) T-shaped acetabular fracture
     (E) Transverse with posterior wall acetabular fracture

Jon A. Jacobson, M.D.

Pelvic Trauma

Questions 35 through 39

Select the one lettered diagnosis (A, B, C, D, or E) for each figure. Each lettered diagnosis should be used once.

35. Figure 8-1A
36. Figure 8-1B
37. Figure 8-1C
38. Figure 8-1D
39. Figure 8-1E

(A) Transverse acetabular fracture
(B) Posterior wall acetabular fracture
(C) Both-column acetabular fracture
(D) T-shaped acetabular fracture
(E) Transverse with posterior wall acetabular fracture

Figure 8-2A (same patient as Figure 8-1A) shows a fracture involving the right acetabulum. The fracture lines disrupt the iliopectineal and ilioischial lines, producing a transverse component relative to the acetabu-

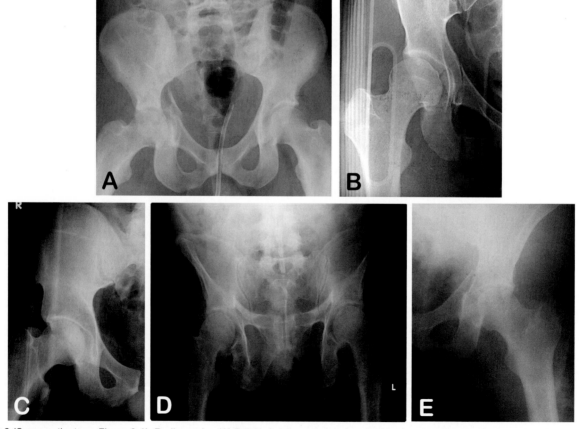

Figure 8-2 (Same patients as Figure 8-1). Radiographs. (A) Pelvis. Anteroposterior view. Both-column acetabular fracture. (B) Right hip. Anteroposterior view. T-shaped acetabular fracture. (C) Right hip. Anteroposterior view. Transverse acetabular fracture. (D) Pelvis. Outlet view. Posterior wall acetabular fracture. (E) Left hip. Anteroposterior view. Transverse with posterior wall acetabular fracture. Detailed discussion and annotated versions of each image appear on the following pages.

lum. In addition, a vertical component disrupts the obturator ring and extends superiorly into the pelvic wing. These findings allow the acetabular fracture to be characterized as a both-column fracture **(Option (C) is the answer to Question 35)**. These findings are also shown on other radiographic views and CT (Figure 8-3).

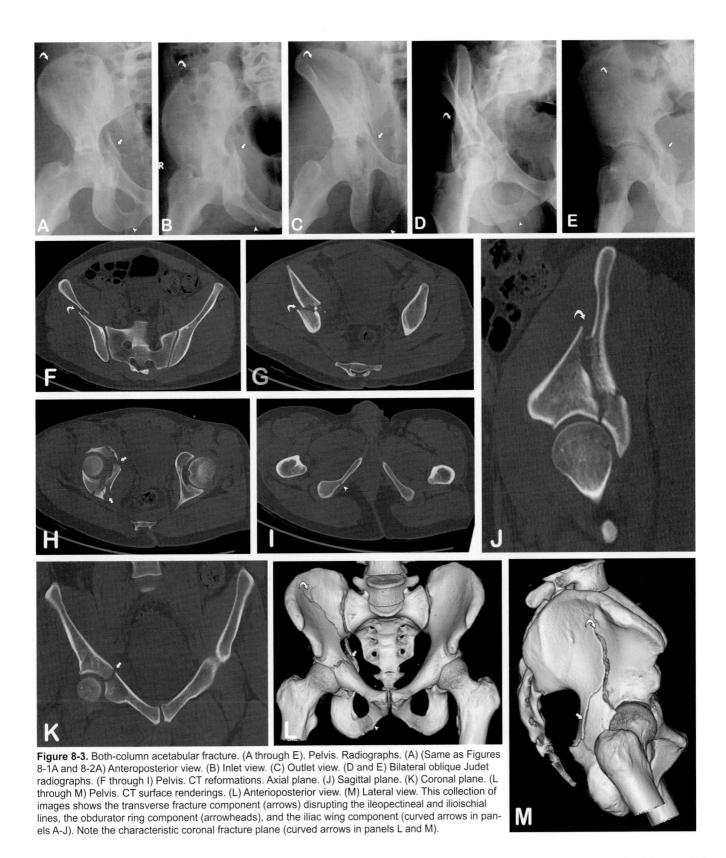

Figure 8-3. Both-column acetabular fracture. (A through E). Pelvis. Radiographs. (A) (Same as Figures 8-1A and 8-2A) Anteroposterior view. (B) Inlet view. (C) Outlet view. (D and E) Bilateral oblique Judet radiographs. (F through I) Pelvis. CT reformations. Axial plane. (J) Sagittal plane. (K) Coronal plane. (L through M) Pelvis. CT surface renderings. (L) Anterioposterior view. (M) Lateral view. This collection of images shows the transverse fracture component (arrows) disrupting the ileopectineal and ilioischial lines, the obdurator ring component (arrowheads), and the iliac wing component (curved arrows in panels A-J). Note the characteristic coronal fracture plane (curved arrows in panels L and M).

Acetabular fractures typically occur after significant trauma, such as a motor vehicle collision, where the proximal femur is impacted into the acetabulum. Characterization of acetabular fractures is accomplished with radiography. A five-view pelvic radiographic series (anteroposterior, left and right [Judet] oblique, inlet, and outlet views) allows visualization of the key structures used to classify the acetabular fracture (Figure 8-3). According to Judet and Letournel, 10 acetabular fractures may be grouped according to their predominant fracture: column, wall, or transverse. The 10 described acetabular fractures include both-column, anterior column, posterior column, transverse, T-shaped, transverse with posterior wall, posterior wall, anterior wall, posterior column with posterior wall, anterior column with posterior hemitransverse. Accurate classification is important to guide operative versus conservative management. Radiographic assessment and characterization of acetabular fractures relies on fracture line identification and subsequent disruption of various normal pelvic structures (Figure 8-4). These structures include the iliopectineal (or iliopubic) line (representing the anterior column of the acetabulum), ilioischial line (representing the posterior column of the acetabulum), posterior wall of the acetabulum, obturator ring, and pelvic wing. Assessment of these structures allows accurate classification of acetabular fractures using pelvic radiographs (Figure

8-5). CT, including multiplanar reformatted images and 3-dimensional surface rendering, can also be used to classify acetabular fractures. CT may show radiographically occult fractures and add information with regard to intraarticular bodies and associated soft tissue injury.

Of the 10 possible acetabular fracture patterns, five patterns comprise nearly 90%. The two most common are the both-column and posterior wall acetabular fractures. An algorithm based on radiographic findings (Figure 8-6) can be followed to accurately characterize the five most common acetabular fractures: both-column, T-shaped, transverse, posterior wall, and transverse with posterior wall. Using this algorithm, if the obturator ring is involved, then both-column and T-shaped fractures should be considered. With a both-column fracture, there is disruption of the iliopectineal line and the ilioischial line, producing the transverse component of the fracture (Figure 8-3). In addition to this component and the fracture line disrupting the obturator ring, the fracture extends in the coronal plane superior to the acetabulum into the pelvic wing. These are the four key components (iliopectineal, ilioischial, obturator ring, and iliac wing) of a both-column fracture as shown in Figures 8-3 and 8-5A. Another feature of a both-column fracture includes what is termed the "spur sign," where a displaced and angulated fracture fragment projects posteriorly just above

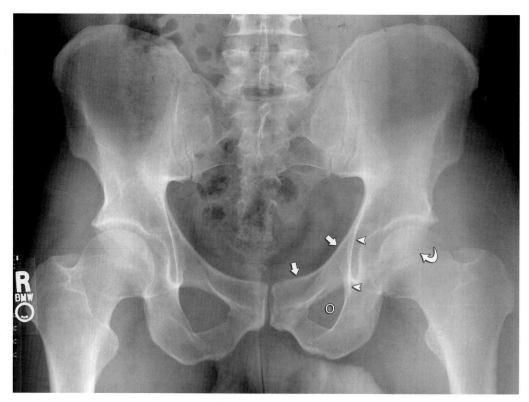

Figure 8-4. Normal pelvis. Radiograph. Anteroposterior view. This view of the pelvis shows the normal iliopectineal line (arrows), the ilioischial line (arrowheads), and the posterior wall of the acetabulum (curved arrow) (O = obturator ring).

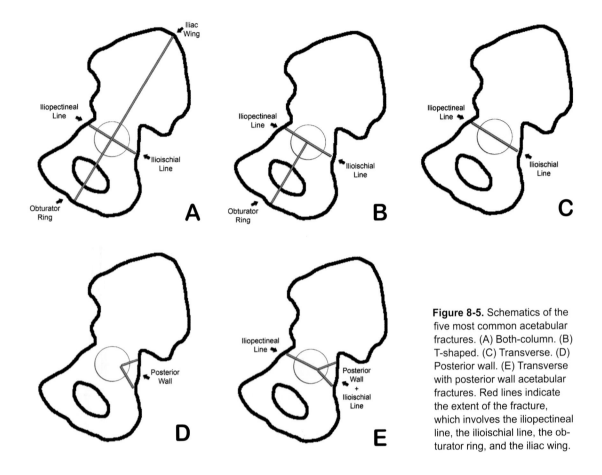

Figure 8-5. Schematics of the five most common acetabular fractures. (A) Both-column. (B) T-shaped. (C) Transverse. (D) Posterior wall. (E) Transverse with posterior wall acetabular fractures. Red lines indicate the extent of the fracture, which involves the iliopectineal line, the ilioischial line, the obturator ring, and the iliac wing.

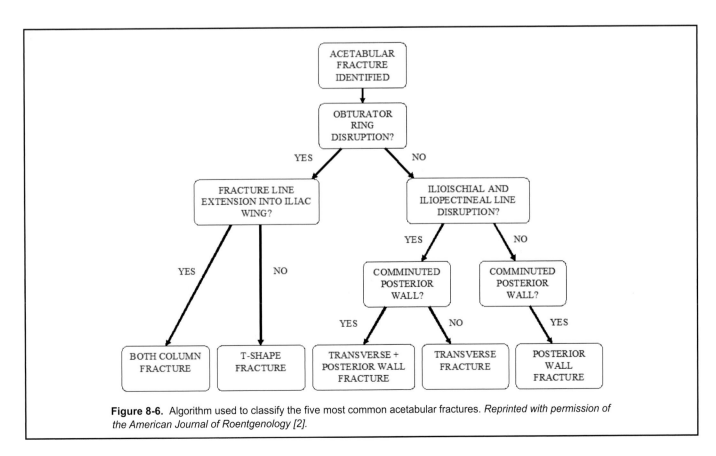

Figure 8-6. Algorithm used to classify the five most common acetabular fractures. *Reprinted with permission of the American Journal of Roentgenology [2].*

the acetabulum on a Judet view. CT of a both-column fracture demonstrates the described radiographic findings with the characteristic fracture plane superior to the acetabulum in the coronal plane (Figure 8-3).

The other common acetabular fracture involving the obturator ring is the T-shaped fracture (Figure 8-7). Like the both-column fracture, there is a transverse component that disrupts the iliopectineal and ilioischial lines and a component that disrupts the obturator ring; however, unlike the both-column fracture, there is no fracture extension into the iliac wing. Figure 8-2B (same as Figure 8-7A) shows these three essential components of a T-shaped fracture (disrup-

tion of iliopectineal line, ilioischial line, and obturator ring) **(Option (D) is the answer to Question 36)**.

The three remaining common acetabular fractures that spare the obturator ring are the transverse, posterior wall, and transverse with posterior wall. A transverse fracture (Figure 8-8) disrupts the iliopectineal and ilioischial lines, creating a fracture plane that is transverse relative to the acetabulum; however, unlike the both-column and T-shaped fractures, the obturator ring is not involved. Figure 8-2C (same patient as Figure 8-8) shows the key components of a transverse acetabular fracture (disrupted iliopectineal and ilioischial lines with spared obturator ring) **(Option (A) is the**

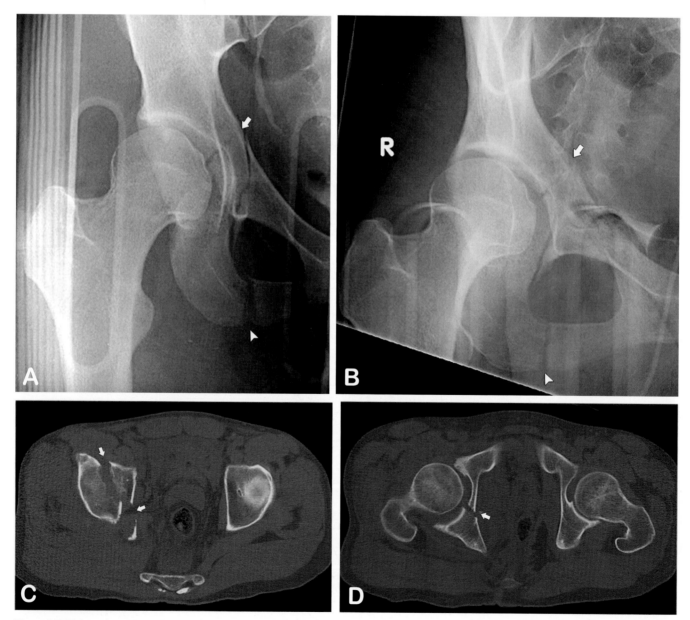

Figure 8-7. T-shaped acetabular fracture. (A) (same as Figures 8-1B and 8-2B) Radiograph. Anteroposterior view. (B) Radiograph. Oblique Judet view. The images show a transverse fracture component (arrows) disrupting the iliopectineal and ilioischial lines, and an obturator ring component (arrowheads). (C and D) CT. Axial plane. Note that the transverse fracture plane is relative to the acetabulum appearing in oblique sagittal plane on CT.

answer to Question 37). CT of a transverse fracture will demonstrate the radiographic findings with the fracture in the oblique sagittal plane, which extends inferior and lateral through the acetabulum.

Another common acetabular fracture that spares the obturator ring is the posterior wall fracture (Figure 8-9). In this scenario, there is a comminuted fracture of the posterior wall of the acetabulum, often with posterior and superior displacement of the fracture fragments. The ilioischial line may be disrupted; how-

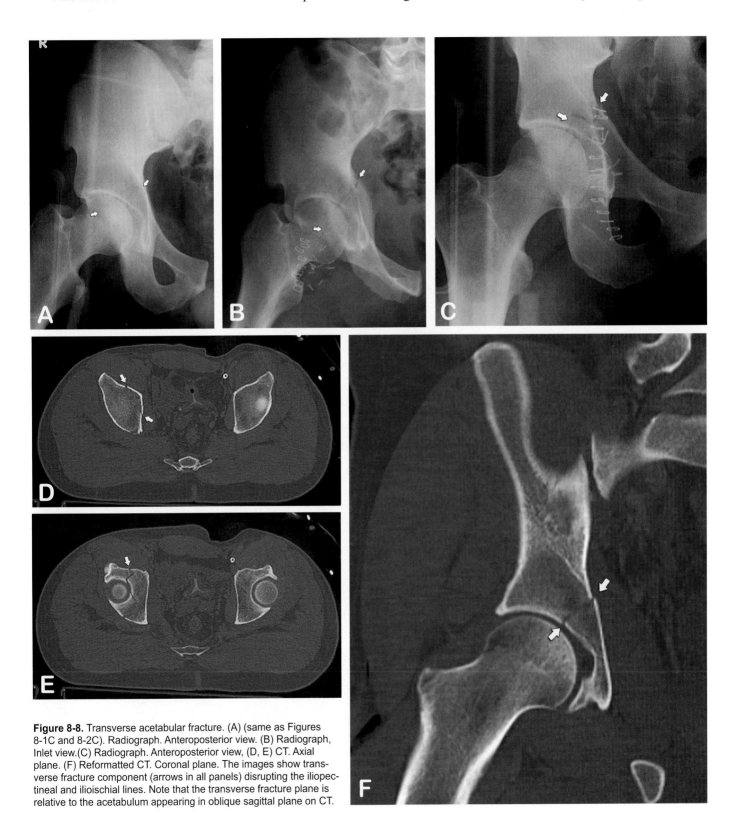

Figure 8-8. Transverse acetabular fracture. (A) (same as Figures 8-1C and 8-2C). Radiograph. Anteroposterior view. (B) Radiograph, Inlet view.(C) Radiograph. Anteroposterior view, (D, E) CT. Axial plane. (F) Reformatted CT. Coronal plane. The images show transverse fracture component (arrows in all panels) disrupting the iliopectineal and ilioischial lines. Note that the transverse fracture plane is relative to the acetabulum appearing in oblique sagittal plane on CT.

ever, the iliopectineal line is intact. Figure 8-2D (same patient as Figure 8-9) shows the key elements of a posterior wall fracture (comminuted fracture involving posterior wall, intact ilioischial line, intact iliopectineal line, and intact obturator ring) **(Option (B) is the answer to Question 38)**. Nondisplaced posterior wall fractures may be difficult to visualize on anteroposterior radiographs because of the superimposed femoral head, and are best seen on oblique views and CT.

Finally, the fifth common acetabular fracture is the transverse with posterior wall fracture (Figure 8-10),

which essentially combines the features of the transverse and posterior wall fractures described above. Figure 8-2E (same patient as Figure 8-10) shows the key elements of a transverse with posterior wall fracture (disrupted iliopectineal and ilioischial lines, posterior wall fracture, intact obturator ring) **(Option (E) is the answer to Question 39)**.

Since acetabular fractures are commonly due to impaction of the femoral head into the acetabulum, it is important to assess for proximal femur fracture as well. Fractures of the femoral head are classified using the

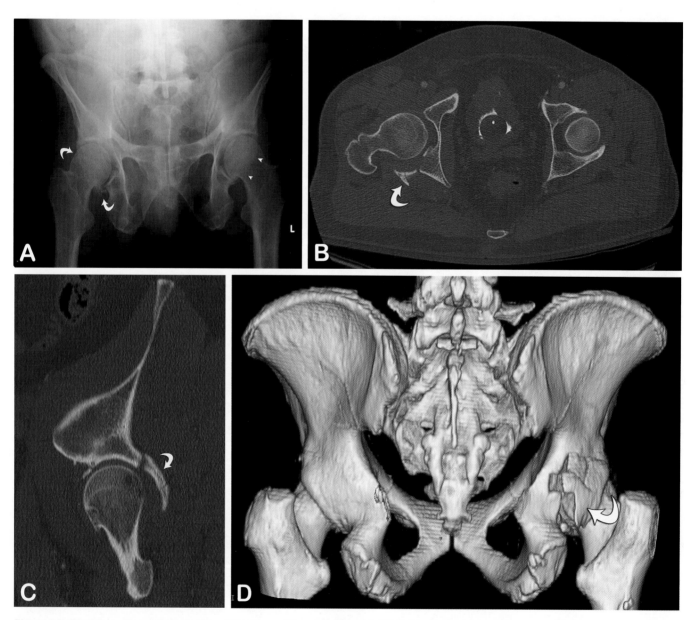

Figure 8-9. Posterior wall acetabular fracture. (A) (same as Figures 8-1D and 8-2D) Pelvis. Radiograph. Outlet view. Note the normal smooth and continuous border of the left acetabular wall (arrowheads). (B) CT. Axial plane, (C) CT reformation. Sagittal plane. (D) CT surface rendering. Posteroanterior view. The images show comminuted and displaced posterior acetabular wall fracture (curved arrows in all panels).

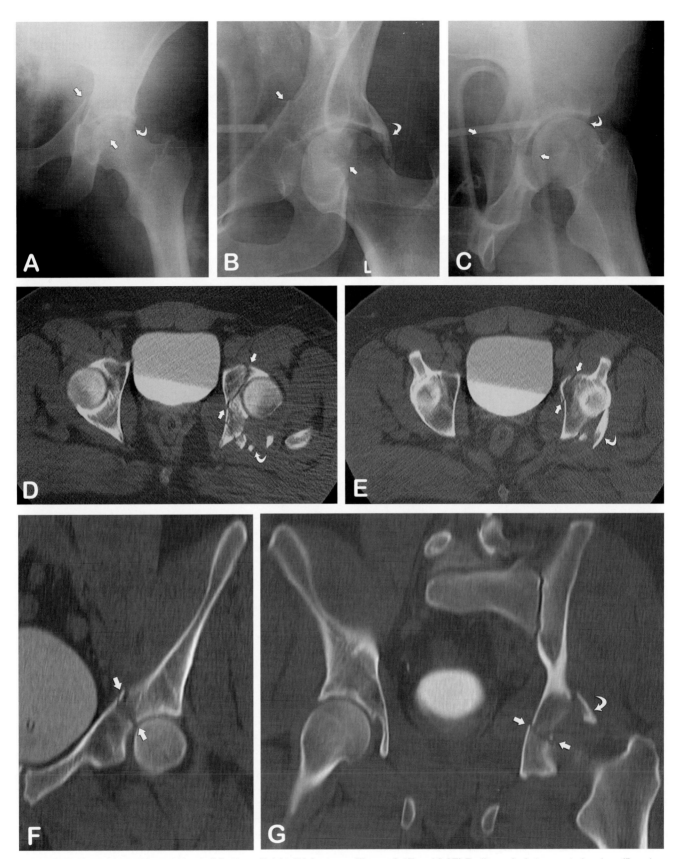

Figure 8-10. Transverse with posterior wall fracture. Pelvis. (A) (same as Figures 8-1E and 8-2E) Radiograph. Anteroposterior view. (B and C) Judet radiographs. Oblique view. (D and E) CT. Axial plane. (F,G) Reformatted CT. Coronal plane. The images show a transverse fracture component (arrows in all panels), disrupting the iliopectineal and ilioischial lines, as well as displaced posterior acetabular wall fracture fragments (curved arrows in all panels).

Pipkin classification. A Pipkin 1 fracture (Figure 8-11) is isolated medial to the fovea centralis, Pipkin 2 is located lateral to the fovea centralis, Pipkin 3 is either a Pipkin 1 or 2 with additional fracture of the femoral neck, and Pipkin 4 is any of the above described femoral head fractures associated with an acetabular fracture. CT is important in assessment for femoral head fractures as well as intraarticular bodies after acetabular fracture. After femoral head impaction injury, subsequent complications include post-traumatic chondrolysis and avascular necrosis.

Also associated with acetabular fractures is dislocation of the hip (Figure 8-12). Approximately 80% to 85% of hip dislocations are posterior. When there is posterior dislocation of the hip, the leg may be internally rotated, and the femoral head usually overlaps the acetabular roof on radiography. Less commonly, the hip may be dislocated anteriorly, where the femoral head is usually seen overlying the obturator ring and the leg may be externally rotated. When a patient undergoes a CT after acetabular fracture, a hip dislocation may have been reduced prior to imaging. In this setting, the presence of an intra-

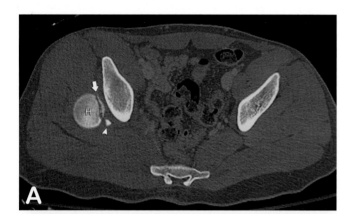

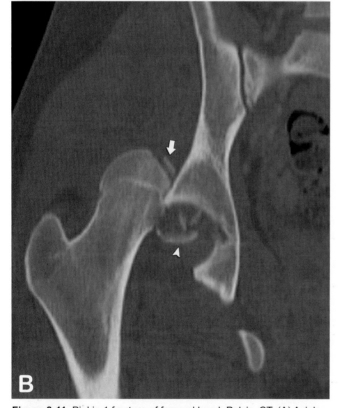

Figure 8-11. Pipkin 1 fracture of femoral head. Pelvis. CT. (A) Axial plane. (B) Reformation. Coronal plane. The images show dislocation of the femoral head (H) with a femoral head fracture (arrows in both panels) and several ossified intraarticular bodies (arrowheads in both panels).

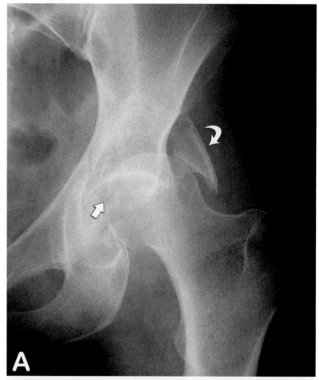

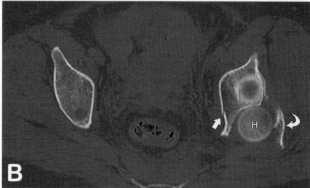

Figure 8-12. Posterior hip dislocation and posterior wall fracture. (A) Hip. Radiograph. Anteroposterior view. Note the intact iliopectineal line. (B) Pelvis. CT. Axial plane. Both images show posterior dislocation of the femoral head (H) with posterior acetabular wall fracture (curved arrows in both panels) causing disruption of the ilioischial line (arrows in both panels).

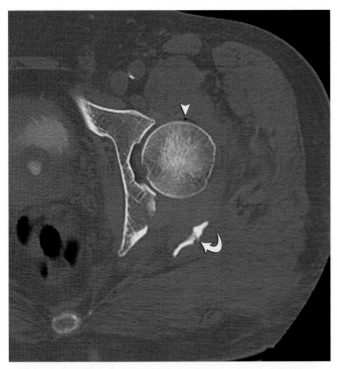

Figure 8-13. Bubble sign. Hip. CT. Axial plane. The image shows the focus of air (arrowhead). Note the displaced posterior wall fracture fragments (curved arrow) from prior posterior hip dislocation.

capsular gas bubble in the hip joint is evidence that a dislocation had been present (Figure 8-13). This gas bubble is essentially vacuum or nitrogen gas formed at the time of the dislocation.

Question 40

Concerning Figure 8-14 (in the Test section), which *one* of the following BEST describes the mechanism of injury producing the radiographic findings?

(A) Lateral compression
(B) Anteroposterior compression
(C) Vertical shear
(D) Complex

In addition to acetabular fracture, pelvic trauma may produce other fracture patterns outside of the acetabulum that can be predicted by the mechanism of injury. One classification system divides the mechanisms of pelvic injury into lateral compression, anteroposterior compression, vertical shear, and mixed or complex. With a lateral compression injury, ipsilateral fracture of the obturator ring is common with associated ipsilateral or contralateral sacral fracture, appearing as a disruption of the arcuate lines on radiography. Figure 8-15 (same patient as Figure 8-14) shows the characteristic findings of a lateral compression mechanism of injury (obturator ring fracture and sacral fracture) **(Option (A) is correct).** Of note, lateral compression injuries may also produce an isolated fracture of the iliac wing (or Duverney fracture), usually associated with minimal displacement and without major hemorrhage (Figure 8-16).

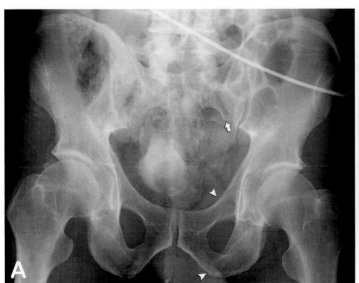
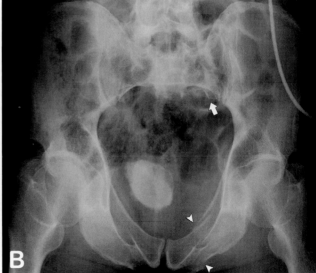

Figure 8-15 (Same as Figure 8-14). Lateral compression injury. Pelvis. (A) Radiograph. Anteroposterior view. (B) Radiograph. Inlet view.

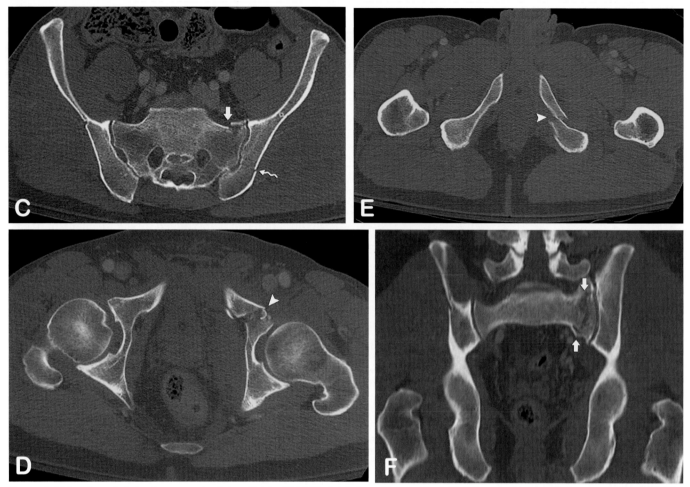

Figure 8-15 (continued). Lateral compression injury. Pelvis. (C-E) CT. Axial plane. Note incidental left ilium fracture (squiggly arrow in panel C). (F) Reformatted CT. The images show obturator ring fractures (arrowheads in panels B, D, and E) and a sagittal fracture of the left sacral ala (arrows in A, B, and F) causing buckling of an arcuate line in (A).

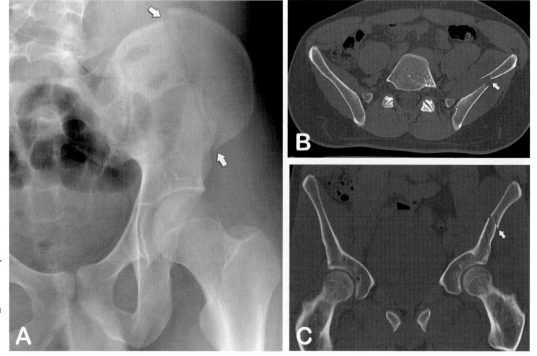

Figure 8-16. Iliac wing fracture. Pelvis. (A) Radiograph. Antero-posterior view. Arrows show an isolate left iliac wing fracture. (B) CT. Axial plane. (C) Reformatted CT. Coronal plane. Both images show isolate left iliac wing fracture (arrows in both panels).

Question 41

Concerning Figure 8-17 (in the Test section), which *one* of the following BEST describes the mechanism of injury producing the radiographic findings?

(A) Lateral compression
(B) Anteroposterior compression
(C) Vertical shear
(D) Complex

Another mechanism of injury-producing pelvic fracture is anteroposterior compression (Figure 8-18). In this setting, a force is directed in the anteroposterior direction, which may cause bilateral superior and inferior pubic rami fractures or diastasis of the pubic symphysis. Normally, the pubic symphysis measures up to 4 mm in men, 5 mm in women, and 6 mm in pregnancy. With anteroposterior compression, sacroiliac joint diastasis and sacral fractures are possible. Figure 8-18 (same as Figure 8-17) shows the characteristic findings of an anteroposterior mechanism of injury **(Option (B) is correct).**

A third mechanism of injury for pelvic trauma is a vertical shear (Figure 8-19). The radiographic findings in this setting are vertical offset of the hemipelvis, with either diastasis of pubic symphysis and/or pubic rami fractures, and diastasis of a sacroiliac joint and/or sacral fracture. Last, a mixed appearance or complex pattern of fractures may be seen that does not cleanly fit into one of the above classification schemes.

SUMMARY: Accurate identification and characterization of pelvic fractures after trauma depends on assessment of specific pelvic structures. When an acetabular fracture is present, assessment of the iliopectineal, ilioischial, posterior wall, iliac wing, and obturator ring is important. The presence of an obturator ring fracture divides the possible acetabular fractures into two categories of common fractures. In addition to acetabular fractures, obturator ring fractures are also seen in lateral compression injuries and possible anteroposterior compression injuries. Arcuate line disruption indicates the presence of sacral fracture. CT can add important information when characterizing finding from pelvic injury.

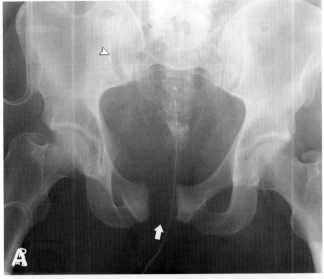

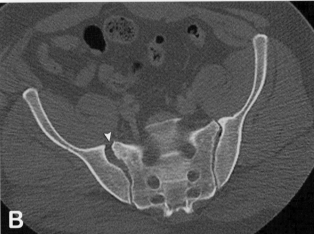

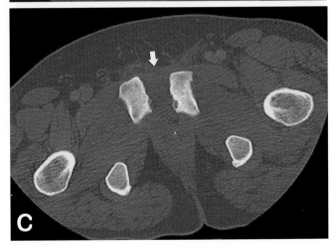

Figure 8-18 (Same as Figure 8-17). Anteroposterior compression injury. Pelvis. (A) Radiograph. Anteroposterior view. (B and C) CT. Axial plane. The images show diastasis of pubic symphysis (arrows) and sacroiliac joint (arrowheads).

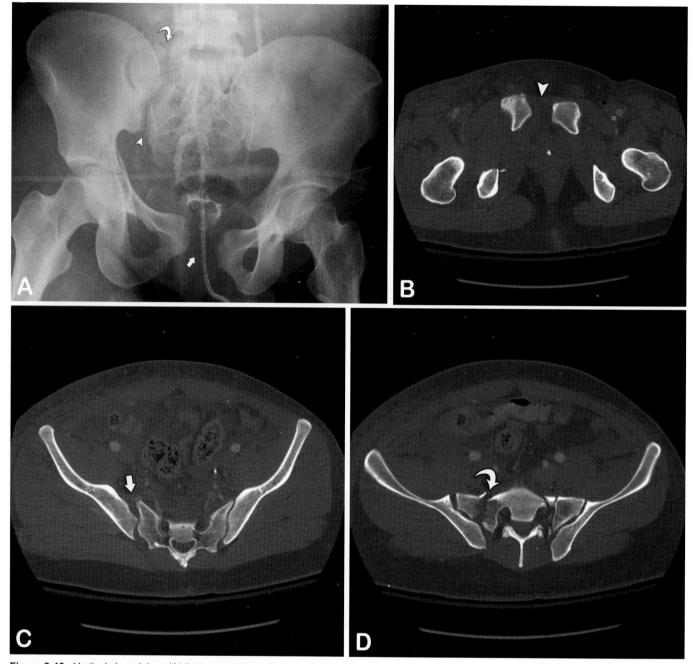

Figure 8-19. Vertical shear injury. (A) Anteroposterior radiograph and (B-D) axial CT images show sacroiliac joint diastasis (arrowhead), sacral fracture (curved arrow), and pubic symphysis diastasis (arrow) causing vertical offset of the right hemipelvis.

Suggested Readings

1. Brandser E, Marsh JL. Acetabular fractures: easier classification with a systematic approach. AJR Am J Roentgenol. 1998;171:1217-1228.

2. Durkee NJ, Jacobson J, Jamadar D, Karunakar MA, Morag Y, Hayes C. Classification of common acetabular fractures: radiographic and CT appearances. AJR Am J Roentgenol. 2006;187:915-925.

3. Fairbairn KJ, Mulligan ME, Murphey MD, Resnik CS. Gas bubbles in the hip joint on CT: an indication of recent dislocation. AJR Am J Roentgenol 1995;164:931-934.

4. Harris JH, Jr., Coupe KJ, Lee JS, Trotscher T. Acetabular fractures revisited: part 2, a new CT-based classification. AJR Am J Roentgenol. 2004;182:1367-1375.

5. Harris JH, Jr., Lee JS, Coupe KJ, Trotscher T. Acetabular fractures revisited: part 1, redefinition of the Letournel anterior column. AJR Am J Roentgenol. 2004;182:1363-1366.

6. Hunter JC, Brandser EA, Tran KA. Pelvic and acetabular trauma. Radiol Clin North Am. 1997;35:559-590.

7. Ohashi K, El-Khoury GY, Abu-Zahra KW, Berbaum KS. Interobserver agreement for Letournel acetabular fracture classification with multidetector CT: are standard Judet radiographs necessary? Radiology. 2006;241:386-391.

Case 9

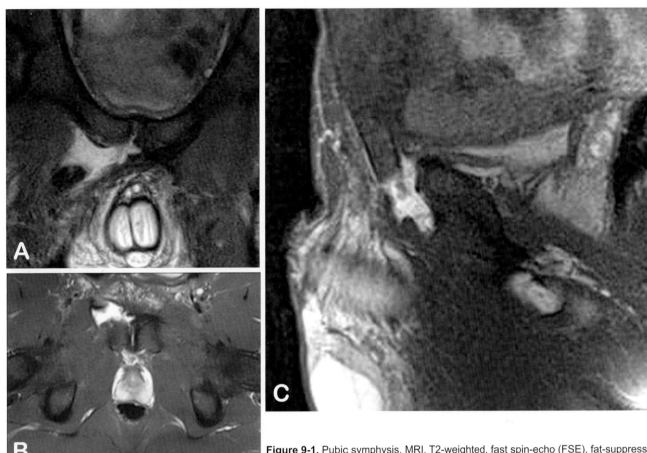

Figure 9-1. Pubic symphysis. MRI. T2-weighted, fast spin-echo (FSE), fat-suppressed. (A) Coronal oblique plane. (B) Axial plane. (C) Sagittal plane.

Question 42

A 24-year-old professional American football player presented with acute onset of left-sided groin pain following a hyperextension and twisting injury at the waist. The patient also suffers from chronic right-sided groin pain. You are shown three images (Figure 9-1) from the patient's T2-weighted, fast spin-echo, fat-suppressed MRI. Which *one* of the following is the MOST likely diagnosis?

(A)   Osteitis pubis
(B)   Traumatic inguinal hernia
(C)   Rectus abdominis/adductor aponeurosis tear
(D)   Adductor tubercle avulsion

Adam C. Zoga, M.D.

Adductor Injury

Question 42

Which *one* of the following is the MOST likely diagnosis?

(A) Osteitis pubis
(B) Traumatic inguinal hernia
(C) Rectus abdominis/adductor aponeurosis tear
(D) Adductor tubercle avulsion

MR images from this patient show a unilateral defect in the tendinous attachments at the anterior pelvis, just lateral to the pubic symphysis (Figure 9-2). On the coronal oblique T2-weighted, fast spin-echo (FSE), fat-suppressed image (Figure 9-2A), the adductor longus and pectineus tendons are avulsed from their origins at the anteroinferior aspect of the superior pubic ramus, and there is reactive muscle edema throughout the adductor compartment. On an axial image with the same parameters acquired at the level of the superior margin of the symphysis (Figure 9-2B), a large defect is seen within the caudal rectus abdominis tendon, extending from its lateral edge. A sagittal T2-weighted FSE fat-suppressed image (Fig-

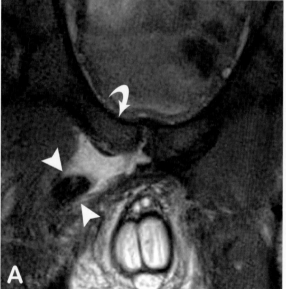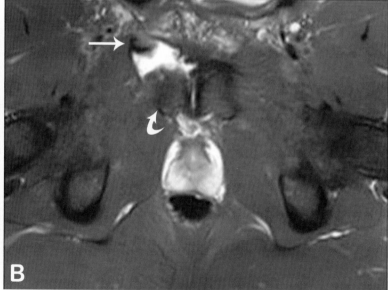

Figure 9-2. Rectus abdominis/adductor aponeurosis tear. Pubic symphysis. MRI. T2-weighted, fast spin-echo (FSE), fat-suppressed. (A) Coronal oblique plane. (B) Axial plane. (C) Sagittal plane. Images of the pubic symphysis region were acquired as a part of an athletic pubalgia MRI protocol in a 24-year-old professional American football player with acute onset chronic right-sided groin pain. There is detachment of the caudal rectus abdominis tendon (arrows in panels B and C) from its superior pubic ramus attachment (curved arrows in all panels) as well as detachment and retraction of the right adductor logus tendon (arrowheads in panels A and C). This confluent but unilateral lesion has been termed the rectus abdominis/adductor aponeurosis disruption.

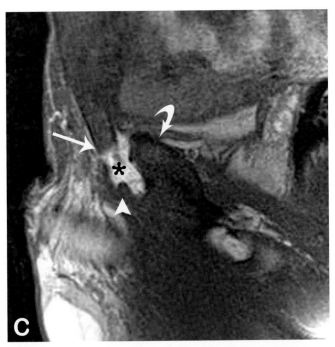

Figure 9-2 (continued). Rectus abdominis/adductor aponeurosis tear. MRI. T2-weighted, FSE, fat-suppressed. (C) Sagittal plane at a level 1 cm lateral to the pubic symphysis. This confluent but unilateral lesion (arrow) has been termed the rectus abdominis/adductor aponeurosis disruption.

ure 9-2C) acquired 1cm lateral to the pubic symphysis nicely shows a large gap confluently spanning the torn ends of the caudal rectus abdominis and cephalad adductor longus tendons, marking the site of injury, the rectus abdominis/adductor aponeurosis **(Option (C) is correct).** Although there may be an element of mild osteitis pubis in this patient, noted by the increased signal intensity, it is a frequent finding with rectus abdominis/adductor aponeurosis injuries. The dominant finding, however, is clearly a unilateral tendinous detachment **(Option (A) is incorrect).** There is no MRI evidence of viscera within the inguinal canal to suggest an inguinal hernia **(Option (B) is incorrect),** and the adductor tendon origins, while torn, are not injured in isolation and show no osseous avulsion **(Option (D) is incorrect).**

Groin pain in athletes has been a common but elusive problem for team physicians and athletic trainers for decades. There are several reproducible patterns of musculoskeletal injury in the area of the pubic symphysis that can be identified on MRI. They are often encountered in patients with clinical athletic pubalgia or "sports hernia." In the setting of athletic pubalgia, MRI is the imaging examination of choice, and a noncontrast study utilizing a dedicated pubalgia protocol (as was used in this case) is recommended. Activity-induced groin pain can be related to osseous or soft

tissue lesions around the pubic symphysis, internal derangements of the hip, or any one of a myriad of other soft tissue lesions between the hip and the symphisis. The MRI protocol should, therefore, include a large field of view that covers the hips and the anterior, superior, and inferior iliac spines and sacroiliac joints, as well as smaller field of view high resolution sequences dedicated to the pubic symphysis region. One way to accomplish this objective is to place a receive-only surface coil over the pubic symphysis, turning it off in favor of the built-in body coil for the large field-of-view sequences and turning it on for the sequences dedicated to the symphysis region. With the surface coil on, a T2-weighted, axial oblique sequence obtained along the anterior iliac wing or the arcuate line of the pelvis from a sagittal localizer can improve sensitivity for rectus abdominis and adductor tendon injuries.

After image acquisition, review should follow a dogmatic algorithm with emphasis on categorizing injuries into syndromes based upon MRI findings and should be directed toward appropriate treatment plans. First, the pubic symphysis articulation should be interrogated for osseous edema, including its location in the bone and any asymmetry as well as any degenerative or erosive arthropathic changes. Frequently, these osseous findings will lead to identification of associated soft tissue lesions. At this point, any MRI equivalent of the secondary cleft should be noted and defined as "inferolateral extension of T2 hyperintense signal from the primary symphyseal cleft," as its situs will serve as a strong indicator of the side of pain. Next, the imager should examine the morphology and signal of the caudal rectus abdominis attachments to the superior pubic rami, assessing symmetry and identifying any detachment or frank tear. Adductor tendon origins should then be reviewed and inguinal canal anatomy carefully examined, with an emphasis on symmetry. Finally, care must be taken to assess more remote structures on the larger field-of-view sequences that might be sources of referred pain, including the sacroiliac joints, the hips, the pelvic apophyses and the visceral pelvis. Using this approach, the majority of patients with true athletic pubalgia can be categorized into a specific MRI injury pattern.

Question 43

Based on your evaluation of Figure 9-3 (in the Test section), which *one* of the following is the *dominant* finding in this 18-year-old soccer player with chronic bilateral groin pain?

(A) Osteitis pubis
(B) Traumatic inguinal hernia
(C) Rectus abdominis / adductor aponeurosis tear
(D) Adductor tubercle avulsion

On MRI, osteitis pubis manifests as bone marrow edema resembling osteoarthritis of other fibrous joints such as the acromioclavicular or upper sacroiliac joints. Figure 9-4 shows bone marrow edema on both sides of the symphysis, extending anterior to posterior in a subchondral location and consistent with osteitis pubis **(Option (A) is correct)**. The findings are distinct from isolated subcortical marrow edema seen in tendinous avulsive stress and linear foci of marrow edema seen in fractures. There is no hernia seen on the MRI **(Option (B) is incorrect)**. Although the adductor tendons are bilaterally enlarged and tendinotic, they are intact **(Option (C) is incorrect)**. The caudal rectus abdominis tendons are somewhat ill-defined, but the dominant MRI finding in this case is within the osseous structures of the symphysis **(Option (D) is incorrect)**.

While bone marrow edema must be present bilaterally in osteitis pubis, it is frequently asymmetric, with more extensive or intense edema on the side of dominant pain. Other findings that can be seen with osteitis pubis in some cases include geode formation, eburnation, and resorption of subchondral bone. These degenerative changes suggest an element of chronicity and repetitive microtrauma at the symphysis. Although osteitis pubis can be an isolated finding seen most commonly in postpartum females with ligamentous laxity, a regional soft tissue injury such as a rectus abdominis/adductor aponeurosis lesion is present in many cases. Such a soft tissue injury in the region of the pubic symphysis may contribute to instability at the symphysis and the subsequent repetitive microtrauma that ultimately leads to the typical subchondral bone marrow reaction seen with osteitis pubis. In the Test case (Figure 9-3 in the Test section), enlargement of both the caudal rectus abdominis tendons and the adductor tendon origins suggest that a previous tendinous injury may have predisposed the patient to osteitis pubis, but the dominant finding by MRI is within the subchondral bone. With both inflammatory and degenerative elements, osteitis pubis often responds to minimally invasive therapies such as fluoroscopy-

guided steroid and anesthetic injections. Symptom recurrence is common, however, and many patients with osteitis pubis ultimately undergo surgical rectus abdominis or pelvic floor repair.

The caudal rectus abdominis muscle and tendon should be evaluated for abnormal T2 hyperintense signal, an indicator of acute injury, or for either hypertrophic or atrophic muscle morphology, a suggestion of a more chronic lesion. Symmetry is key in the assess-

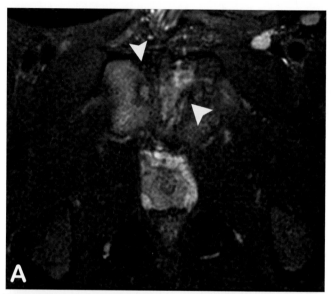

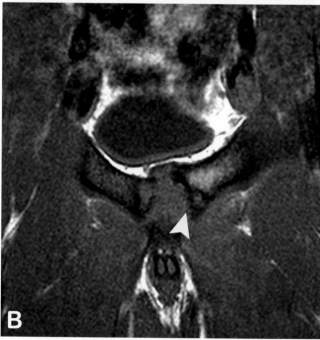

Figure 9-4 (same as Figure 9-3). Severe osteitis pubis. Pubic symphysis. MRI. (A) T2-weighted FSE, fat-suppressed. Axial plane. (B) Proton-density-weighted FSE. Coronal oblique plane. Both images from an 18-year-old male soccer player with refractory bilateral groin pain show extensive subchondral bone marrow edema and osseous resorption at the pubic symphysis (arrowheads in both panels).

ment of the rectus abdominis, as an insertional injury may manifest simply as diminution of the tendon on coronal and axial sections. Specific attention should be directed to the elongated tenoperiosteal attachment of the caudal rectus abdominis tendon on the anteroinferior aspect of the superior pubic ramus, because a disruption here is frequently a cause of pain that can also lead to instability at the pubic symphysis and secondary osteitis pubis. Distally, the lateral edge of the most caudal portion of the rectus abdominis tendon helps to reinforce the posteromedial aspect of the superficial inguinal canal. An injury in this location may mimic a hernia on physical examination, as the examiner elicits pain with pressure on the superficial inguinal ring. In other cases, the distal rectus abdominis tendons are symmetric in morphology, but there is unilateral tenoperiosteal detachment best identified on sagittal, T2-weighted, fat-suppressed sequences that span the area between the symphysis and the lateral edges of the rectus abdominus/adductor aponeuroses. Some rectus abdominis lesions extend confluently into either the ipsilateral adductor longus tendon origin or the pubic attachment of

the contralateral rectus abdominis. Variations in injury to this location include detachment without tear (where the tendons are intact but detached from bone), myotendinous strain (where there is peritendinous edema), and frank tear (or tendinous disruption).

Question 44

In the setting of athletic pubalgia, which *one* of the following is the MOST common adductor tendon injured?

    (A)   Adductor longus
    (B)   Adductor brevis
    (C)   Adductor magnus
    (D)   Gracilis

In some patients with groin pain and athletic pubalgia, lesions are isolated to the thigh adductor compartment, involving one or more tendons or muscles. On MRI, proximal adductor tendinopathies, can appear analogous to other tendinopathies, such as those of the distal supraspinatus or Achilles (Figure 9-5). Again, symmetry is important, because tendinosis on MRI can present as enlargement, peritendinous edema, or heterogeneity in signal. Other acute adductor injuries visible on MRI include proximal myotendinous strains, and soft tissue or osseous avulsions at the origins of the tendon. Chronic tendinopathies in the adductor compartment may be due to mucoid degeneration and even calcific tendinosis. While any tendon or muscle in the adductor compartment can be injured, the adductor longus origin is the one most frequently involved in athletes with refractory groin pain **(Option (A) is correct)**. The adductor brevis is often secondarily, and less severely injured in the setting of adductor longus strain **(Option (B) is incorrect)**. The adductor magnus is most frequently injured at its mid to distal muscle belly, some distance from the pubic symphysis **(Option (C) is incorrect)**. While gracilis strains can present with groin pain, there is rarely tenderness in the anterior or inguinal regions and so patients do not typically present with athletic pubalgia **(Option (D) is incorrect)**. Numerous adductor longus variants have been described in the surgical literature, and most can be seen at MRI. Isolated adductor tendon compartment injuries are most frequently treated conservatively, with other therapeutic options including minimally invasive procedures such as directed steroid injections, ultrasound-guided tenotomy, and prolotherapy with platelet-rich solutions. More distal adductor compartment strains are the most common injury in patients

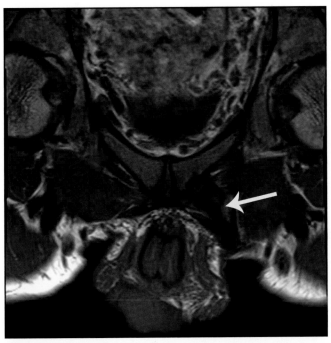

Figure 9-5. Chronic hypoxic adductor longus tendinosis. Left groin. MRI. Proton-density-weighted, FSE. Coronal oblique view. The image shows asymmetric enlargement and ill definition of the left adductor longus tendon origin (arrow). This case demonstrates just one of numerous lesions isolated to the thigh adductor compartment in clinical athletic pubalgia. The patient is a 40-year-old kick boxer with refractory left-sided groin pain.

with recurrent groin pain after a surgical pelvic floor repair. Occasionally, a myotendinous junction strain will lead to herniation of muscle through its surrounding epimysium, and subsequent painful fibrosis. This scenario can be a surgical indication and has been termed "baseball pitcher, hockey goalie syndrome."

Question 45

The patient in Figure 9-6 (in the Test section) is a runner with bilateral groin pain whose MRI findings show a lesion that can be referred to as which *one* of the following?

(A) Adductor longus strain
(B) Rectus abdominis/adductor aponeurotic plate disruption
(C) Bilateral inguinal hernia
(D) Gilmore groin

At the pubic symphysis, the most caudal rectus abdominis fibers blend with the adductor longus tendon origin as well as the anterior and arcuate ligaments of the pubic symphysis, the symphyseal capsule, and the periosteum of the pubic rami. This aponeurosis is a common location for soft tissue injury in the athlete with

groin pain. It is uncommon for the caudal rectus abdominis to be torn in isolation. In fact, an injury to the most distal aspect of the rectus abdominis almost invariably involves the ipsilateral adductor longus origin. When describing these injuries on MR review, it is difficult to distinguish the rectus abdominis from the adductor longus and the pubic symphysis ligaments. Thus, descriptive terms based upon MRI appearance have been used in an effort to guide therapy. When a region of the distal rectus abdominis is detached from the pubic ramus confluently with partial or complete avulsion of the adductor longus origin, it can be described as an ipsilateral rectus abdominis/adductor detachment. A frank tear involving both of these structures is most commonly located at the level of the anteroinferior aspect of the superior pubic ramus, one to two centimeters lateral to the pubic symphysis. Another common injury pattern is one in which the rectus abdominis detaches from the pubis along a line spanning the midline to involve both the left and right sides, creating the appearance of a platelike delamination. This pattern clearly reflects a bilateral lesion, and can be called a rectus abdominis/adductor aponeurotic plate disruption **(Option (B) is correct)**. The adductor tendon origins are symmetric without evidence for a traumatic strain **(Option (A) is incorrect)**. There

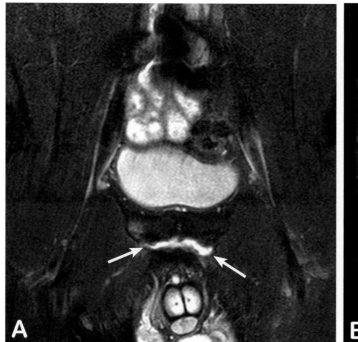
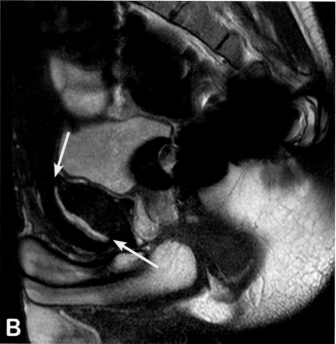

Figure 9-7 (same as Figure 9-6). Pubic symphysis. MRI. T2-weighted, fat-suppressed FSE. (A) Coronal oblique plane. (B) Sagittal plane. The images of the pubic symphysis region in this collegiate football player with chronic bilateral groin pain show confluent bilateral detachment of the caudal rectus abdominis tendons (arrows in both panels). This pattern with the rectus abdominis/adductor aponeurosis lifted from the pubic symphysis has been termed a rectus abdominis/adductor aponeurotic plate disruption, and requires a bilateral treatment plan.

are no MRI findings to suggest extrusion of visceral pelvis through the inguinal rings **(Option (C) is incorrect).** "Gilmore groin" is a term that has been used for unilateral painful lesions in the setting of athletic pubalgia, but MRI findings have not been clearly established **(Option (D) is incorrect).** With these patterns, the presence and morphology of an MRI secondary cleft can be very helpful. A *unilateral* secondary cleft generally indicates an ipsilateral rectus abdominis/adductor detachment or tear. A confluent, *bilateral* secondary cleft indicates a rectus abdominis/adductor aponeurotic plate disruption.

If surgical pelvic floor repair is a therapeutic option, distinguishing bilateral lesions from unilateral ones is exceedingly important, as a unilateral repair in the setting of a bilateral lesion may simply lead to contralateral symptoms.

In 2009, MRI plays a primary and integral role in the evaluation of active patients with groin pain. Several reproducible patterns of injury have been described at MRI in the setting of clinical athletic pubalgia, and a dedicated noncontrast athletic pubalgia protocol (Table 9-1) is advocated.

Table 9-1. Thomas Jefferson University Hospital 1.5 Tesla noncontrast athletic pubalgia MRI protocol								
Sequence	*Coil*	*FOV*	*TR/TE*	*Fat Sat*	*Matrix*	*Slice/Gap*	*NEX*	*ETL*
COR STIR	body	32	max/25	IR	172/256	4/1	2	8
COR T1	body	32	750/15	no	256/256	4/1	1.5	-
AX T2 FSE	body	32	2000/55	freq	172/256	4/1	2	8
COR oblique T2 FSE	5" disc	20	2000/50	freq	256/256	4/.5	2	8
COR oblique PD FSE	5" disc	20	2000/15	no	256/256	4/.5	3	4
SAG T2 FSE	5" disc	20	2000/50	freq	256/256	4/.5	2	8

Suggested Readings

1. Brennan D, O'Connell MJ, Ryan M, et al. Secondary cleft sign as a marker of injury in athletes with groin pain: MR image appearance and interpretation. Radiology. 2005;235:162–167.

2. Caudill P, Nyland J, Smith C, Yerasimides J, Lach J. Sports hernias: a systematic literature review. Br J Sports Med. 2008;42:954–964.

3. Cunningham PM, Brennan D, O'Connell M, MacMahon P, O'Neill P, Eustace S. Patterns of bone and soft-tissue injury at the symphysis pubis in soccer players: observations at MRI. AJR Am J Roentgenol. 2007;188:W291–296.

4. Meyers WC, Foley DP, Garrett WE, Lohnes JH, Mandlebaum BR. Management of severe lower abdominal or inguinal pain in high-performance athletes. PAIN (Performing Athletes with Abdominal or Inguinal Neuromuscular Pain Study Group). Am J Sports Med. 2000;28:2–8.

5. Meyers WC, Lanfranco A, Castellanos A. Surgical manage-ment of chronic lower abdominal and groin pain in high-performance athletes. Curr Sports Med Rep. 2002; 1:301–305.

6. Meyers WC, McKechnie A, Philippon MJ, Horner MA, Zoga AC, Devon ON. Experience with "sports hernia" spanning two decades. Ann Surg. 2008;248:656–665.

7. Omar IM, Zoga AC, Kavanagh EC, et al. Athletic pubalgia and "sports hernia": optimal MR imaging technique and findings. RadioGraphics. 2008;28:1415–1438.

8. Robinson P, Barron DA, Parsons W, Grainger AJ, Schilders EM, O'Connor PJ. Adductor-related groin pain in athletes: correlation of MR imaging with clinical findings. Skeletal Radiol. 2004;33:451–457.

9. Shortt CP, Zoga AC, Kavanagh EC, Meyers WC. Anatomy, pathology, and MRI findings in the sports hernia. Semin Musculoskelet Radiol. 2008;12:54–61.

10. Zoga AC, Kavanagh EC, Omar IM, et al. Athletic pubalgia and the "sports hernia": MR imaging findings. Radiology. 2008;247:797–807.

Case 10

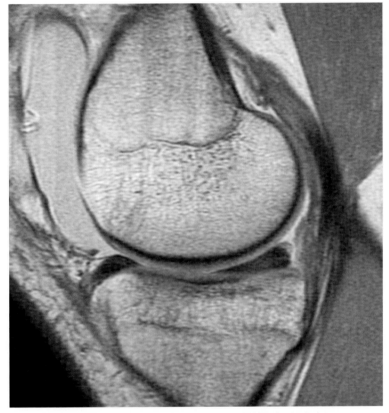

Figure 10-1. Knee. MRI. Fast spin-echo (FSE). Sagittal plane.

Question 46

You are shown a single sagittal fast spin-echo MR image (Figure 10-1) of the knee. The patient is a 33-year-old woman who presented status post trauma. Which *one* of the following is the MOST likely diagnosis?

(A)   Meniscocapsular injury/separation
(B)   Parameniscal cyst
(C)   Medial collateral ligament bursitis
(D)   Joint effusion with fluid in the joint recess
(E)   Meniscal flounce

Gerson E. Alvarez, M.D.

Meniscocapsular Injury

Question 46

Which *one* of the following is the MOST likely diagnosis?

    (A) Meniscocapsular injury/separation
    (B) Parameniscal cyst
    (C) Medial collateral ligament bursitis
    (D) Joint effusion with fluid in the joint recess
    (E) Meniscal flounce

A single image from a sagittal fast spin-echo MRI of the knee (Figure 10-2) shows abnormal fluid signal along the posterior margin of the posterior horn of the medial meniscus. The fluid is located at the menisco-capsular junction, abutting the entire posterior surface of the meniscus. The meniscus is otherwise intact. There is a large joint effusion, which contains a fluid-fluid level. This is one form of meniscocapsular separa-tion **(Option (A) is correct).**

Paramensical cysts result from fluid extrusion through a peripheral meniscal tear. The diagnosis is thus more likely if a peripheral cyst demonstrates con-tinuity with a horizontal or complex meniscal tear. A recent study demonstrated that in patients with menis-cal cysts, MRI evidence of direct communication of the cyst with a meniscal tear was present in 98% of

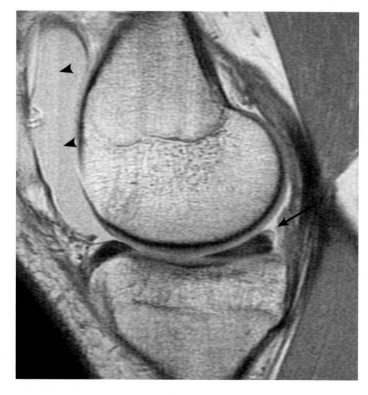

Figure 10-2 (same as Figure 10-1). Knee. MRI. Fast spin-echo (FSE). Sagittal plane. There is abnormal fluid signal along the poste-rior margin of the posterior horn. The fluid can be seen at the menis-cocapsular junction (arrow), abutting the entire posterior surface of the meniscus, which is otherwise intact. A large joint effusion contains a fluid-fluid level (arrowheads).

cases (Figure 10-3). Neither situation is seen in the test image **(Option (B) is incorrect).** On the medial side, parameniscal cysts are most commonly located adjacent to the posterior horn. On the lateral side, they are most commonly associated with the anterior horn and body of the meniscus and may become very large due to the relatively loose surrounding connective tissues compared to those of the medial side.

The medial collateral ligament (MCL) bursa is located in the middle third of the medial side of the knee, between the superficial MCL and the deep MCL. Fluid in the bursa tends to be well defined (Figure 10-4). This is not seen in the test image **(Option (C) is incorrect).** The posterior margin of the bursa is formed by the junction of the superficial and deep portions of the MCL. Thus, fluid in the MCL bursa should not extend to the posterior third of the medial knee. Proposed etiologies for MCL bursitis include osteoarthrosis, likely directly related to mechanical deformity of the capsule from large marginal osteophytes, and friction, which may result from activities such as horseback or motorcycle riding.

In the setting of a large joint effusion, fluid can accumulate in the posterior capsular recesses of the knee. When excess fluid is present, it may simulate fluid in the meniscocapsular junction. However, fluid in the joint recess should not completely extend between the meniscus and the joint capsule **(Option (D) is incorrect).**

Meniscal flounce refers to a wavy or S-shape of the meniscus (Figure 10-5). It was first described in ar-

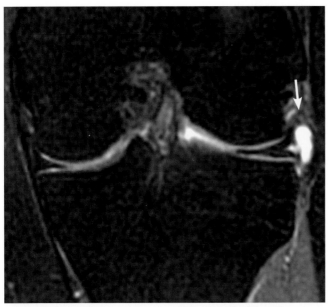

Figure 10-3. Parameniscal cyst. Knee. MRI. T2-weighted, fat-suppressed. Coronal plane. There is a horizontal tear of the body of the lateral meniscus extending to the far periphery. A rounded lesion, representing a parameniscal cyst (arrow), abuts the peripheral aspect of the tear.

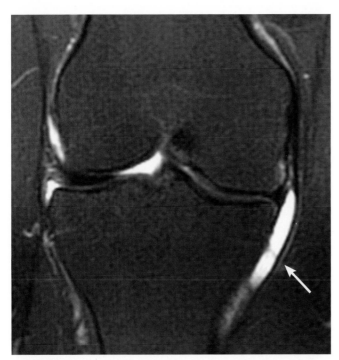

Figure 10-4. MCL bursitis. Knee. MRI. T2-weighted, fat-suppressed. Coronal plane. There is a well-defined fluid collection between the deep and superficial fibers of the MCL (arrow). A small septation is noted within. The medial meniscus is intact.

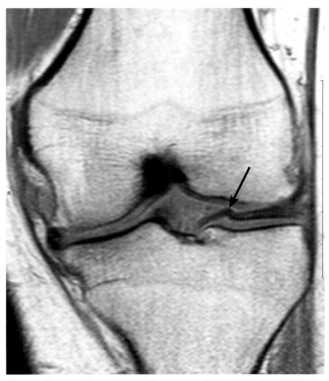

Figure 10-5. Meniscal flounce. Knee. MRI. Proton-density-weighted. Coronal plane. The image shows buckling of the anterior horn of the lateral meniscus in a wavy or S-shape (arrow).

throscopy, and it was thought to be positional, induced by external forces. It has been postulated that in the absence of external forces, as is the case on MR imaging, meniscal flounce may be caused by joint laxity, ligamentous injuries, a large joint effusion, or external rotation in the surface coil. In a recent study Park et al concluded that meniscal flounce is a transient physiologic distortion that can be changed by altering the anatomic knee position.

Question 47

Concerning meniscocapsular separation, which *one* of the following is true?

(A) It is most common on the lateral side.
(B) Prognosis is poor without surgical treatment.
(C) MRI is highly accurate in the diagnosis of meniscocapsular separation.
(D) Fluid between deep and superficial fibers of MCL is diagnostic.
(E) Irregularity of posterior meniscal margin on sagittal images is one sign of meniscocapsular separation on MRI.

Meniscocapsular separation (MCS) refers to detachment of the joint capsule from the periphery of the meniscus. MCS has a spectrum of appearances, with milder forms representing injuries to the meniscocapsular junction without frank disruption, and more severe forms representing complete separation. Clinically, the lesion may become significant if hypermobility of the meniscus results. Meniscocapsular separation most commonly involves the medial side **(Option (A) is false).** The meniscocapsular region is well vascularized given its close proximity to the perimeniscal capillary plexus. Therefore, healing is possible if close approximation is achieved, even without surgical intervention **(Option (B) is false).** There is a high association between medial meniscocapsular separation and anterior cruciate ligament (ACL) tears.

De Maeseneer et al examined artificially created MCS in eight cadaveric knee specimens with standard MRI, MR arthrogram, sonography, and arthroscopy. The study found that fluid or contrast interposed between the meniscus and the MCL, an irregular meniscal outline, and increased distance between the meniscus and the MCL correlated with meniscocapsular separation.

Unfortunately, the accuracy of MRI in the diagnosis of meniscocapsular separation has been shown to be poor **(Option (C) is false).** A retrospective study that correlated the MRIs of 52 patients with arthroscopic

results showed a positive predictive value of 9% on the medial side and 13% on the lateral side. None of the specific signs described in the literature were found to be reliable in the diagnosis of meniscocapsular separation **(Option (D) is false).** A large prospective clinical study is needed.

MR criteria described in the literature include perimeniscal fluid (Figure 10-6), meniscal displacement relative to the tibia, irregular meniscal margins (Figure 10-7) **(Option (E) is true),** meniscal corner tears (Fig-

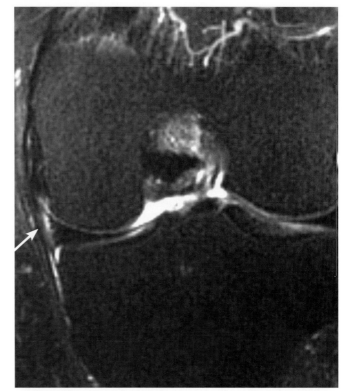

Figure 10-6. Meniscocapsular separation. Knee. MRI. T2-weighted, fat-suppressed. There is a band of fluid signal along the periphery of the body of the meniscus (arrow).

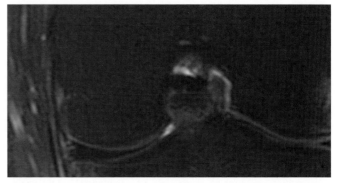

Figure 10-7. Meniscocapsular separation. Knee. MRI. Coronal fat-suppressed T2-weighted image demonstrates irregularity along the periphery of the body of the medial meniscus. This has been described in patients with meniscocapsular separation.

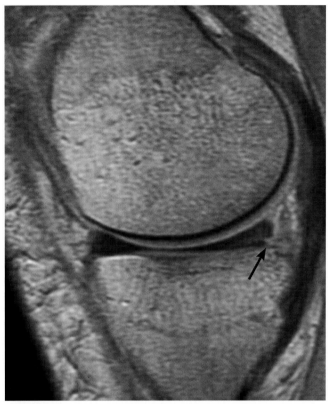

Figure 10-8. Corner tear. Medial meniscus. Knee. MRI. Proton-density-weighted. Sagittal plane. The image demonstrates a corner tear involving the posterior horn of the medial meniscus. This has been described in patients with meniscocapsular separation (arrow).

ure 10-8), and tears of the meniscofemoral or meniscotibial arms of the deep MCL.

Question 48

Concerning the anatomy of the meniscus:

 (A) The lateral meniscus is larger than the medial meniscus.
 (B) The circumferential fibers resist hoop stress and are concentrated in the inner third.
 (C) The medial meniscus is relatively mobile compared to the lateral meniscus.
 (D) The peripheral two thirds of the menisci are supplied by the perimeniscal capillary plexus.
 (E) Functions of the menisci include distribution of synovial fluid.

The menisci are C-shaped or semilunar fibrocartilaginous structures located in the knee joint. On cross section, the menisci are triangular in shape, widest at the periphery with the apex pointing towards the center of each compartment. The superior articular surface is concave to accommodate the convex femoral condyle,

whereas the inferior articular surface is flat and rests on the articular surface of the tibia. The peripheral surface is for the most part continuous with the joint capsule.

Each meniscus is divided in thirds: the anterior horn, the body, and the posterior horn. On the medial side the posterior horn is two to three times larger in anteroposterior dimension than the anterior horn. On the lateral side, the posterior and anterior horns are roughly equal in size. The medial meniscus is larger than the lateral meniscus **(Option (A) is false)**; however, the medial meniscus covers 50% of the tibial surface compared to 70% on the lateral side.

The menisci are primarily composed of collagen, particularly type I fibers. On electron microscopy three distinct layers can be visualized. A superficial layer of randomly oriented meshlike fibers is seen along the superior and inferior articular surfaces. Deep to it, a thin layer of radially oriented fibers is present. The third and thickest layer is located in the mid-substance and consists primarily of circumferential collagen bundles, parallel to the long axis of the meniscus. These fibers are concentrated in the peripheral third of the meniscus **(Option (B) is false).** Their orientation provides tensile strength, allowing the meniscus to resist hoop or compressive forces. Interspersed between the longitudinal fibers are radially oriented fibers, which extend from the periphery to the apex and serve as tie fibers to resist longitudinal splitting.

The menisci are attached to the tibial surface anteriorly and posteriorly at the roots. These are relatively consistent in location, and well demonstrated on MRI. The anterior root of the medial meniscus has the greatest footprint surface area, located just anterior to the tibial attachment of the anterior cruciate ligament. The posterior horn is attached to the tibia just posterior to the insertion of the posterior cruciate ligament. A radial tear through the posterior root is a common injury and easily missed if attention is not given to the coronal images. The lateral meniscus has a tighter C-shape. Therefore, the anterior and posterior roots are closer to each other. The anterior root is located lateral to the ACL insertion and the posterior horn is attached between the tibial intercondylar eminence and the posterior medial meniscus. The meniscal roots are very strong structures, and along with the peripheral circumferential collagen fibers, they help resist compressive forces.

The medial meniscus is firmly attached to the joint capsule peripherally. The attachment is especially strong at the level of the medial collateral ligament, where distinct meniscofemoral and meniscotibial ligaments are present as part of the deep capsular ligament or deep MCL. The lateral meniscus is less firmly attached to the capsule **(Option (C) is false)**, especially posterolaterally, where the popliteus tendon courses through the hiatus.

At birth, the menisci are well vascularized. This changes as the body ages, and at 10 years of age only the peripheral 5% to 30% of the meniscus is vascularized. This distribution is largely unchanged in the adult meniscus **(Option (D) is false)**. Vascular supply predominantly originates from the superior and inferior branches of the medial and lateral genicular arteries, which form the perimeniscal capillary plexus. This is of paramount importance from a surgical standpoint, as nonvascularized tissue will not heal even after surgical intervention. Tears involving the central two thirds of the menisci are thus treated with partial meniscectomy.

Although the menisci were once thought to represent remnants of intraarticular leg muscles, their importance is well established. Functions of the menisci include increasing congruity and contact area, stabilization, load sharing, shock absorption, and contribution to joint lubrication. It has been shown that the menisci transmit at least 50% of axial load in extension and up to 85% in knee flexion. Absence of menisci greatly increases the load per unit area and results in damage and degeneration of the articular cartilage. In addition, the viscoelastic properties of the menisci help attenuate the loading of the knee during walking. Studies have shown that meniscectomy reduces the shock absorption capacity of a normal knee by 20%. The importance of the menisci as stabilizers has been studied. For one, the menisci increase the congruence of the knee joint, deepening the articular surfaces and stabilizing the joint. Moreover, in the ACL-deficient knee, the posterior horn of the medial meniscus serves as a restraint to anterior tibial translation, and its absence results in up to 58% increase in tibial translation at 90 degrees flexion.

It has been suggested that the menisci are proprioceptive structures, providing a feedback mechanism for joint position sense. This has been inferred from the observation of type-I and type-II nerve endings in the anterior and posterior horns of the menisci. The improved congruity also helps to distribute the fluid that is expressed from the articular cartilage, thereby facilitating joint lubrication and nutrition **(Option (E) is true)**.

Question 49

Concerning meniscal tears:

(A) The lateral meniscus is most frequently involved.
(B) Grade II signal is linear and extends to the articular surface.
(C) MRI sensitivity is higher for lateral meniscal tears.
(D) Medial meniscal tears are more common in the setting of an acute ACL tear.
(E) The incidence of meniscal tears in asymptomatic patients with radiographic evidence of OA has been found to be as high as 60%.

Meniscal tears may be degenerative or traumatic. Degenerative tears result from normal forces on a degenerated meniscus. Traumatic tears result from excessive force on a normal meniscus. Tears are more common in the medial meniscus **(Option (A) is false)**, in part due to its less mobile nature. Tears of the lateral meniscus are more common in younger patients and are usually traumatic in etiology.

There are three basic types of meniscal tears. A horizontal cleavage tear divides the meniscus in superior and inferior segments (Figure 10-9). When these segments are displaced, a flap tear results. Horizontal tears are not amenable to repair and can be treated with partial meniscectomy. A vertical longitudinal tear occurs along the circumferential collagen bundles and divides the meniscus in central and peripheral segments (Figure 10-10). The tear remains equidistant from the edge

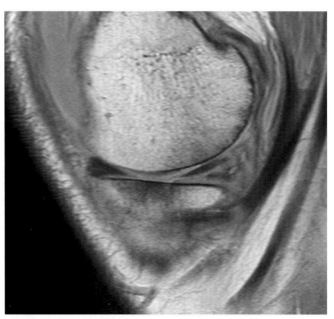

Figure 10-9. Horizontal tear. Knee. MRI. Proton-density-weighted. Sagittal plane through the medial compartment in a patient with osteoarthrosis. The horizontal tear is seen as linear signal in the posterior horn of the medial meniscus, which extends to the inferior articular surface and divides the meniscus in inferior and superior segments.

of the meniscus along its course. Vertical longitudinal tears occur in the vascularized portion of the meniscus and are thus amenable to surgical repair. It is important

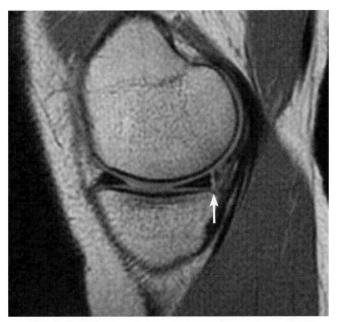

Figure 10-10. Longitudinal vertical tear. Knee. MRI. Proton-density-weighted. Sagittal plane through the medial meniscus. Linear signal can be seen in the peripheral third of the posterior horn. The tear is vertical in orientation, dividing the meniscus in central and peripheral segments (arrow).

to note the longitudinal length of the tear as long tears may displace, resulting in bucket handle tears. The third basic type of meniscal tear is the radial tear (Figure 10-11). It is perpendicular to the long axis of the meniscus, dissecting the circumferential collagen bundles. It may be incomplete, involving only the inner margin of the meniscus, or complete. Clinically, a patient with a complete radial tear behaves similar to a patient status post complete meniscectomy. The ability of the meniscus to resist hoop stresses is compromised. Oblique tears display a radial component along the inner margin of the meniscus and a vertical longitudinal component (Figure 10-12). When viewed in consecutive images, the vertical component does not remain equidistant from the meniscal margin due to its oblique orientation. They have been referred to as parrot beak tears.

On MRI, the menisci are hypointense on T1- and T2-weighted images. Intrasubstance intermediate signal in not necessarily abnormal, however. In children, intrasubstance signal may relate to the increased vascularity of the meniscus. In middle age and in the elderly, intrasubstance intermediate signal is seen as part of aging. Lotysch et al developed a grading system based on the configuration and location of the intrameniscal signal. Grade I signal is defined as punctate or globular intrasubstance signal with no articular extension. It cor-

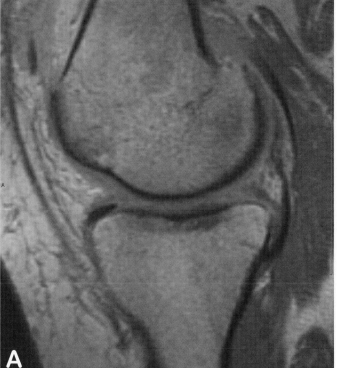

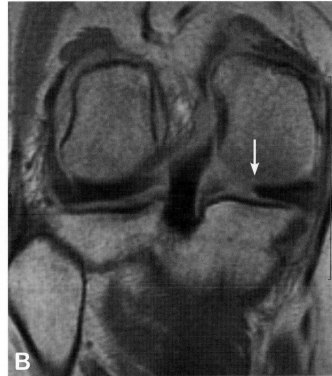

Figure 10-11. Radial tear. Knee. MRI. (A) Proton-density-weighted. Sagittal plane through the medial compartment of the knee, near the meniscal root. The posterior horn of the meniscus is not visualized. This has been described as the "ghost meniscus." (B) Proton-density-weighted. Coronal plane through the posterior horn. The image demonstrates abrupt blunting of the meniscus near the root (arrow).

responds to foci of mucinous degeneration. Grade II signal is also intrameniscal but linear in nature **(Option (B) is false)**. It corresponds to degeneration that is located

in the central portion of the meniscus (layer 3) along the radially oriented collagen bundle. It should not extend to an articular surface. Grade III signal is defined as any

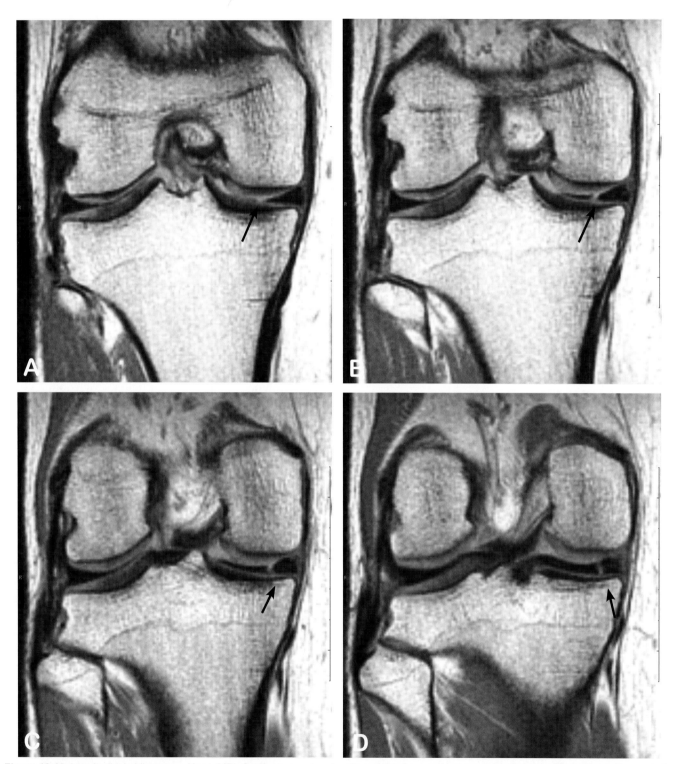

Figure 10-12. Longitudinal oblique tear. Knee. MRI. Contiguous proton-density-weighted coronal images extending from the bodies to the posterior horns of the menisci (A to D). (A) There is subtle blunting of the inner margin of the body of the medial meniscus (arrow). This represents the radial component of the oblique tear. (B) Coronal plane through the junction of the body and posterior horn. The tear now demonstrates a vertical orientation involving the inner third of the meniscus (arrow). (C) Coronal plane through the posterior horn. The longitudinal oblique tear is shown approaching the periphery of the meniscus as it moves posteriorly (arrow). (D) The tear further approaches the periphery of the meniscus, now involving the outer third (arrow). This is a typical feature of longitudinal oblique tears.

intrameniscal signal that extends to an articular surface. Histologically, discrete cleavage planes are present.

For the diagnosis of meniscal tear to be made, at least one of two criteria must be met: there must either be abnormal signal extending to the articular surface of the meniscus or an abnormality in the shape of the meniscus.

De Smet et al first proposed the "two-slice touch rule" after the analysis of 200 patients showed a decrease in the accuracy of MR when Grade III signal was only identified in one cut. Specifically, the study found a low frequency (less than 9%) of tears in menisci without signal surface contact, a moderate frequency (56% medial and 30% lateral) in menisci with surface contact in one image, and a high frequency (greater than 90%) in menisci with surface contact in more than one image. A recent study by the same author confirmed the original findings, with an increase in positive predictive value from 91% to 94% for medial meniscal tears and from 83% to 96% for lateral meniscal tears, when utilizing the "two-slice touch rule." The author suggests that the diagnosis of a meniscal tear should only be made with certainty when abnormal signal extends to the articular surface in two cuts, which need not be consecutive or in the same plane. When articular contact is only seen on one slice, the examination should be interpreted as a possible tear.

Magnetic resonance is highly accurate in the evaluation of meniscal tears, its sensitivity ranging from 80% to 100%. It has been well established that the sensitivity of MRI is higher for the medial meniscus, compared to the lateral meniscus **(Option (C) is false).** Possible reasons for the discrepancy include the more complex anatomy of the posterior horn of the lateral meniscus, arterial pulsation artifact, magic angle artifact and obliquity of the posterior horn near the root.

In patients with an acute ACL injury, lateral meniscal tears are more frequent **(Option (D) is false).** Most of these tears are longitudinal vertical tears involving the posterior horn. A particular type of lateral meniscal tear has been described in patients with an acute ACL tear. It relates to the attachment of the meniscofemoral ligaments to the posterior horn of the lateral meniscus. As a result of anterior tibial translation, the meniscofemoral ligament may partially avulse the posterior horn of the lateral meniscus, resulting in a longitudinal tear known as the Wrisberg Rip (Figure 10-13). A recent study suggested that the diagnosis should be considered whenever a far lateral meniscofemoral insertion is seen on sagittal images (4 or more cuts lateral to the PCL on 3mm images).

In patients with chronic ACL deficient knees, medial meniscal tears are more common. This is explained by the role of the posterior horn of the medial meniscus as a stabilizer in the absence of a normal ACL, leading to increasing shear forces.

Meniscal tears are very common in patients with osteoarthrosis. Englund et al studied the menisci in the right knee on MRI scans obtained from 991 random subjects, 50 to 90 years of age. Among persons with radiographic evidence of osteoarthritis, the prevalence of a meniscal tear was 63% among those with knee pain, aching, or stiffness on most days and 60% among those without these symptoms **(Option (E) is true).**

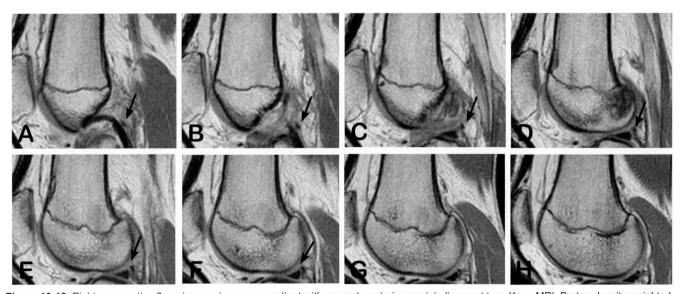

Figure 10-13. Eight consecutive 3mm images in a young patient with an acute anterior cruciate ligament tear. Knee MRI. Proton-density-weighted. Sagittal plane. There is apparent far lateral insertion of the meniscofemoral ligament of Wrisberg, 8 images lateral to the posterior cruciate ligament. This is consistent with a longitudinal tear, also known as the Wrisberg Rip (arrows).

Suggested Readings

1. Campbell SE, Sanders TG, Morrison WB. MR imaging of meniscal cysts: Incidence, location, and clinical significance. AJR Am J Roentgenol. 2001;177:409–413.

2. Catherine L. McCarthy, Eugene G. McNally. The MRI appearance of cystic lesions around the knee. Skeletal Radiol. 2004;33:187–209.

3. Chew FS. Medial meniscal flounce: demonstration on MR imaging of the knee. AJR Am J Roentgenol. 1990;155:199.

4. DeHaven KE. Meniscus repair. The American Journal of Sports Medicine,Vol. 27, No. 2.

5. Dehaven KE, Arnoczky SP. Repair part I: Basic science. Indictions for repair and open repair. J Bone Joint Surg Am. 1994;76:140–152.

6. De Maeseneer M, Lenchik L, Starok M, Pedowitz R, Trudell D, Resnick D. Normal and abnormal medial meniscocapsular structures: MR imaging and sonography in cadavers. AJR Am J Roentgenol. 1998;171:969–976.

7. De Maeseneer M, Shahabpour M, Vanderdood K, Van Roy F, Osteaux M. Medial meniscocapsular separation: MR imaging criteria and diagnostic pitfalls. European Journal of Radiology. 2002;41:242–252.

8. De Maeseneer M, Shahabpour M, Van Roy P, et al. MR imaging of the medial collateral ligament bursa: findings in patients and anatomic data derived from cadavers. AJR Am J Roentgenol. 2001;177:911–917.

9. De Maeseneer M, Van Roy P, Shahabpour M, Gosselin R, De Ridder F, Osteaux M. Normal anatomy and pathology of the posterior capsular area of the knee: Findings in cadaveric specimens and in patients. AJR Am J Roentgenol. 2004;4:182.

10. De Smet AA, Norris MA, Yandow DR, Quintana FA, Graf BK, Keene JS. Diagnosis of meniscal tears of the knee: Importance of high signal in the meniscus that extends to the surface. AJR Am J Roentgenol. 1993;161:101–107.

11. De Smet AA, Tuite MJ. Use of the "two-slice-touch" rule for the MRI diagnosis of meniscal tears. AJR Am J Roentgenol. 2006;187:911–914.

12. Deutsch AL, Mink JH, Fox JM, et al. Peripheral meniscal tears: MR findings after conservative treatment or arthroscopic repair. Radiology. 1990;176:485–488.

13. Fox MG. Imaging of the meniscus: Review, current trends, and clinical implications. Radiol Clin N Am. 2007;45:1033–1053.

14. Greis PE, Bardana DD, Holmstrom MC, Burks RT. Meniscal injury: I. Basic science and evaluation. J Am Acad Orthop Surg. 2002;10:168–176.

15. Grossman JW, De Smet AA, Shinki K. Comparison of the accuracy rates of 3-T and 1.5-T MRI of the knee in the diagnosis of meniscal tear. AJR Am J Roentgenol. 2009;193:509–514.

16. Lotysch M, Mink J, Crues JV, Schwartz SA. Magnetic resonance imaging in the detection of meniscal injuries. Magn Reson Imaging. 1986;4:185.

17. McDermott ID, and Amis AA. The consequences of meniscectomy. J Bone Joint Surg Br. 2006;88-B:1549–1556.

18. Oei EHG, Nikken JJ, Verstijnen ACM, Ginai AZ, Myriam Hunink, MG. MR imaging of the menisci and cruciate ligaments: A systematic review. Radiology. 2003;226:837–848.

19. Park JS, Ryu KN, and Yoon KH. Meniscal flounce on knee MRI: Correlation with meniscal locations after positional changes. AJR Am J Roentgenol. 2006;187:364–370.

20. Rath E, Richmond JC. The menisci: basic science and advances in treatment. Br J Sports Med. 2000;34:252–257.

21. Rubin DA, Britton CA, Towers JD, Harner CD. Are MR signs of meniscocapsular separation valid? Radiology. 1996;201:829–836.

22. Stoller DW et al. Magnetic Resonance Imaging in Orthopaedics and Sports Medicine. vol 1. 2nd ed. Philadelphia PA: J.B. Lippincott; 1997: 203–442.

23. Stoller DW, Martin C, Crues III JV, et al: Meniscal tears: Pathologic correlation with MR imaging. Radiology. 1987;163:731.

24. Tschirch FTC, Schmid MR, Pfirrmann CWA, Romero J, Hodler J, and Zanetti M. Prevalence and size of meniscal cysts, ganglionic cysts, synovial cysts of the popliteal space, fluid-filled bursae, and other fluid collections in asymptomatic knees on MR imaging. AJR Am J Roentgenol. 2003;180:1431–1436.

25. Tyson LL, Daughters TC Jr, Ryu RKN, Crues JV III. MRI appearance of meniscal cysts. Skeletal Radiol. 1995;24:421–424.

26. Yu JS, Cosgarea AJ, Kaeding CC, Wilson D. Meniscal flounce MR imaging. Radiology. 1997;203:513–515.

Case 11

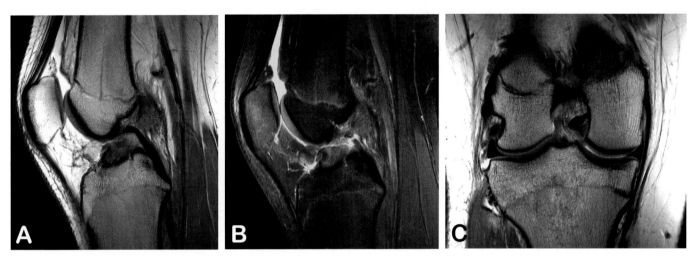

Figure 11-1. Knee. MRI. (A) Intermediate-weighted. Sagittal plane. (B) Fluid-sensitive. Sagittal plane. (C) Intermediate-weighted. Coronal plane.

Question 50

A 19-year-old woman presents with knee pain. You are shown (A) sagittal intermediate-weighted, (B) sagittal fluid-sensitive, and (C) coronal intermediate-weighted MR images of her knee (Figure 11-1). Which *one* of the following is the MOST likely diagnosis?

(A)   Normal anterior cruciate ligament
(B)   Partial-thickness tear of anterior cruciate ligament
(C)   Full-thickness tear of anterior cruciate ligament
(D)   Mucoid degeneration of anterior cruciate ligament
(E)   Cyclops lesion (localized arthrofibrosis)

Jon A. Jacobson, M.D.

Full-Thickness Tear of the Anterior Cruciate Ligament

Question 50

Which *one* of the following is the MOST likely diagnosis?

(A) Normal anterior cruciate ligament
(B) Partial-thickness tear of anterior cruciate ligament
(C) Full-thickness tear of anterior cruciate ligament
(D) Mucoid degeneration of anterior cruciate ligament
(E) Cyclops lesion (localized arthrofibrosis)

Figure 11-2 shows abnormal increased signal and no intact ligament fibers between the femur and tibia in the expected location of the anterior cruciate ligament (ACL), findings consistent with full-thickness ACL tear **(Option (C) is correct)**. In addition to nonvisualization of the ACL, another finding that may be seen with ACL tear is abnormal horizontal orientation of the distal aspect of a torn ACL in the sagittal plane (Figure 11-3). ACL tears can be diagnosed with MR imaging with accuracies over 95%. Most tears involve the middle as-

pect of the ACL (90%), followed by femoral (7%) and tibial (3%) attachments.

ACL tears represent the most common of knee ligament injuries. There are several mechanisms of injury that can produce an ACL tear. The most common mechanism of injury is that of internal rotation of the tibia relative to the femur, or external rotation of the femur relative to the tibia. This usually occurs with the knee near full extension, often during deceleration, and often is associated with valgus stress. This pivot shift mechanism of injury results in anterior translation of the lateral aspect of the tibia relative to the femur and valgus angulation. Other possible mechanisms of injury include hyperextension of the knee, as well as varus angulation with external rotation of the tibia. Most ACL tears occur as a noncontact injury, often during sporting or recreational activities such as skiing, football, or soccer. ACL tears are three times more common among

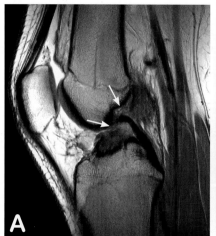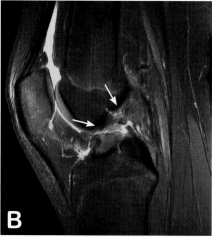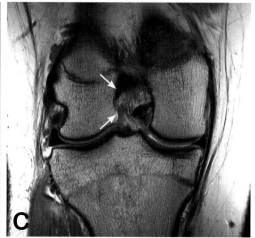

Figure 11- 2 (Same as Figure 11- 1). Full-thickness tear of ACL. Knee. MRI.(A) Intermediate-weighted. Sagittal plane. (B) Fluid-sensitive. Sagittal plane. (C) Intermediate-weighted. Coronal plane. All three images show abnormal signal and discontinuity of the ACL (arrows) consistent with full-thickness tear.

females than among males. The physical examination findings that are present with ACL tear include abnormal anterior tibial translation relative to the femur (Lachman and anterior drawer tests).

MR imaging can be used to assess ACL integrity, although it is most important for evaluation of other associated knee injuries. ACL tears are associated with meniscal tears, some of which are unique. One such tear is a peripheral longitudinal tear of the posterior horn of the lateral meniscus (Figure 11-4). On MR imaging, it is

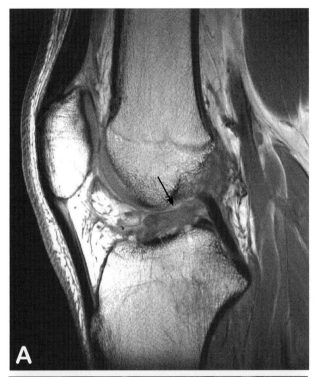

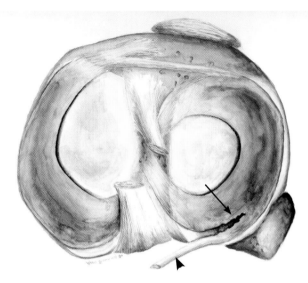

Figure 11- 4. Tear of the posterior horn of the lateral meniscus. An axial illustration at the level of the menisci shows peripheral vertical longitudinal tear (arrow) of the posterior horn of the lateral meniscus at the attachment of the meniscofemoral ligament (arrowhead). *Illustration reproduced with kind permission of Springer Science and Business Media [#9].*

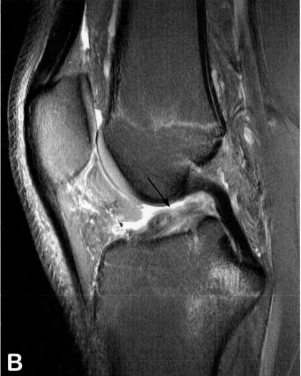

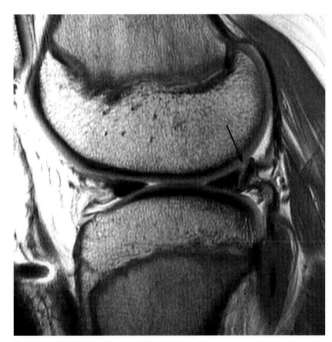

Figure 11-3. Full-thickness tear of the ACL. MRI. (A) Intermediate-weighted. (B) Fluid-sensitive. Sagittal plane. The MR images show discontinuity of the ACL with abnormal horizontal orientation of the distal aspect (arrow in each panel).

Figure 11-5. Tear of the posterior horn of the lateral meniscus. MRI. Intermediate-weighted. Sagittal plane. The image shows a longitudinal vertical tear of the posterior horn of the lateral meniscus (arrow).

important not to mistake this coronal meniscal tear for a variation in the attachment of the meniscofemoral ligament (Figure 11-5). The normal meniscofemoral ligaments should completely attach to the posterior horn of the lateral meniscus within 14 mm lateral to the margin of the posterior cruciate ligament (PCL); a persistent cleft beyond this measurement would indicate posterior horn lateral meniscus tear. Another type of meniscal tear associated with ACL tear is a peripheral tear of the posterior horn of the medial meniscus, often associated with meniscocapsular separation. Other types of meniscal tears are also possible. Tibial collateral ligament injury may also be seen, and the combination of ACL tear, tibial collateral ligament tear, and medial meniscal tear has been termed "O'Donoghue triad."

With MR imaging, the normal ACL will appear as continuous low signal fibers extending from the posterior aspect of the femur to the anterior aspect of the tibia (Figure 11-6) **(Option (A) is incorrect).** The ACL consists of a thin anteromedial band, which is taut in knee flexion, and a thicker posterolateral band, which is taut in knee extension. On T1-weighted and intermediate-weighted MR images, the ligament fibers may

be less defined compared to fluid-sensitive sequences. The thickness of the normal ligament should be fairly uniform, although the fibers somewhat broaden at the tibial attachment. The inferior aspect of the normal ACL may have increased intrasubstance signal at the

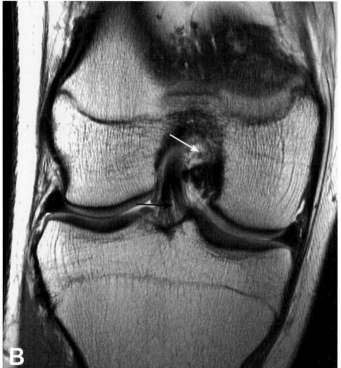

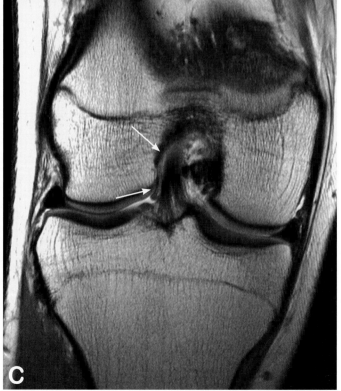

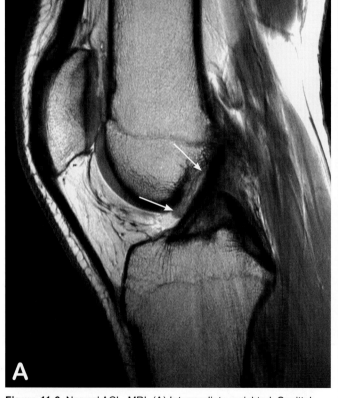

Figure 11-6. Normal ACL. MRI. (A) Intermediate-weighted. Sagittal plane. (B) Fluid-sensitive. Sagittal plane. (C) Intermediate-weighted. Coronal plane. All images show a normal intact ACL (arrows in all panels).

tibial insertion. On MR images in the sagittal plane, an angle formed by the ACL and the intercondylar line of Blumensaat (a line paralleling the intercondylar roof) is approximately 7.5 degrees.

The diagnosis of partial-thickness tear of the ACL can be difficult, as associated hemorrhage and edema may make the intact fibers indistinct; however, unlike a full-thickness ACL tear, some intact fibers should be identified connecting the femur to the tibia on both coronal and sagittal images **(Option (B) is incorrect).** Mucoid degeneration would not appear as complete ligament fiber loss **(Option (D) is incorrect).** Similarly, cyclops lesion would also not have the appearance of complete ligament fiber loss as demonstrated in Figures 11-1 and 11-2 **(Option (E) is incorrect).**

Question 51

This ancillary imaging finding supports the diagnosis of anterior cruciate ligament tear:

- (A) Lateral compartment bone marrow edema
- (B) Lateral femoral notch sign
- (C) Anterior tibial translation
- (D) Buckling of posterior cruciate ligament
- (E) Posterior tibial plateau avulsion fracture

There are a number of indirect or secondary MR imaging findings that support the diagnosis of ACL tear in addition to the primary findings related to the ACL tear itself. Such secondary signs are a reflection of the mechanism of injury that caused the ACL tear. Because the mechanism of internal tibial rotation and valgus is most common, the indirect signs associated with this mechanism are also common. One such finding is lateral compartment bone marrow edema, which characteristically involves the central aspect of the lateral femoral condyle and the posterior aspect of the lateral (and possibly medial) aspects of the tibial plateau (Figure 11-7) **(Option (A) is true).** The lateral femoral condyle bone marrow edema is located at the condylopatellar sulcus immediately adjacent to the anterior horn of the lateral meniscus when the knee is in extension. The bone marrow edema is subchondral in location, and may be associated with an adjacent cartilage abnormality and low signal subchondral fracture line. The location of these findings is related to anterior translation of the lateral aspect of the tibia relative to the femur and impaction between the posterior tibia and the lateral femur. If this force is great enough, there can be an impaction fracture that is visible on MR imaging and radiography, termed the "lateral femoral notch sign" **(Option (B) is true).** On a lateral radiograph of the knee (as well as

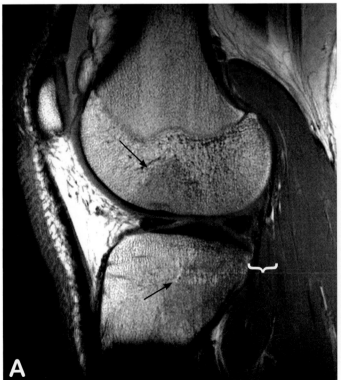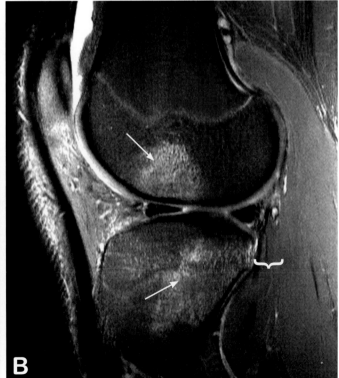

Figure 11-7. Indirect signs of ACL tear. MRI. Sagittal plane. (A) Intermediate-weighted. Note the anterior translation of the tibia relative to the femur (bracket). (B) Fluid-sensitive. Both images show bone marrow edema (arrows) of the lateral femoral condyle and tibial plateau.

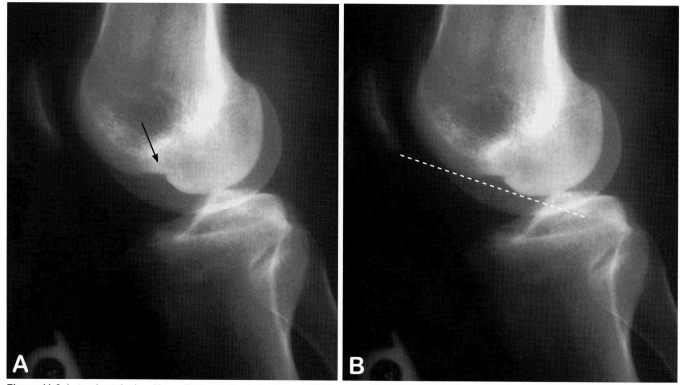

Figure 11-8. Lateral notch sign. Knee. Radiographs. Lateral view. (A) There is a deep condylopatellar sulcus (arrow). (B) The sulcus seen in panel A measures greater than 1.5 mm in depth relative to a line tangential to the lateral femoral condyle (dotted line).

sagittal MR images), if one draws a line tangential to the lateral femoral condyle, deepening of the normal condylopatellar sulcus or lateral notch greater than 1.5 mm is an indirect sign of ACL tear (Figure 11-8).

Another indirect sign of ACL tear related to internal tibial rotation and valgus stress is anterior tibial translation **(Option (C) is true).** Also called the anterior drawer sign, this finding is present on sagittal MR im-

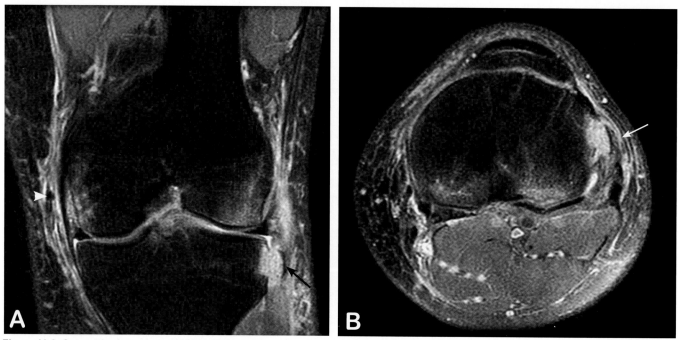

Figure 11-9. Segond fracture. Knee. (A) MRI. Fluid-sensitive. Coronal plane. Note the avulsion fracture fragment (arrow) and tibial collateral ligament injury (arrowhead). (B) MRI. Fluid-sensitive. Axial plane.

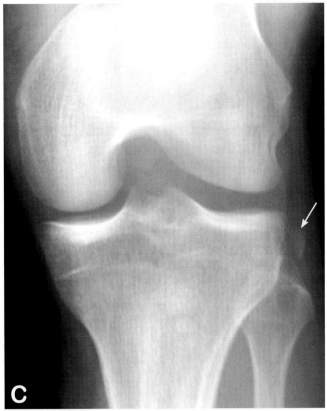

Figure 11-9 (continued). Segond fracture. Knee. (C) Radiograph. Anteroposterior view. An avulsion fracture can be seen at the lateral tibia (arrow).

ages centered over the lateral femoral condyle. At this location, if a line drawn superiorly from the posterior tibial cortex is greater than 5 mm anterior to the posterior aspect of the femur, then anterior tibial translation is present (Figure 11-7). The two indirect signs of lateral compartment bone marrow edema and anterior tibial translation have been shown to be of value in the diagnosis of ACL tear, with a reported sensitivity of 82% and specificity of 90%. Related to anterior translation of the tibia are other secondary findings, such as buckling of the PCL **(Option (D) is true)** and uncovering of the posterior horn of the lateral meniscus. The presence of posterior tibial avulsion fracture is described with injuries related to avulsion at the tibial attachment of the PCL **(Option (E) is false).**

Other indirect signs of ACL injury may also be present, also specific to mechanism of injury. For example, when an ACL tear is due to hyperextension, bone contusions may be seen involving the anterior aspects of the distal femur and proximal tibia due to direct impaction during the injury. If the mechanism of injury involves varus angulation and knee rotation, an avulsion fracture of the lateral margin of the tibia (Segond fracture) may be seen at the attachment of iliotibial tract and anterior oblique band fibers, associated with ACL tears in 75% to 100% of patients (Figure

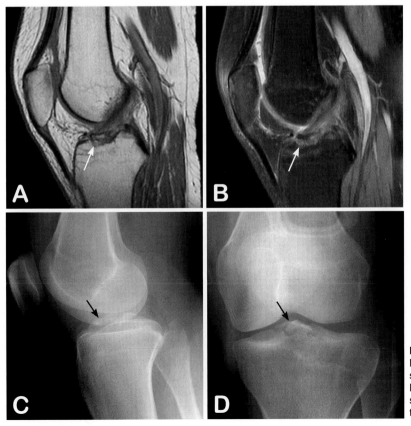

Figure 11-10. Anterior tibial eminence avulsion. Knee. (A) MRI. Intermediate-weighted. Sagittal plane. (B) MRI. Fluid-sensitive. Sagittal plane. (C) Radiograph. Lateral view. (D) Radiograph. Anteroposterior view. On all 4 images, an avulsion fracture (arrow) can be seen at the tibial attachment of the ACL.

11-9). Anterior tibial eminence avulsion at the tibial attachment of the ACL is most commonly seen in children (Figure 11-10), and may be difficult to identify on a lateral radiograph.

Question 52

Concerning mucoid degeneration of the anterior cruciate ligament:

(A) It can be misinterpreted as ligament tear.
(B) It is also called "celery stalk" anterior cruciate ligament.
(C) It is associated with adjacent ganglion cysts.
(D) It is associated with anterior cruciate ligament laxity.
(E) It may be overlooked at arthroscopy.

Another pathologic condition of the ACL is mucoid degeneration. On MR imaging, this condition is characterized by intermediate to fluid signal abnormality extending through the ACL in between intact ACL fibers (Figure 11-11). On T1 and intermediate-weighted MR images, the indistinctness of the ligament fibers may simulate ACL tear **(Option (A) is true).** However, on fluid-sensitive sequences, intact ACL fibers are seen

connecting the femur and tibia, excluding ligament tear. In addition, the fluid signal appearance extending between the intact ACL fibers creates what has been called a "celery stalk" appearance **(Option (B) is true).** It has been shown that mucoid degeneration is associated with intraligamentous ganglia, as well as adjacent ganglion cysts in the femur, tibia (Figure 11-11), and soft tissues (Figure 11-12) **(Option (C) is true).** Clinically, patients with mucoid degeneration of the ACL

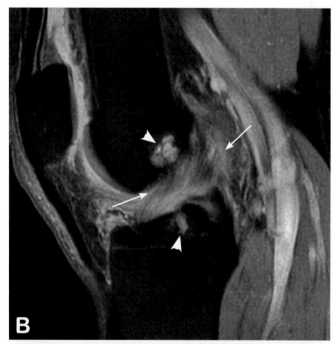

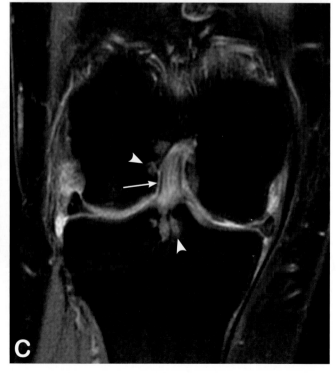

Figure 11-11. Mucoid degeneration of ACL. Knee. MRI. (A) Intermediate-weighted. Sagittal plane. (B) Fluid-sensitive. Sagittal plane. (C) Intermediate-weighted. Coronal plane. All images show intermediate signal throughout the ACL (arrows) with adjacent intact ligament fibers. Note adjacent intraosseous ganglia (arrowheads in all panels).

usually do not have ACL ligament laxity, which can be helpful information when interpreting MR images **(Option (D) is false).** In addition, the ancillary or indirect signs of ACL tear (such as lateral compartment bone marrow edema, anterior tibial translation, etc.) are absent with isolated mucoid degeneration of the ACL, which further helps to exclude the possibility of ACL tear. At knee arthroscopy using a standard anterior portal, mucoid degeneration of the ACL may be

overlooked unless the ACL is probed, often requiring a posterior portal approach **(Option (E) is true).**

Question 53

Concerning cyclops lesion (or localized anterior arthrofibrosis):

    (A) It is a complication after anterior cruciate ligament repair.
    (B) It is asymptomatic.
    (C) It characteristically is seen anterior in the intercondylar notch.
    (D) It is usually uniformly low signal on MRI.
    (E) Synovial sarcoma should be strongly considered in the differential diagnosis.

The cyclops lesion represents localized anterior arthrofibrosis as a potential complication after ACL tear and surgical reconstruction **(Option (A) is true).** The term was given as it appears as a round mass-like structure extending anteriorly from the ACL repair site at arthroscopy using an anterior portal, which resembles an eye. Symptomatic cyclops lesions have been reported in up to 2% of patients after ACL reconstruction. Histologically, a cyclops lesion represents fibrous granulation tissue at the anterior aspect of the ACL graft, originating from the residual ACL stump, adjacent fat pad metaplasia, intercondylar fibrosis, or possibly the ACL graft. Its location anteriorly can cause symptoms, such as limita-

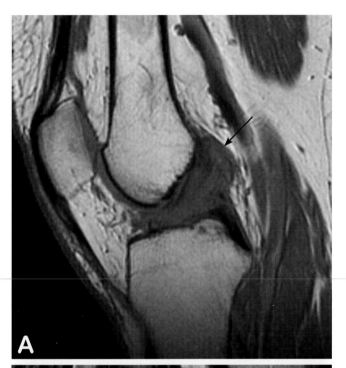

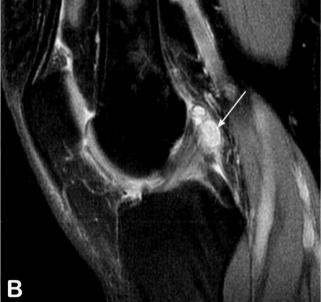

Figure 11-12. Mucoid degeneration of the ACL. Knee. MRI. Sagittal plane.(A) Intermediate-weighted. (B) Fluid-sensitive. Both images show intermediate signal throughout the ACL, representing mucoid degeneration, with associated posterior ganglion cysts (arrow in each panel).

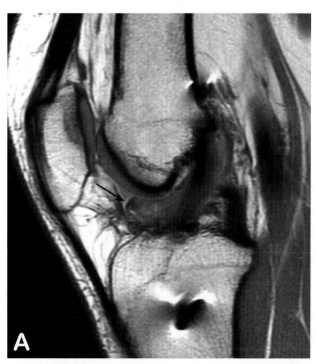

Figure 11-13. Cyclops lesion (localized arthrofibrosis). Knee. MRI. (A) Intermediate-weighted. Sagittal plane.

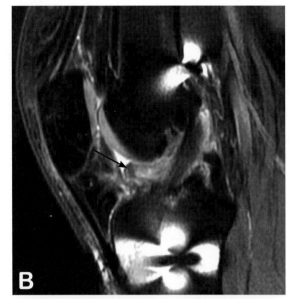

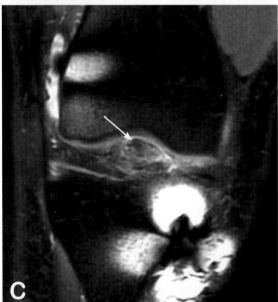

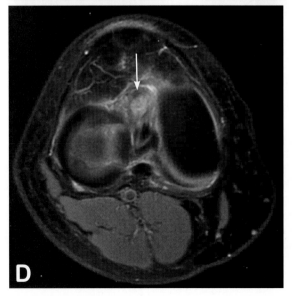

tion of knee extension **(Option (B) is false).** On MR imaging, a cyclops lesion appears as a heterogeneous round mass-like area extending anteriorly from the intercondylar notch, often best appreciated on axial images (Figure 11-13) **(Option (C) is true).** The diagnosis of a cyclops lesion may be difficult, as the signal intensity is not uniformly low but rather is heterogeneous and often similar in intensity to or slightly brighter than hyaline cartilage **(Option (D) is false).** In evaluation after ACL reconstruction, MR imaging is effective in the diagnosis of full-thickness ACL graft tear, but less effective with partial-thickness tears. Small amounts of increased signal within an intact ACL graft can be seen and is of little clinical significance. Full-thickness tear is diagnosed when the ACL graft is discontinuous, best appreciated in the coronal and sagittal planes. The differential diagnosis for a cyclops lesion is essentially other forms of synovitis, such as focal nodular synovitis or a form of pigmented villonodular synovitis. Synovial sarcoma should not realistically be considered in the differential diagnosis **(Option (E) is false).** Synovial sarcoma most commonly originates near but outside of a joint and despite its name does not arise from synovium. Synovial sarcoma is extremely rare in an intraarticular location, where it would appear more aggressive than the findings shown in Figure 11-13. Association with ACL reconstruction graft further supports the diagnosis of localized anterior arthrofibrosis. A cyclops lesion may also rarely occur in the setting of a native ACL tear, where the proximal stump of a native ACL tear may displace anteriorly with fibrosis causing entrapment (Figure 11-14).

Figure 11-13 (continued). Cyclops lesion (localized arthrofibrosis). Knee. MRI. (B) Fluid-sensitive. Sagittal plane. (C) Intermediate-weighted. Coronal plane. (D) Fluid-sensitive. Axial plane. The images show cyclops lesion (arrow in each image), which is heterogeneous, shows intermediate signal intensity, and is located anterior to the intercondylar notch. Note the adjacent intact ACL reconstruction graft.

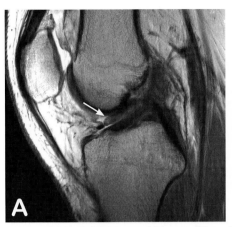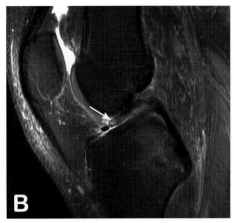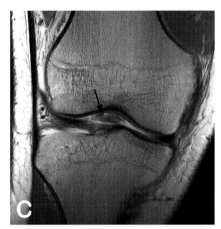

Figure 11-14. Full-thickness ACL tear with cyclops lesion. Knee. MRI. (A) Intermediate-weighted. Sagittal plane. (B) Fluid-sensitive. Sagittal plane. (C) Intermediate-weighted. Coronal plane. The images all show an entrapped stump of the torn ACL (arrow in each panel) anterior to the intercondylar notch.

Suggested Readings

1. Bergin D, Morrison WB, Carrino JA, Nallamshetty SN, Bartolozzi AR. Anterior cruciate ligament ganglia and mucoid degeneration: coexistence and clinical correlation. AJR Am J Roentgenol. 2004;182:1283–1287.

2. Bradley DM, Bergman AG, Dillingham MF. MR imaging of cyclops lesion. AJR Am J Roentgenol. 2000;174:719–726.

3. Brandser EA, Riley MA, Berbaum KS, El-Khoury GY, Bennett DL. MR imaging of anterior cruciate ligament injury: independent value of primary and secondary signs. AJR Am J Roentgenol. 1996;167:121–126.

4. Campos JC, Chung CB, Lektrakul N, Pedowitz R, et al. Pathogenesis of the Segond fracture: anatomic and MR imaging evidence of an iliotibial tract or anterior oblique band avulsion. Radiology. 2001;219:381–386.

5. Horton LK, Jacobson JA, Lin J, Hayes CW. MR imaging of anterior cruciate ligament reconstruction graft. AJR Am J Roentgenol. 2000;175:1091–1097.

6. Huang GS, Lee CH, Chan WP, Lee HS, Chen CY, Yu JS. Acute anterior cruciate ligament stump entrapment in anterior cruciate ligament tears: MR imaging appearance. Radiology. 2002;225:537–540.

7. McIntyre J, Moelleken S, Tirman P. Mucoid degeneration of anterior cruciate ligament mistaken for ligamentous tears. Skeletal Radiol. 2001;30:312–315.

8. Murphey MD, Gibson MS, Jennings BT, et al. From the archives of the AFIP: imaging of synovial sarcoma with radiologic-pathologic correlation. RadioGraphics. 2006;26:1543–1565.

9. Park LS, Jacobson JA, Jamadar DA, Caoili E, Kalume-Brigido M, Wojtys E. Posterior horn lateral meniscal tears simulating meniscofemoral ligament attachment in the setting of ACL tear: MRI findings. Skeletal Radiol. 2997;36:399–403.

10. Remer EM, Fitzgerald SW, Friedman H, Rogers LF, Hendrix RW, Schafer MF. Anterior cruciate ligament injury: MR imaging diagnosis and patterns of injury. RadioGraphics. 1992;12:901–915.

11. Saupe N, White LM, Chiavaras MM, et al. Anterior cruciate ligament reconstruction grafts: MR imaging features at long-term follow-up—correlation with functional and clinical evaluation. Radiology. 2008;249:581–590.

12. Umans H, Wimpfheimer O, Haramati N, Applbaum YH, Adler M, Bosco J. Diagnosis of partial tears of the anterior cruciate ligament of the knee: value of MR imaging. AJR Am J Roentgenol. 1995;165:893–897.

Case 12

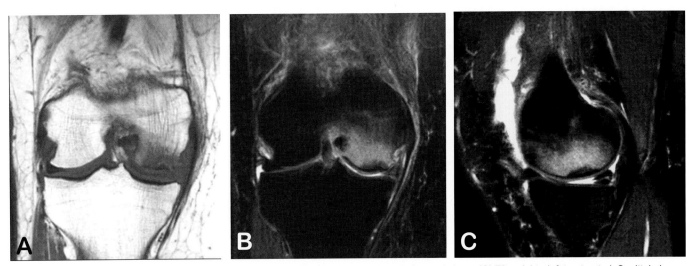

Figure 12-1. Knee. MR. (A) T1-weighted. Coronal plane. (B) T2-weighted, fat-saturated. Coronal plane. (C) T2-weighted, fat-saturated. Sagittal plane.

Question 54

You are shown coronal T1-weighted, coronal T2-weighted, fat-saturated (FS), and sagittal T2-weighted, fat-saturated MR images of the knee of a 53-year-old woman. With which *one* of the following are the findings MOST consistent?

(A)   Osteomyelitis
(B)   Subchondral insufficiency fracture
(C)   Cartilage loss
(D)   Osteochondritis dissecans
(E)   Acute fracture

William B. Morrison, M.D.

Subchondral Insufficiency Fracture

Question 54

With which *one* of the following are the findings MOST consistent?

(A) Osteomyelitis
(B) Subchondral insufficiency fracture
(C) Cartilage loss
(D) Osteochondritis dissecans
(E) Acute fracture

Option (B) is correct. Subchondral insufficiency fracture of the knee is most common in middle-aged women. Patients often present with acute severe pain and are unable to bear weight, typically without significant precedent injury. Many patients present shortly after arthroscopic surgery. Subchondral insufficiency fracture most commonly occurs at the weight-bearing aspect (i.e., central aspect) of the medial femoral

condyle, but can occur at the medial tibial plateau, or at the lateral aspect of the knee. Because the line of force across the knee usually passes through the medial joint, lateral insufficiency fractures are less common.

Radiographs in the early stages are rarely contributory. An effusion may be seen, and osteopenia with lack of established osteoarthritis is common. CT does not add much to the radiographic evaluation. Bone scan reveals intense uptake, but lack of morphological correlation leads to a nonspecific diagnosis. MRI is the test of choice in this setting, revealing the characteristic appearance and enabling a specific diagnosis (Figure 12-2). Findings include a low signal linear or crescentic focus of low signal on T1-weighted and T2-weighted images within the subchondral bone at the

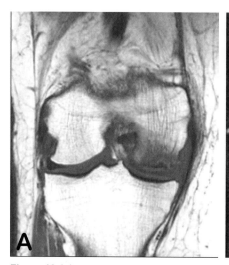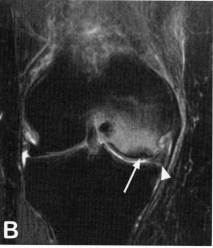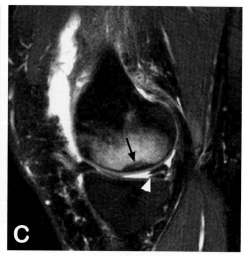

Figure 12-2 (same as Figure 12-1). Subchondral insufficiency fracture. Knee. MR. (A) T1-weighted. Coronal plane. (B) T2-weighted, fat-saturated. Coronal plane. (C) T2-weighted, fat-saturated. Sagittal plane. Note the low-signal crescent (arrows in panels B and C) in the subchondral bone with surrounding marrow edema representing insufficiency fracture. The underlying meniscal tear is evident (arrowheads in panels B and C).

central ("weight-bearing") aspect of the compartment, with marrow edema extending to the epimetaphysis and intercondylar region (or if tibial, to the tibial spines). There is generally an unstable tear of the meniscus (especially a complex or radial tear) with extrusion (peripheral displacement) or recent partial meniscectomy. There is also a distinct lack of osteophytes and bone sclerosis, although there is often overlying cartilage loss.

Osteomyelitis is not correct for a number of reasons including lack of appropriate signs and symptoms of infection and lack of generalized findings such as diffuse marrow edema and marginal erosions **(Option (A) is incorrect)**.

This brings up the differential diagnosis. Although subchondral marrow edema is common in the setting of cartilage loss, the edema pattern is more focal, less pronounced, and more "flame-shaped" rather than confluent **(Option (C) is incorrect)**. Similarly, an osteochondral lesion (the modern name for osteochondritis dissecans, another anachronistic term) is focal, tends to be rounded, rarely presents with extensive marrow edema, and rarely occurs at the weight-bearing aspect of the joint **(Option (D) is incorrect)**. Acute fracture, especially osteochondral impaction injury (from pivot-shift mechanism, for example) can be seen on MRI as crescentic or linear signal in the subchondral bone with collapse of the articular surface and extensive marrow edema, but these injuries occur in predictable locations (e.g., the terminal sulcus of the lateral femoral condyle, the posterolateral tibial plateau) and have associated injuries (e.g., ACL tear); more importantly, there is a defined history of trauma rarely seen with insufficiency fracture **(Option (E) is incorrect)**.

Question 55

SONK (spontaneous osteonecrosis of the knee) is an outdated term because:

(A) It is not spontaneous.
(B) It does not necessarily progress to osteonecrosis.
(C) It does not involve the knee.
(D) Both (A) and (B).

Option (D) is correct. The term "SONK" arose based on radiographic appearance in the late stages of disease, when the subchondral bone became sclerotic, often collapsing and resulting in secondary osteoarthritis, without evident cause such as steroid use. Patients experienced severe pain, and surgeons became nervous,

especially since many cases appeared following arthroscopic meniscal debridement. The obvious (but incorrect) conclusion was that prolonged tourniquet time during surgery (to prevent blood loss) predisposed some patients to avascular necrosis (AVN). Historical literature discusses proper treatment of this condition including core decompression (similar to the treatment for AVN of the femoral head) and total knee arthroplasty. However, as MRI evaluation of patients with this condition became more commonplace, it was noticed that a uniform pattern presented itself that was not consistent with classic avascular necrosis. In fact, the findings fit well with the MR appearance of stress fracture in other locations. When stress fractures occur in the subchondral bone they tend to have a crescentic shape; these appear similar regardless of location and have been described in the hip (also known as "transient osteoporosis of the hip"), the ankle and the foot. These lesions typically exhibit extensive bone marrow edema. In the knee, the edema extends to the intercondylar region; in the hip, edema extends to the intertrochanteric region. Other entities have also been proposed as representing stress injury, including "osteitis pubis" and "distal clavicular osteolysis." Note that these names also describe the radiographic appearance and are nebulous at best, misleading at worst. MRI has led to recognition that many of these subchondral abnormalities are related to a mechanical disturbance of the joint (e.g., meniscal tear) which in the appropriate setting (e.g., osteoporosis) and with superimposed stress can result in convergent pathology. The term "SONK" has become so entrenched in the medical nomenclature that it is difficult to erase.

Question 56

Subchondral insufficiency fracture of the knee is associated with:

(A) Lack of osteoarthritis
(B) Meniscal tear
(C) Meniscal debridement
(D) Osteopenia
(E) All of the above

(Option (E) is true). One of the functions of the normal meniscus is to distribute the weight-bearing forces uniformly across the articular surface, thereby relatively offloading the central aspect of the femoral condyle and tibial surface. One can think of SONK as a "perfect storm." Meniscal tear (and/or partial meniscectomy) causes alteration of weight bearing **(Options**

(B) and (C) are true) with concentration of force into a small area of the articular surface (Figures 12-2 and 12-3). If the individual does not have the additional buttressing supplied by established osteoarthritis, and if they have a tendency to develop bone stress (due to osteopenia) the stage is set to form a subchondral stress fracture **(Options (A) and (D) are true)**. Because they have abnormal bone, and pathology occurs from normal activities, this is termed an "insufficiency" fracture.

As one can expect, treatment for a stress fracture is very different from that for osteonecrosis. If the radiologist correctly identifies this entity and communicates the significance and implications (avoiding use of the term "SONK") of the findings, patients can receive a trial of conservative therapy (limited weight-bearing) rather than aggressive treatments proposed previously. However, it must be acknowledged that approximately 50% of all cases progress to true osteonecrosis, with collapse of the articular surface, gross incongruity and secondary osteoarthritis. When the subchondral bone becomes black on T1-weighted images or when it collapses, osteonecrosis should be suggested.

Question 57

Subchondral insufficiency fracture can occur at the tibia as well as the femoral condyle. *True or False?*

The answer is "True." (Figure 12-3). Other terms had been proposed for this variation, including "SONT" (spontaneous osteonecrosis of the tibia), but because the etiology is the same as for the femur, efforts at creating a new term for this condition have faded. Also, although the medial femoral condyle is most commonly involved, the lateral condyle can also be affected.

Question 58

Subchondral insufficiency fracture at the knee can heal spontaneously. *True or False?*

The answer is "True." In an estimated 50% of cases, the stress fracture can heal, resulting in little to no sequelae (Figure 12-4). However, this leaves a significant proportion that do progress, resulting in necrosis and collapse of the articular surface (and subse-

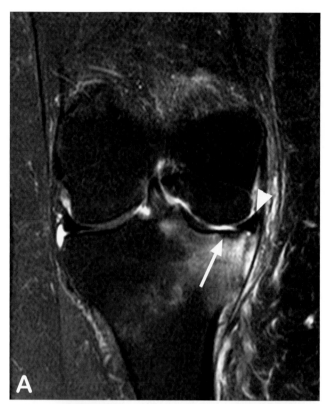

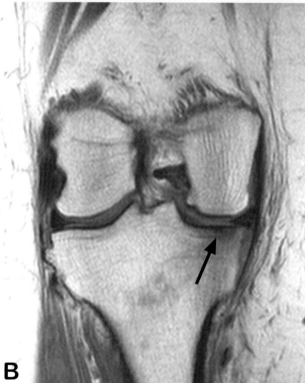

Figure 12-3. Tibial subchondral stress fracture. Knee. MRI. Coronal plane. Fat-suppressed. (A) T1-weighted. (B) T2-weighted. The images show a characteristic tibial subchondral stress fracture. Note the low signal subchondral line (arrows) at the medial plateau with surrounding edema. Also note the major extrusion (displacement marked by an arrowhead) of the medial meniscus, suggesting the presence of an unstable tear and resulting in altered forces leading to the stress fracture.

quent osteoarthritis). Factors leading to healing versus progression have not yet been determined.

Suggested Readings

1. Gil HC, Levine SM, Zoga AC. MRI findings in the subchondral bone marrow: a discussion of conditions including transient osteoporosis, transient bone marrow edema syndrome, SONK, and shifting bone marrow edema of the knee. Semin Musculoskeletal Radiol. 2006;10:177-186.

2. Yao L, Stanczak J, Boutin RD. Presumptive subarticular stress reactions of the knee: MRI detection and association with meniscal tear patterns. Skeletal Radiol. 2004;33:260-264.

3. Robertson DD, Armfield DR, Towers JD, Irrgang JJ, Maloney WJ, Harner CD. Meniscal root injury and spontaneous osteonecrosis of the knee: an observation. J Bone Joint Surg Br. 2009;91:190-195.

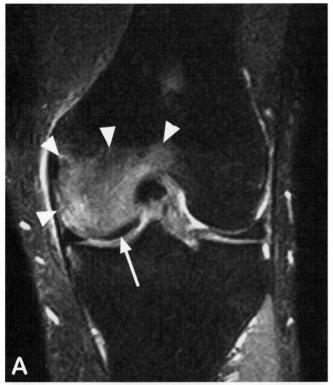

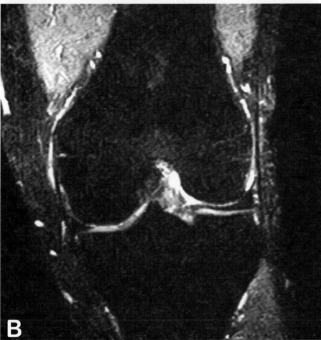

Figure 12-4. Healing of a subchondral stress fracture of the medial femoral condyle (arrow). Knee. MRI. Short-tau inversion recovery (STIR). Coronal plane. (A) This image, obtained at initial presentation, shows a subchondral stress fracture of the medial femoral condyle (arrow), with characteristic surrounding marrow edema (arrowheads). There is no collapse of the articular surface to suggest necrosis. (B) A follow-up image after 8 months shows complete resolution of findings.

Case 13

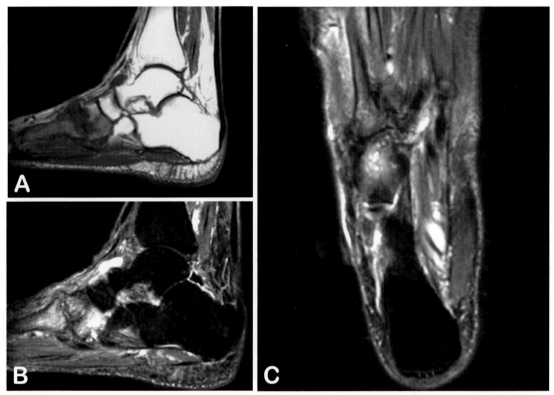

Figure 13-1. Ankle and mid-foot. MR. (A) T1-weighted. Sagittal plane. (B) STIR. Sagittal plane. (C) T2-weighted, fat-saturated. Axial plane.

Question 59

You are shown three MR images acquired in a diabetic patient who presented with a swollen, erythematous foot. Radiographs were nonspecific. CBC is normal. There is a small skin ulcer. Which *one* of the following is MOST accurate?

(A)   Findings are most consistent with osteomyelitis.
(B)   Findings are most consistent with neuropathic osteoarthropathy.
(C)   MRI cannot differentiate infection from neuropathic disease.
(D)   A bone biopsy should be performed through the ulcer.

William B. Morrison, M.D.

Neuropathic Osteoarthropathy of the Foot

Question 59

Which *one* of the following is MOST accurate?

(A) Findings are most consistent with osteomyelitis.
(B) Findings are most consistent with neuropathic osteo-
arthropathy.
(C) MRI cannot differentiate infection from neuropathic
disease.
(D) A bone biopsy should be performed through the ulcer.

(Option (B) is correct). The images (Figure 13-2)
show intense bone marrow edema centered at the Lisfranc joint. There are discrete subchondral cysts within
the edema. Although there is surrounding soft tissue
edema, the subcutaneous fat is preserved. Osteomyelitis is common in the feet of diabetic patients due to a
constellation of factors. Peripheral neuropathy causes
relative lack of sensation leading to skin breaks, often
related to punctures or toenail cutting. Ischemia due

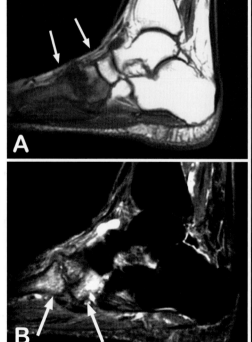

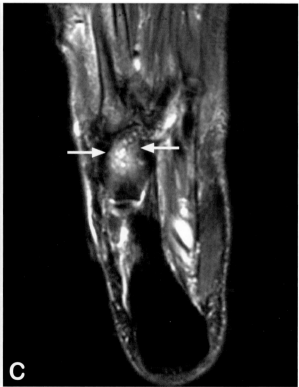

Figure 13-2 (same as
Figure 13-1). Neuropathic
osteoarthropathy. Ankle
and mid-foot. MRI. (A) T1-
weighted. Sagittal plane.
Note preservation of the
subcutaneous fat (arrows).
(B) Short-tau inversion
recovery (STIR). Sagit-
tal plane. Extensive bone
marrow edema (arrows) is
present around the Lisfranc
joint, but there is no evidence of contiguous spread
through the soft tissues. (C)
T2-weighted, fat-saturated.
Axial plane. There are
degenerative subchondral
cysts (arrows), which,
along with the bone mar-
row edema seen in panel
B, supports a diagnosis of
neuropathic osteoarthropathy and argues against superimposed infection.

to combined large and small vessel disease results in slow healing and poor response to bacterial invasion. Underlying immunosuppression contributes to progression of infection. Tendinopathy occurs, especially in the posterior tibialis. Altered weight-bearing related to a deforming arthropathy (neuropathic osteoarthropathy) and posterior tibialis tendon dysfunction leads to collapse of the arch of the foot, and, in more severe cases, a "rocker-bottom" deformity. Deformities can also occur at the ankle and the toes (e.g., "clawtoe" deformity). These deformities result in overlying callus formation. The callus can break down and form an ulcer. Contiguous spread of infection then occurs through the soft tissues, forming sinus tracts and abscesses, eventually contacting bone or a joint and leading to osteomyelitis and septic arthritis.

The subcutaneous fat is preserved, and there is no evidence of contiguous spread through the soft tissues. Cystic degenerative change is present at the edematous subchondral bone of the Lisfranc joint. These findings favor neuropathic disease and argue against superimposed infection **(Option (A) is incorrect).**

Infection by contiguous spread is by far the most common form in the feet of diabetic patients. Although hematogenous implantation is the most common way to acquire osteomyelitis in general, it is relatively uncommon in the foot in this population. Contiguous spread leads to a characteristic appearance on MR images; interruption of the skin signal representing ulceration is seen, often with granulation tissue at the base if chronic. Surrounding cellulitis in active infection results in replacement of soft tissue fat signal on T1-weighted images and soft tissue edema on fluid-sensitive (T2-weighted, fat-suppressed or short-tau inversion recovery (STIR) images; however, edema alone is a nonspecific finding that can be seen with other conditions such as trauma, ischemia, and dependent edema from venous insufficiency. To complicate things further, diabetic patients often have underlying muscle atrophy, the early manifestation of which is muscle hyperintensity on fluid-sensitive sequences. Therefore, it is important to acquire and evaluate at least one non–fat-suppressed T1-weighted sequence, preferably in a plane perpendicular to the ulcer. Preservation of subcutaneous fat around the bones argues against a marrow abnormality representing contiguous spread of infection. Using these guidelines, MRI can be useful for evaluating pedal complications in diabetic patients and can (with approximately 90% accuracy) differentiate neuropathic osteoarthropathy from infection **(Option (C) is incorrect).** In positive cases, MRI provides a useful surgical "roadmap" to determine location and extent of disease. In indeterminate cases, MRI can help guide percutaneous biopsy.

Although the most direct route (bone biopsy through the skin ulceration) seems most convenient, it is possible that the bone was not infected (note that bone marrow edema is not specific for infection). However, breaching the cortex through infected tissue will assure that the bone becomes infected. Therefore, unless the bone is unequivocally infected, care should be taken to avoid infected soft tissue in acquiring bone samples **(Option (D) is incorrect).**

Question 60

Findings on MRI that help differentiate neuropathic osteoarthropathy from infection include:

(A) Subchondral cysts
(B) Sinus tract to bone
(C) Fluid collections
(D) Bone marrow edema
(E) Both A and B

(Option (E) is true). Neuropathic osteoarthropathy can be thought of as an aggressive form of osteoarthritis (OA) and instability. Osteoarthritis is characterized by spurs, cartilage loss and subchondral cysts, and osteoarthropathy related to neuropathic disease is no exception. In fact, unless there is chronic disease or acute infection superimposed on long-standing arthritis, subchondral cysts would not be expected at a septic joint. In joints with established osteoarthritis and superimposed infection, cysts disappear as the cortical surface erodes. Therefore, subchondral cysts are a common sign in OA but not in neuropathic osteoarthropathy **(Option (A) is true).** However, since osteophytes do not disappear with superinfection, presence of spurs is not a good discriminator for infection versus no infection.

Since osteomyelitis in diabetic patients is mainly due to spread via skin ulceration, a sinus tract visualized communicating with a bone that has abnormal marrow signal is highly suggestive of infection **(Option (B) is true).** However, fluid collections in the soft tissues are not necessarily abscesses and are often seen in patients with neuropathic disease due to injury and friction-related bursitis **(Option (C) is false).** Subchondral edema is also nonspecific and can be seen with a number of processes including infection and arthritis **(Option (D) is false).** Since neuropathic disease is associated with joint instability, marrow edema can be extensive, especially if there is unrecognized fracture ("neuropathic fracture").

Fractures can occur at insensate joints, with continued weight-bearing resulting in intense marrow and soft tissue edema. This is more commonly seen in diabetic patients in the tarsal bones and the posterior tubercle of the calcaneus at the Achilles tendon insertion. Patients may not report injury, leading to presentation with an acute swollen, erythematous foot. When there is very intense bone marrow edema, always look for underlying fracture that may be responsible.

Question 61

The BEST single test for evaluation of the foot in a diabetic with ulceration and clinical concern for infection is:

(A) Three-phase bone scan
(B) Radiographs
(C) MRI
(D) Labeled white blood cell scan
(E) Ultrasound

Radiographs are excellent for evaluation of the deformity, disorganization, debris and preservation of density (the "four Ds") that characterize chronic neuropathic osteoarthropathy **(Option (C) is correct).** They are useful as a widely available, inexpensive modality for follow-up of findings and for correlation of anatomy and deformity with other imaging exams. Signs of infection are delayed on radiographs, however, and patients who present with suspicious symptoms should get advanced imaging regardless of radiographic findings. If radiographs are negative for infection, there could be early involvement, and if radiographs are suspicious for infection, advanced imaging is important for characterizing extent of bone and soft tissue involvement to guide appropriate treatment. Advanced imaging should not be delayed, since infection can spread rapidly. Radiographic signs of osteomyelitis include soft tissue swelling, joint space narrowing and erosions, cortical rarefaction and frank bone destruction. Soft tissue swelling is seen early but is nonspecific. Advanced findings of bone destruction can be delayed by as much as two weeks following inoculation of the bone **(Option (B) is incorrect).**

Three-phase technetium-99m methylene diphosphonate (Tc-99m-MDP) bone scan is sensitive for detection of osteomyelitis, showing uptake on early, vascular phases with concentration in the bone on subsequent blood pool and delayed phases. Yet uptake may be delayed or weak, or not be seen at all in the setting of pedal ischemia. Also, neuropathic osteoarthropathy is commonly associated with hyperemia (which can be extreme when there is underlying fracture) resulting in a false positive exam. Specificity may be enhanced by correlation with a labeled WBC scan (using In-111 or Tc-99m-MDP), showing uptake in the same region positive on three-phase bone scan. However, if the exam(s) is/are negative for osteomyelitis, the extent of soft tissue involvement (including size and location of abscess and septic tenosynovitis) remains an important question. If positive for osteomyelitis, the extent in bone and involvement of adjacent joints must be mapped for surgical management. Therefore, whenever MR imaging is available, it has largely supplanted nuclear medicine exams for evaluating complications of neuropathic disease and infection in the diabetic foot **(Option (A) and Option (D) are incorrect).**

MR imaging provides excellent anatomic detail and can be used not only to diagnose osteomyelitis and differentiate infection from neuropathic disease but also to define the extent of bone and soft tissue involvement, including abscess, sinus tract, septic arthritis and septic tenosynovitis. Since diabetic foot infection is typically initiated through a skin ulcer, early findings include soft tissue edema and replacement of subcutaneous fat signal on T1-weighted images. This finding helps differentiate infection from dependent edema, which is very common in diabetic feet. As the ulceration and infection progresses through the soft tissues, underlying tendons can become involved; complex fluid within a tendon sheath that passes through an infected zone should be considered suspicious for septic tenosynovitis. Abscess formation can occur, leading to focal fluid collections in the infected soft tissues; often these communicate and drain to the skin via sinus tracts. As infection reaches the cortex, reactive subcortical edema may be seen; this finding, if directly contiguous with soft tissue infection, should be considered suspicious for early osteomyelitis. Occasionally, periosteal reaction (linear T2 hyperintensity along the cortex) occurs, but this may not be apparent in the tarsal bones and small phalanges. As infection progresses, bone marrow signal abnormality (as evidenced by edema on T2-weighted images and low signal with replacement of marrow fat on T1-weighted images) extends beyond the subcortical bone into the medullary space.

Ultrasound can be used for documentation of soft tissue fluid collections, joint effusion and tenosynovitis, with power Doppler for vascularity related to inflammation. Periosteal reaction can be seen with osteomyelitis; however, lack of overview and evaluation of extent of bone involvement limit the value of this modality for

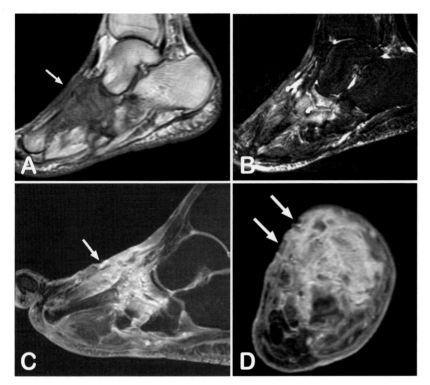

Figure 13-3. Osteomyelitis in a diabetic patient. Foot. MRI. (A) T1-weighted. Sagittal plane. (B) Single tau inversion recovery (STIR). Sagittal plane. (C) Postcontrast T1-weighted, fat-suppressed. Sagittal plane. (D) Postcontrast. T1-weighted, fat-suppressed. Coronal plane. This diabetic patient has MRI findings that overlap those of the patient from Question 59, including low T1 signal and marrow edema at the midfoot with an adjacent fluid collection. However, in this case there is shallow dorsal ulceration with loss of subcutaneous fat signal (arrows) contiguous with the marrow, suggesting infectious spread. Also note the lack of subchondral cystic change that was present on the Figure 13-2 example with neuropathic osteoarthropathy.

assessment of suspected diabetic foot infection **(Option (E) is incorrect).**

Question 62

Regarding sequences, the *one* LEAST useful for diagnosis of osteomyelitis is:

(A) STIR
(B) T1-weighted, spin-echo
(C) Proton density
(D) T2-weighted, fast spin-echo, fat-suppressed
(E) Gradient-recalled echo (GRE)

An important part of diagnosis of infection in soft tissues or the marrow cavity deals with absence of fat signal or presence of edema signal. Proton density sequences are excellent for acquiring high resolution images, since fat and fluid are both bright, leading to a signal-rich image that can be acquired at high matrix without significant loss of signal-to-noise. However, proton density images can hide important pathology such as fractures, tumors, and infection **(Option (C) is correct).**

Fluid-sensitive sequences such as STIR (A) and T2-weighted, fast spin-echo, fat-suppressed imaging (D) are essential for detection of edema in the soft tissues and marrow associated with inflammation **(Options (A)**

and (D) are incorrect). Similarly, T1-weighted spin-echo images are essential for evaluation of replacement of fat in the soft tissues and marrow seen with infection **(Option (B) is incorrect).** Gradient-recalled echo (GRE) images can be T1-weighted or fluid-weighted, but these images are prone to magnetic susceptibility artifact. Calcium creates "blooming" artifact; therefore signal in the marrow can be influenced by trabecular density. As a result, GRE images are of limited use in evaluation of osteomyelitis, unless acquired before and after intravenous administration of contrast, with difference in signal indicating hyperemia **(Option (E) is incorrect).**

Question 63

Regarding use of gadolinium contrast for diagnosis of osteomyelitis on MRI:

(A) It is essential to check creatinine clearance/glomerular filtration rate prior to contrast administration in diabetic patients and patients over 60.
(B) Contrast should only be given when absolutely necessary.
(C) Contrast can help delineate areas of necrosis, abscesses, and sinus tracts, and can differentiate inflammation from "bland" soft tissue edema.
(D) Contrast is best reserved for preoperative cases.
(E) All of the above.

Option (E) is true. Due to emergence of nephrogenic systemic fibrosis, recommendations regarding contrast usage for diabetic foot infection have recently changed. Current ACR recommendations on screening are available on www.acr.org. These include patients with:

- Renal disease (including solitary kidney, renal transplant, renal tumor)
- Age greater than 60
- History of hypertension
- History of diabetes
- History of severe hepatic disease/liver transplant/pending liver transplant

Based on the ACR screening recommendations [go to www.acr.org and enter "Manual on Contrast Media v6" in the search box], **(Options (A) and (B) are true).** Contrast-enhanced imaging sequences remain an important method for delineating inflammatory tissue (to differentiate from bland or dependent edema), sinus tracts, abscesses and areas of devitalization **(Option (C) is true).** This information is particularly useful for planning surgical intervention; therefore, contrast is best reserved for patients status preoperative for diabetic foot complications, if they have adequate renal function **(Option (D) is true).**

Suggested Readings

1. Russell JM, Peterson JJ, Bancroft LW. MR imaging of the diabetic foot. Magn Reson Imaging Clin N Am. 2008;16:59–70.

2. Ledermann HP, Morrison WB. Differential diagnosis of pedal osteomyelitis and diabetic neuroarthropathy: MR Imaging. Semin Musculoskelet Radiol. 2005;9:272–283.

3. Ahmadi ME, Morrison WB, Carrino JA, Schweitzer ME, Raikin SM, Ledermann HP. Neuropathic arthropathy of the foot with and without superimposed osteomyelitis: MR imaging characteristics. Radiology. 2006;238:622–231.

Case 14

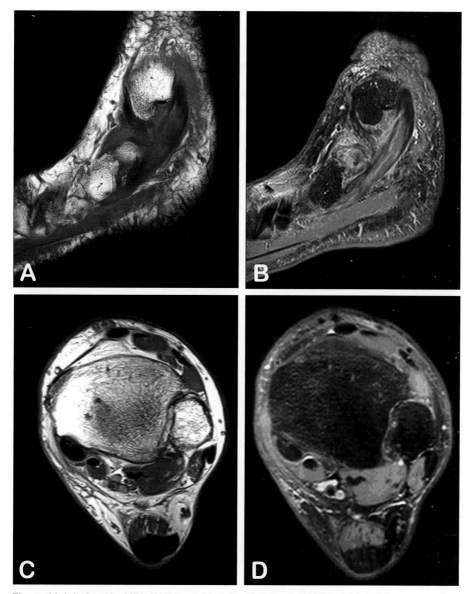

Figure 14-1. Left ankle. MRI. (A) T1-weighted. Sagittal plane. (B) T2-weighted, fat-suppressed. Sagittal plane. (C) T1-weighted. Axial plane. (D) T2-weighted, fat-suppressed. Axial plane.

Question 64

You are shown four images (Figure 14-1) from the left ankle MRI examination of a 56-year-old woman who presented with a history of chronic left ankle pain. Which *one* of the following is the MOST likely diagnosis?

(A) Medial malleolar fracture
(B) Flexor hallux longus tear
(C) Posterior tibialis dysfunction
(D) Ankle joint arthropathy

Teik C. Oh, M.B. and Mark E. Schweitzer, M.D.

Posterior Tibialis Tendon Dysfunction

Question 64

Which *one* of the following is the MOST likely diagnosis?

(A) Medial malleolar fracture
(B) Flexor hallux longus tear
(C) Posterior tibialis dysfunction
(D) Ankle joint arthropathy

The patient's MRI of the ankle shows abnormality of the posterior tibialis tendon. It is markedly thickened on both the sagittal (Figure 14-2A & 14-2B) and axial (Figure 14-2C & 14-2D) planes. All images also show areas of heterogeneous signal within the tendon substance. On the short tau inversion recovery (STIR) sequence (Figure 14-2B), the tendon contains lines of increased signal intensities indicating longitudinal splits within the tendon. The findings are most compat-ible with posterior tibialis tendon tearing and dysfunc-tion **(Option (C) is correct).**

Posterior tibialis tendon (PTT) dysfunction occurs more commonly in women who are middle-aged or el-derly. Classically, two thirds of spontaneous ruptures oc-cur in women in their fifth or sixth decade of life. There are systemic risk factors which predispose to this condi-tion, the most important of these being hypertension, obesity, lupus, gout, rheumatoid arthritis, and, somewhat less commonly Reiter's syndrome, now termed reactive arthritis. Because of these first two risk factors, PTT dys-function is sometimes referred to as the cardiovascular disease of the foot. Tears are likely related to chronic synovitis, which most often is mechanical but is also seen in patients with rheumatoid arthritis and reactive arthritis.

Ninety percent of cases have unilateral disease. The initial presentation is either related to tendon

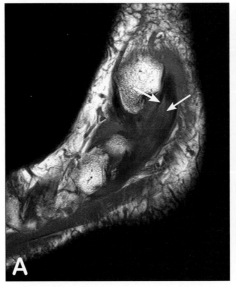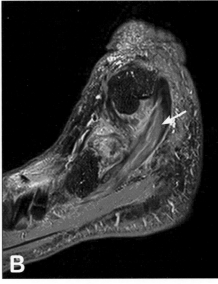

Figure 14-2. (Same as Figure 14-1) MRI. Left ankle. (A) T1-weighted. Sagittal plane. The expanded tendon shows heterogeneous signal within (arrows). (B) T2-weighted, fat-suppressed. Sagittal plane. This image shows similar appearances with vertical high-er signal lines (arrow) indicating tears.

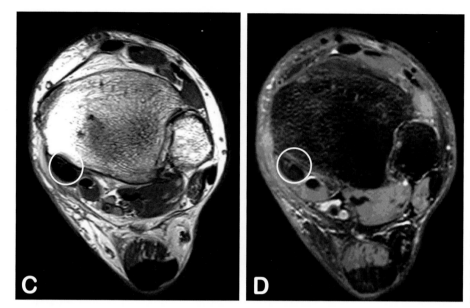

Figure 14-2 (continued). MRI. Left ankle.(C) T1-weighted. Axial plane (D) T2-weighted, fat-suppressed. Axial plane. Both panels show increased signal within the posterior tibial tendon (circles). Note that there is no significant fluid around the tendon in this case.

symptoms, most commonly pain along the course of the tendon. In a surprisingly high percentage of cases symptoms are a manifestation of altered mechanics such as weakness of the ankle and pes planus (flatfoot deformity) with the latter due to loss of the medial longitudinal arch or even lateral pain from overuse or secondary articular changes. Clinical examination tends to reveal weakness of inversion, difficult toe raises, and a lack of heel varus. These clinical findings are more a manifestation of motor dysfunction than they are a relation to the PTT itself.

Conventional radiographs are not usually diagnostic although they can help exclude underlying fractures or may show end-stage disease. In later stages of disease, however, they may show the mechanical alterations with forefoot valgus, talar plantar flexion, and lateral impingement with secondary articular disease. Ultrasound or MRI imaging is more useful to reveal the earlier, presalvage stages of disorders of the posterior tibialis tendon.

In order to evaluate this condition on MRI of the ankle, it is important to appreciate some idiosyncrasies

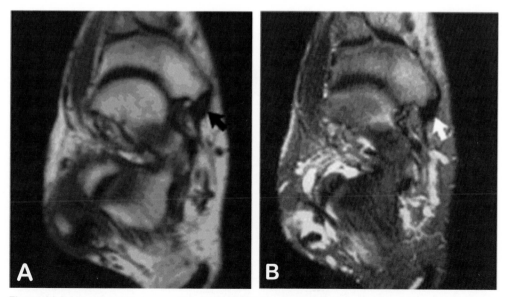

Figure 14-3. Normal appearances of the posterior tibial tendon. MRI. (A) T1-weighted. Axial plane. Note the diffuse internal signal in the posterior tibialis tendon (arrow). (B) T2-weighted, fat-suppressed. Axial plane. The T2-weighted image reveals internal signal intensity in the posterior tibialis tendon that fades on long TE images, consistent with "magic angle" artifact (arrow).

of imaging. On MRI imaging, the posterior tibialis tendon is normally black (as are tendons in general) without any internal signal intensity, unless the echo time (TE) is lower then 1. One notable exception to this is the magic angle artifact seen as tendons curve with respect to B0 of the magnet (Figure 14-3). In the PTT, this occurs as the tendon curves around the medial malleolus. Unlike the Achilles tendon, the distal posterior tibialis tendon has no normal internal signal intensity; however, there is variability of signal intensity distally related to volume averaging of the spring ligament (extremely distally), tibionavicular, and the tibiotalar components of the deltoid ligament (slightly more proximally).

On sagittal images, the PTT should have a smooth curve around the medial malleolus to limit focal compression and impingement. A small (1-2 mm) amount of partially surrounding incomplete rim of low signal on T1 (Figure 14-2A & 14-2C) and high signal on T2 (Figure 14-2C & 14-2D) indicates normal fluid within the synovial sheath of the posterior tibialis tendon. When this fluid becomes completely circumferential, and especially when it is seen distally, this is a sign of synovitis, usually chronic. When excessive fluid is seen around the PTT, care should be taken to exclude an ankle joint effusion, as occasionally this joint can communicate with the PTT. In this situation there is usually excessive fluid in the flexor hallucis tendon sheath and often in the flexor digitorum tendon sheath, as well.

Posterior tibialis tendon dysfunction may initially present as synovitis or paratendonitis. The term synovitis should be used to describe this disorder only when it occurs more proximally, because fluid is not normally present distally around the posterior tibialis tendon on MR imaging (Figure 14-4). If apparent synovitis is seen distally, it is anatomically a paratendonitis and often reveals fluid slightly lower in signal intensity. The tendon itself is normal and should not show intratendinous signal at this stage of the disorder. The MR imaging appearance of this paratendonitis shows partially circumferential high signal intensity, slightly hypointense to fluid, located distally around the posterior tibialis tendon.

Figure 14-2 shows normal bone marrow signal with no evidence of cortical breaks to indicate any fractures present **(Option (A) is incorrect)**. The flexor hallucis longus (FHL) is visible on axial scans, lying posterior and medial to the posterior tibialis tendon. It is not seen on the sagittal scans. Normal low signal is seen on both sequences, with no evidence of any tears **(Option (B) is incorrect)**.

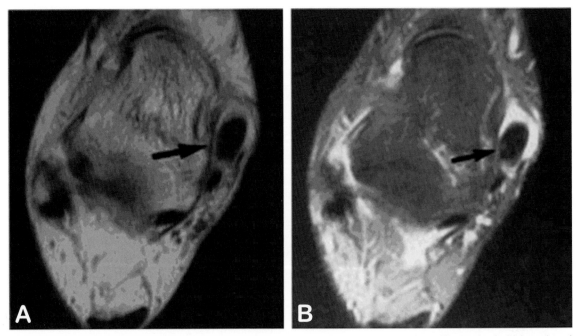

Figure 14-4. Synovitis of posterior tibialis tendon. MRI. (A) Proton density-weighted. Axial plane. The tendon is thickened, and there is surrounding fluid (arrow). (B) T2-weighted, fat-suppressed. Axial plane. Multifocal, speckled internal signal intensity can be seen, surrounded by excessive synovial fluid (arrow).

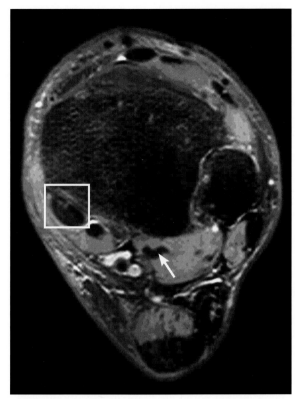

Figure 14-5. Hypertrophied posterior tibialis tendon (square). Ankle. MRI. T2-weighted, fat-suppressed. Axial plane. An arrow shows the normal flexor halllucis longus (FHL) lying behind the medial side of the tibia, posterior and medial to the hypertrophied posterior tibialis tendon and normal flexor digitorum. Even though the tendon is abnormal, no synovitis is present.

Although this is not a contrast-enhanced scan, there is normal appearance of the joint spaces and no significant joint effusion or thickened synovium present. The findings on the test case images are not consistent with evidence of arthropathy **(Option (D) is incorrect).**

Question 65

Regarding MRI use in fractures:

    (A) It is useful in detecting stress fractures.
    (B) A rim of fluid signal around an osteochondral fragment indicates that it is a stable fragment.
    (C) Signal changes within surrounding bone marrow are due to hemorrhage.
    (D) There are no specific distinguishing features of new compared to old fractures.

MRI can help clarify occult fractures when they are not clearly identified on radiographs. As such, MRI can detect fractures earlier than conventional radiographs, especially in bones that have fractures such as scaphoid or dome-of-talus, which do not appear on radiographs

early. However, while secondary findings like marrow edema may be present to suggest underlying fracture, cortical breaks may not always be visible on MRI.

Stress fractures may not always be apparent on plain radiographs. MRI is useful to detect stress fractures, as there is often extensive surrounding marrow edema to indicate their presence. **(Option (A) is true).** (Figure 14-6A).

MRI is very useful at detecting osteochrondral fragments. Osteochondral fragments may contain a rim of high signal on T2-weighted scans, indicating fluid sig-

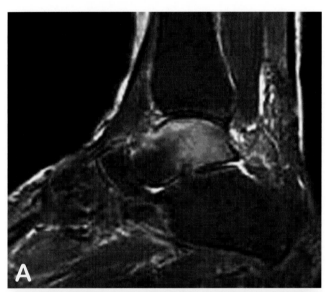

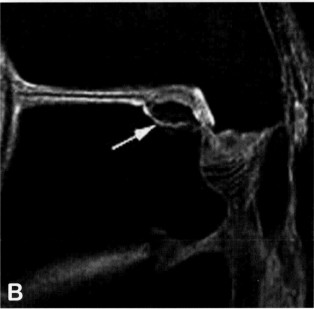

Figure 14-6. Osteochondral defect. Ankle. MRI. (A) T2-weighted, fat-suppressed. Note the linear hypointense subchondral region of stress fracture with surround hyperintense marrow edema. (B) T2-weighted fat-suppressed. The talar dome osteochondral fragment with a surrounding rim of hyperintense fluid signal (arrow) indicates an unstable fragment.

nal, which means the fragment is fully detached. This is an unstable fragment and usually requires fixation. **(Option (B) is false)** (Figure 14-6B).

The extensive marrow signal intensity on T2-weighted, fat-suppressed (Figure 14-6A) MR images is due to edema rather than hemorrhage **(Option (C) is false)**.

Acute fractures show linear hypointensity surrounded by generalized hyperintense marrow edema. More established and old fractures tend to show low intensity line due to the sclerosis that occurs after fracture healing. The marrow returns to normal signal after the edema has resolved. So, there are features to distinguish acute from established fractures. This is especially useful in vertebral body fractures. **(Option (D) is false)** (Figure 14-7A&B).

Question 66

Regarding flexor hallucis longus (FHL) tendon:

(A) Complete tears are common in patients with active lifestyles.
(B) The mechanism of injury is constant repetitive extension movement, which stretches the tendon.
(C) Long-standing inflammation may lead to hallux rigidus.
(D) Fluid in the synovial sheath is always abnormal and indicates that pathology is present.

Though the pathology of FHL tendon can present in various ways, actual complete tears are rare, being less

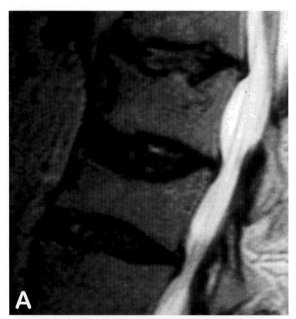

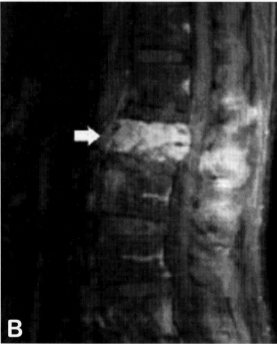

Figure 14-7. Old versus new fractures. Spine. MRI. (A) T2-weighted. Sagittal plane. Established vertebral fractures of L1 and L2. Note normal marrow signal. (B) Proton-density-weighted, fat-suppressed. Extensive edema in the fractured L2 vertebra can be seen (arrow). Surrounding signal changes of ligamentous damages are also visible.

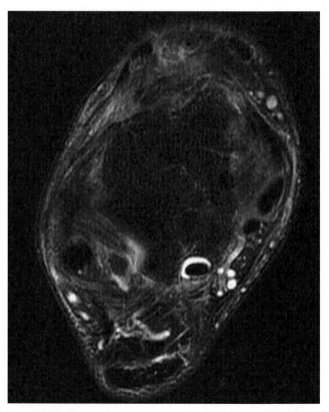

Figure 14-8. Suggestive for tenosynovitis. MRI. T2-weighted, fat-suppressed. Axial plane. The FHL lies posterior and medial to both the posterior tibialis tendon and the flexor digitorum longus. There is fluid around the FHL tendon, which is suggestive but not diagnostic of tenosynovitis.

than 4% of acute cases reported **(Option (A) is false)**. Injuries to the FHL tendon are usually due to constant repetitive flexion movement **(Option (B) is false)**. It is therefore often described in patients who use frequent push-off maneuvers of the forefoot such as those required by dancing, climbing, and soccer. FHL tenosynovitis is infrequently seen in association with other conditions, such as diabetes, rheumatoid arthritis, lupus, and seronegative spondyloarthropathies.

The tendon can also become inflamed and, over time, become nodular, resulting in great toe triggering (hallux saltans) which may progress to hallux rigidus **(Option (C) is true)**. The FHL may also become entrapped by enlarged os trigonum or calcaneal fracture-dislocations or from scarring postoperatively. The former is not infrequent and is a type of mechanical stenosing tendonitis; however, these types of disorders occur posteriorly.

The FHL is best seen just lateral to the posterior tibialis tendon as it curves around the sustentaculum tali. It is the most lateral muscle of the deep compartment of the calf, originating from the lower two thirds of the posterior surface of the shaft of the fibula to insert on the distal phalanx of the great toe.

Tenosynovitis may be present either alone or in combination with FHL tendinopathy. While isolated fluid in the synovial sheath may indicate tenosynovitis, this is not specific and can be a normal variant in up to 20% of cases **(Option (D) is false)** (Figure 14-8). The term "normal variant" here uses a little poetic license, as most often this is a manifestation of a prior or current ankle joint effusion. For this reason we sometimes call the FHL tendon sheath the "Baker's cyst of the ankle."

Question 67

Regarding ankle joint arthropathy:

(A) In neuropathic arthropathy, T1-weighted images demonstrate high signal intensity.
(B) It is a more common site of involvement by rheumatoid arthritis than is the forefoot.
(C) Hemophilic arthropathy results in low signal foci throughout the synovium.
(D) Most cases due to osteoarthritis do not have a specific cause.

Neuropathic arthropathy (Charcot joint) is the term used for bone and joint changes secondary to loss of sensation due to a variety of causes, as first described by Charcot in 1868. Changes seen include destruction of articular surfaces, subchondral sclerosis, debris within the

joint, deformity, and dislocation. Early radiographic imaging is usually normal, but the bone scan is invariably hot on all three phases. In this early, preradiographic stage, MR images usually show marrow edema without deformity.

In midstage Charcot, it is difficult to distinguish the radiographic changes from osteoarthritis. Late radiographic changes with associated soft tissue changes and subsequent subluxations and dislocations are more characteristic. However, Charcot joints may continue to look like osteoarthritis, and sometimes the term "osteoarthritis with a vengeance" is used. More characteristic, however, is frequent bone atrophy, termed "a bag of bones."

Ultrasound is sometimes used to evaluate complications such as fluid collections. Such soft tissue collections can be seen with both neuropathic feet and infections.

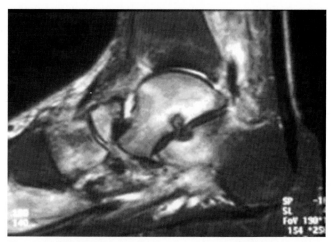

Figure 14-9. Diabetic foot. MRI. Fat-suppressed. Sagittal plane. Neuropathic changes of the patient's midfoot with marrow edema can be seen. Minimal joint fluid is present in this case.

CT findings are not specific in early stages, as CT merely shows the radiographic changes to greater detail. CT may identify early fragmentation, however. Radionuclide and MRI imaging is used primarily to distinguish soft tissue infection from osteomyelitis. On T1-weighted images, generalized low signal intensity is present **(Option (A) is false)** (Figure 14-9). Fat-suppressed sequences may detect the high-signal marrow edema, but this can be difficult to distinguish from osteomyelitis. Secondary signs of osteomyelitis such as ulcer and sinus formation, focal bony destruction, or large collections adjacent to ulcers are most helpful. This is particularly important as over 90% of osteomyelitis cases in diabetic patients are often associated with secondary to local spread. MRI is more useful in overall assessment of extent of disease and the presence of soft tissue infection.

Rheumatoid arthritis can frequently involve the foot and ankle. Patients usually, but not invariably, have hand and wrist changes as well. Rheumatoid arthritis more commonly involves the forefoot (metatarsal and phalangeal joints) than the ankle joint **(Option (B) is false).** The ankle is usually the last joint in this region to be affected but when involved, it can be painful and cause deformity. In the ankle there is a characteristic fibula notch sign secondary to synovitis of the syndesmotic recess. Imaging features are similar to rheumatoid joints

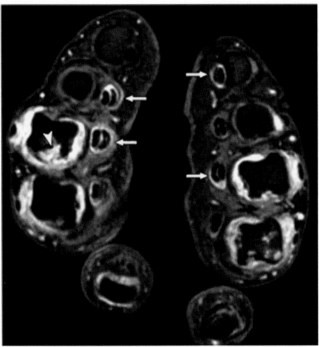

Figure 14-10. Early detection of rheumatoid arthritis. Bilateral hands. MRI. Fat-suppressed, contrast-enhanced. Axial plane. Bilateral synovitis of 2nd and 3rd metacarpals is seen, with supporting erosion of the radial aspect of the 3rd metacarpal bone (arrowhead). Flexor digitorum tenosynovitis is present bilaterally (arrows).

elsewhere, including effusion, synovitis, and erosions, with later features of joint subluxation somewhat more common. Overall, though, MR imaging of the ankle is less important than imaging of the other joints, because by the time the ankle joint is affected, the diagnosis of rheumatoid arthritis is often well established.

Contrast-enhanced MRI of the hands in patients who have normal radiographs and blood tests but whose clinical symptoms arouse suspicion for rheumatoid arthritis can help detect early disease and lead to earlier treatment. Detection of synovitis with marrow edema or erosions has a sensitivity of 100% in one study. Supporting features of tenosynovitis and bursitis can also be helpful (Figure 14-10).

Patients with hemophilia are prone to having multiple recurrent episodes of hemarthoses, i.e. hemorrhage into joints. This occurs in about 80% of patients. The bleeding originates in the synovial vessels and can be spontaneous or result from minor trauma. Chronic and

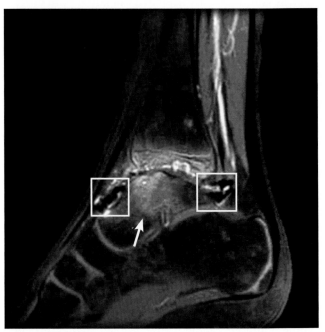

Figure 14-11. Hemophilic arthropathy. MRI. Increased signal intensity within tibial metaphysis and talar dome. Subchondral cystic changes evident of arthropathy. Note the presence of low signal synovium due to hemosiderin deposits (squares). An arrow marks the reactive marrow edema.

repeated episodes can lead to destruction of the joint and hemosiderin deposition in the tissues adjacent to the joint as well as the synovium, a condition known as hemophilic arthropathy. MRI is now the standard of imaging for most accurate assessment of this disorder.

MRI of hemophiliac arthropathy shows low intensity foci throughout the synovium **(Option (C) is true).** These are due to the hemosiderin deposits that are invariably found in this condition. An important distinction is that the hemosiderin deposits are not nodular and thus can usually be differentiated from pigmented villonodular synovitis. In the acute phase, reactive marrow edema is evident (Figure 14-11). MRI can also detect erosions and subchondral cysts as well as the often dark, joint effusions.

Osteoarthritis can affect the ankle, just like other joints. However, the majority of these cases are secondary to previous trauma, often associated with instability **(Option (D) is false).** The injury may have happened many years before any clinical or radiological evidence of osteoarthritis is present. The cartilage injury may be related directly to the osteoarthritis or may be related indirectly by affecting the mechanics of the ankle joint. Other risk factors that can contribute to osteoarthritis include obesity and congenital altered foot mechanics such as pes planus (flat feet) resulting in added stress to ankle joint.

Radiologically, the appearance of ankle osteoarthritis is similar to that of osteoarthritic features elsewhere. (Figure 14-12). These include nonuniform joint space loss, osteophyte formation, cyst formation, and subchondral sclerosis. The osteophytes tend to predominate anteriorly, and the cysts are usually seen in the talus. MRI also can be helpful in evaluating cartilage loss but often is unnecessary because conventional radiography provides adequate information. MRI studies should not be routinely performed in diagnosing osteoarthritis unless additional pathology, such as posttraumatic injuries, malignancy, or infectious process is suspected.

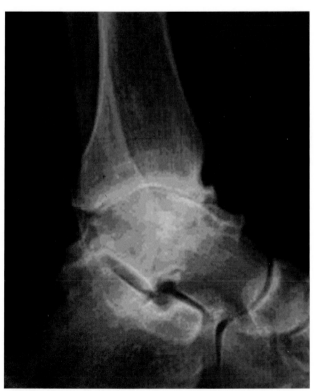

Figure 14-12. Osteoarthritis. Ankle. Radiograph. Lateral view. The image shows nearly complete loss of joint space with subchondral sclerosis of the ankle joint.

Suggested Readings

POSTERIOR TIBIALIS TENDON DYSFUNCTION

1. Bluman EM. Stage IV posterior tibial tendon rupture. Foot Ankle Clin. 2007;12:341–362.
2. Foster AP. Rupture of the tibialis posterior tendon: an important differential in the assessment of ankle injuries. Emerg Med J. 2005;22:915–916.
3. Funk DA et al. Acquired adult flat foot secondary to posterior tibial-tendon pathology. J Bone Joint Surg Am. 1986;68:95–102.
4. Hogan J. Posterior tibial tendon dysfunction and MRI. J Foot Ankle Surg. 1993;32:467–472.
5. Kong A, Van Der Vliet A. Imaging of tibialis posterior dysfunction. Br J Radiol. 2008;81:826–836. Epub 2008 Jun 30.
6. Lim P, Schweitzer M, Deely D, et al. Posterior tibial tendon dysfunction: Secondary MR signs. Foot Ankle Int. 1997;18:658–663.
7. Mendicino SS. Posterior tibial tendon dysfunction. Diagnosis, evaluation and treatment. Clin Podiatr Med Surg. 2000;17:33–54.
8. Nabil J. MR Imaging of posttibial tendon dysfunction. AJR Am J Roentgenol. 1996;167,1996.
9. Schweitzer ME, Karasick D. MR Imaging of Disorders of the Posterior Tibialis Tendon. AJR Am J Roentgenol. 2000; 175:627–635.
10. Zehava S. et al. MR Imaging of the Ankle and Foot. Radio-Graphics. 2000;20:S153–S179.

MR APPEARANCES OF FRACTURES

11. Campbell SE, Warner M. MR imaging of ankle inversion injuries. Magn Reson Imaging Clin N Am. 2008;16:1–18, v. Review.
12. Cerezal L et al. MR arthrography of the ankle: indications and technique. Radiol Clin North Am. 2008 Nov;46:973–994, v. Review.
13. Mandalia V, Henson JH. Traumatic bone bruising--a review article. Eur J Radiol. 2008;67:54–61. Epub 2008 Jun 4. Review.
14. Martin B. Ankle sprain complications: MRI evaluation. Clin Podiatr Med Surg. 2008;25(2):203–247, vi. Review.
15. Naran KN, Zoga AC. Osteochondral lesions about the ankle. Radiol Clin North Am. 2008;46:995–1002, v. Review.
16. Oda H. et al. Bone bruise in magnetic resonance imaging strongly correlates with the production of joint effusion and with knee osteoarthritis. J Orthop Sci. 2008;13:7–15. Epub 2008 Feb 16.
17. Potter HG, Chong le R, Sneag DB. Magnetic resonance imaging of cartilage repair. Sports Med Arthrosc. 2008;16:236–245. Review.
18. Winalski CS, Alparslan L. Imaging of articular cartilage injuries of the lower extremity. Semin Musculoskelet Radiol. 2008;12:283–301. Epub 2008 Nov 18.
19. Yamato M. et al. MR appearance at different ages of osteoporotic compression fractures of the vertebrae. Radiat Med. 1998;16:329–334.

FLEXOR HALLUCIS LONGUS TEARS

20. Bureau NJ, et al. Posterior ankle impingement syndrome: MR imaging findings in seven patients. Radiology. May 2000;215:497–503.

21. Boruta PM. et al. Partial tear of the flexor hallucis longus at the knot of Henry: presentation of three cases. Foot Ankle Int. 1997 Apr;18:243–246.

22. Inokuchi S, Usami N. Closed complete rupture of the flexor hallucis longus tendon at the groove of the talus. Foot Ankle Int. 1997;18:47–49.

23. Entrapment of the flexor hallucis longus tendon after fibular fracture. Foot Ankle Int. 1995;16:232.

24. Lo LD, Schweitzer ME, Fan JK, et al. MR imaging findings of entrapment of the flexor hallucis longus tendon. AJR Am J Roentgenol. 2001;176:1145–1148.

25. Sammarco GJ, Cooper PS. Flexor hallucis longus tendon injury in dancers and nondancers. Foot Ankle Int. 1998;19:356–362.

26. Schweitzer ME, van Leersum M, Ehrlich SS, Wapner K. Fluid in normal and abnormal ankle joints: amount and distribution as seen on MR images. AJR Am J Roentgenol. 1994;162:111–114.

27. Trepman E. et al. Partial rupture of the flexor hallucis longus tendon in a tennis player: a case report. Foot Ankle Int. 1995;16:227–231

ANKLE ARTHROPATHY

28. Boutry N. MR imaging appearance of rheumatoid arthritis in the foot. Semin. Musculoskeletal Radiology. 2005;9:199–209.

29. Dobon M, Lucia JF et al: Value of magnetic resonance imaging for the diagnosis and follow-up of haemophilic arthropathy. Haemophilia. 2003;9:76–85.

30. Doria AS et al. Reliability and construct validity of the compatible MRI scoring system for evaluation of haemophilic knees and ankles of haemophilic children. 2006;12:503–513.

31. Friscia DA. Pigmented villonodular synovitis of the ankle: a case report and review of the literature. Foot Ankle Int. 1994;15:674–678.

32. Funk MB et al. Modified magnetic resonance imaging score compared with orthopaedic and radiological scores for the evaluation of haemophilic arthropathy. Hemophilia. 2002;8:98–103.

33. Lundin B et al. New magnetic resonance imaging scoring method for assessment of haemophilic arthropathy. Hemophilia. 2004;10:383–389.

34. Maillefert JF et al. Magnetic resonance imaging in the assessment of synovial inflammation of the hindfoot in patients with rheumatoid arthritis and other polyarthritis. Eur J Radiol. 2003;47:1–5.

35. Ng WH, Chu WC, et al: Role of imaging in management of hemophilic patients. AJR Am J Roentgenol. 2005;184:1619–1623.

36. Morrison WB, Ledermann HP, Schweitzer ME. MR imaging of inflammatory conditions of the ankle and foot. Magn Reson Imaging Clin N Am. 2001;9:615–637, xi-xii.

37. Schweitzer ME, Morrison WB. MR imaging of the diabetic foot. Radiol Clin North Am. 2004;42:61–71, vi.

38. Uri O, Haim A. Ankle joint arthritis—etiology, diagnosis and treatment. Harefuah. 2008;147:897–900, 940, 939.

39. Winalski CS et al. Imaging of articular cartilage injuries of the lower extremity. Semin Musculoskeletal Radiology. 2008;12:283–301. Epub 2008 Nov 18

Case 15

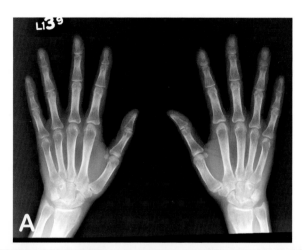

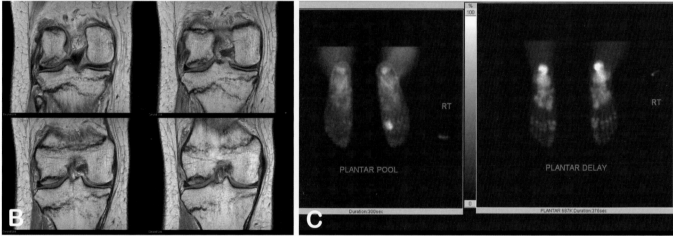

Figure 15-1. (A) Radiograph. Right and left hands. Posteroanterior view. (B) MRI. Right knee. Proton-density-weighted. Coronal view. (C) Three-phase technetium-99m methylene diphosphonate (Tc-99m MDP) bone scan. Plantar view. Pool- and delayed-phase images.

Question 68

A 44-year-old woman had a 3-year history of pain in her back and throughout her lower extremities. She used a walker and had been on disability for 2 years. Evaluation included an electromyogram and a thigh muscle biopsy, both of which yielded negative results. You are shown a posteroanterior radiograph of both hands (Figure 15-1A), a coronal MR image of the knee (Figure 15-1B), and a bone scan (Figure 15-1C). Which *one* of the following is the MOST likely diagnosis?

(A)   X-linked hypophosphatemia
(B)   Fanconi syndrome
(C)   Oncogenic osteomalacia
(D)   Autosomal dominant hypophosphatemic rickets
(E)   Hypophosphatasia

Brandon M. Schooley, M.D.

Oncogenic Osteomalacia

Question 68

Which *one* of the following is the MOST likely diagnosis?

(A) X-linked hypophosphatemia
(B) Fanconi syndrome
(C) Oncogenic osteomalacia
(D) Autosomal dominant hypophosphatemic rickets
(E) Hypophosphatasia

Figure 15-2A, a posteroanterior radiograph of both hands, revealed lucencies involving the distal phalanx of each of the right second through fourth and the left second and third digits; these lucencies were suggestive of pseudofractures. Figure 15-2B, a coronal proton-density-weighted MR image of the right knee, revealed multiple hypointense curvilinear foci representing nondisplaced insufficiency fractures in the distal femoral and the proximal tibial metadiaphyses and in the lateral femoral condyle. Identical findings were present on the left (not shown). Pool- and delayed-phase images from a three-phase technetium-99m methylene diphosphonate (Tc-99m MDP) bone scan (Figure 15-2C) revealed a focus of increased radiotracer uptake adjacent to the first metatarsophalangeal joint on the pool phase but not on the delayed phase. Flow images (not shown) also revealed increased uptake. This constellation of findings suggests tumor, cellulitis, or other focal soft-tissue process.

Oncogenic osteomalacia is an unusual paraneoplastic syndrome that is not well known to many primary

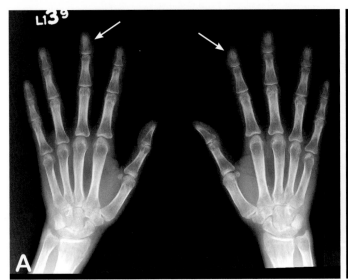
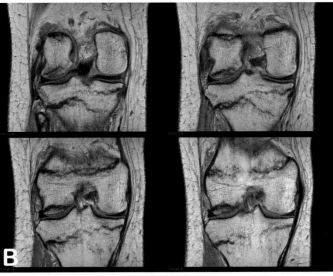

Figure 15-2 (Same as Figure 15-1). Oncogenic osteomalacia. (A) Radiograph. Posteroanterior view. Right and left hands. The image shows lucencies involving the distal phalanx of each of the right second through fourth and the left second and third digits, findings that suggest pseudo-fractures. (B) Proton-density-weighted MRI. Coronal view. Right knee. The image shows multiple hypointense curvilinear foci representing nondisplaced insufficiency fractures in the distal femoral and the proximal tibial metadiaphyses and in the lateral femoral condyle. Identical findings were present on the left (not shown).

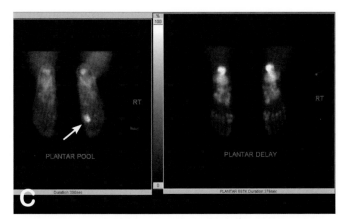

Figure 15-2 (Same as Figure 15-1). Oncogenic osteomalacia. (C) Three-phase Tc-99m MDP bone scan. Plantar view. Pool- and delayed-phase images. A focus of increased radiotracer uptake adjacent to the first metatarsophalangeal joint is seen on the pool phase but not on the delayed phase. Flow images (not shown) also demonstrated increased uptake. This constellation of findings suggests tumor, cellulitis, or other focal soft-tissue process.

and subspecialty physicians and that is attributable to a circulating substance secreted by the inducing neoplasm. Although the disorder is within the spectrum of hypophosphatemic osteomalacia, it is unique in that the symptoms resolve and the laboratory values normalize after the surgical removal of the inciting tumor. Since the first case report, by McCance in 1947, approximately 110 cases have been reported in the medical literature as of May 2007. This small number of reported cases may be attributable to the poor recognition of this disorder in the clinical community. Most cases involve patients more than 40 years old, although a small number of cases have been reported in children and teenagers. The male-to-female distribution has been reported to be 1:1.

The causative tumor is often a small, slowly growing, and clinically insignificant benign mesenchymal tumor (Figure 15-3). Symptoms often precede tumor detection by months to years for these reasons, with reported cases of the tumor being found up to 19 years after the development of initial manifestations and the mean period from symptom onset to diagnosis being approximately 5 years. Although the tumor itself is usually not apparent and clinically insignificant, the generalized debilitating symptoms are of concern to patients. Bone pain, usually involving the lower back, pelvis, hips, and legs, is a predominant symptom. Patients can experience pain, atrophy, and weakness of the proximal muscles; some patients are unable to rise from a seated position. Significant gait disturbances can also occur **(Option (C) is correct)**

In general, bone pain, difficulty walking, and insufficiency fractures in a typical distribution (i.e., bilateral and symmetric) are suggestive of a metabolic bone

disease. The clinical workup begins with a laboratory evaluation of metabolic and endocrinologic factors. Levels of calcium, phosphorus, and alkaline phospha-

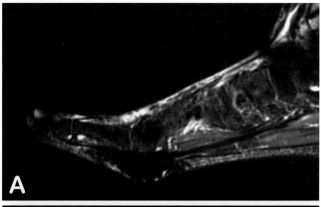

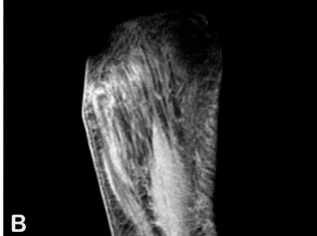

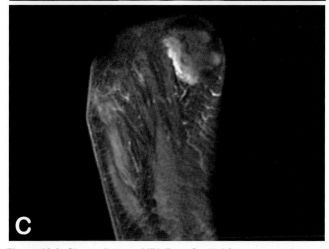

Figure 18-3. Giant cell tumor. MRI. Foot. Sagittal fat-suppressed T2-weighted (A) and axial pregadolinium (B) and postgadolinium (C) fat-suppressed spoiled gradient-recalled (SPGR) images of plantar tissues show a soft-tissue mass abutting or arising from the flexor tendon of the first digit. The mass is hypointense on the T2-weighted image, isointense relative to muscle on the precontrast SPGR image, and shows a moderate degree of homogeneous enhancement on the postcontrast image. The findings suggest hemangiopericytoma or giant cell tumor (likely of the tendon sheath). Surgery revealed that the lesion was not attached to nor did it arise from the tendon. Pathologic evaluation led to a diagnosis of giant cell tumor.

tase in serum should be determined, and standard physiologic measurements, such as complete blood count, glucose levels, renal function, and liver enzyme levels, should be obtained. For further investigation, the levels of 25-hydroxyvitamin D (the inactive form of vitamin D), 1,25-dihydroxyvitamin D (the active form), and calcium and phosphorus in urine, along with a variable known as the tubular maximum for phosphate corrected for the glomerular filtration rate, which is a factor independent of both plasma phosphate and renal function and which evaluates renal phosphate processing, are useful. A more detailed workup to further narrow the differential diagnosis should include levels of parathyroid hormone (PTH), PTH-related hormone, calcitonin, creatine phosphokinase, antinuclear antibodies, and rheumatoid factor; serum protein electrophoresis; and levels of glucose, amino acids, and Bence Jones proteins in urine.

Osteomalacia is defined as a disorder of bone that is characterized by inadequate or delayed mineralization of osteoid into mature cortical and spongy bone and that is attributable to a deficiency of calcium, phosphorus, or vitamin D. The initial workup of suspected osteomalacia should include a detailed clinical history focusing on whether the patient has a dietary, genetic or inherited, or environmental etiology as the cause of the deficiency. In the initial laboratory evaluation, obtaining levels of PTH in serum can assist in determining which of these deficiencies is the root of the problem. The levels of PTH increase when calcium, vitamin D, or both are deficient but typically is normal in the presence of a phosphorus deficiency. A vitamin D deficiency is the most common etiology of osteomalacia and can be attributable to decreased intake, malabsorption (including iatrogenic causes, such as gastrectomy and small-bowel resection), decreased sun exposure (because of cultural factors, such as the wearing of burkas in the Middle East, or living in areas with less sunlight or shorter days), or a combination of these. It has been proposed that about 25% of the older population in the United States may have hypovitaminosis D because of a combination of diet, geography, insufficient sun exposure, and the decrease in gastrointestinal absorption that occurs with age. Other etiologies of vitamin D deficiency–induced osteomalacia, all of which are commonly seen in the older population, include the long-term usage of antiseizure medications and as a side effect of nonabsorbable antacids and bisphosphonates, such as etidronate. In the past, vitamin D deficiency–induced osteomalacia was a frequent sequela of renal osteodystrophy, which is also not uncommon in the older population. The occurrence of this etiology has decreased recently because of oral supplementation with vitamin D. According to DiMeglio et al, isolated dietary phosphate deficiency is exceedingly rare in Western countries because most residents have high-phosphate diets; however, the use of phosphate-binding antacids can cause chronic hypophosphatemia. Additionally, acute hypophosphatemia can result from intracellular phosphate shifts in conditions such as carbohydrate refeeding of malnourished patients and the treatment of diabetic ketoacidosis.

Presenting findings in osteomalacia include diffuse bone pain (especially in the spine, ribs, pelvis, and shoulder girdles), proximal muscle weakness, and polyarthralgias. Some patients have a family history of X-linked hypophosphatemia (XLH). Many patients have normal levels of calcium and 1,25-dihydroxyvitamin D in serum but decreased levels of phosphorus. The multiple overlapping symptoms and radiographic findings seen in osteomalacia can lead to much confusion about the underlying etiology. On a nuclear medicine bone scan, multiple areas of increased radiotracer uptake can be seen because a bone scan is more sensitive to changes in bone metabolism than other methods. These foci of increased uptake represent sites of active osteomalacia and its associated reparative bone formation but can be misinterpreted as sites of osseous metastatic disease, multiple myeloma, or other etiologies (Figure 15-4). Osteomalacia can be misdiagnosed as osteoporosis, because the pseudofractures of osteomalacia can be subtle, missed, or both; the only radiographic finding may be the decreased bone density. Pseudofractures, also known as Looser zones, are lucencies that appear perpendicular to the cortex of the bone because of persistent nonmineralized osteoid with surrounding sclerosis (essentially representing a poorly mineralized callus).

Because of complaints of myalgias and bone pain mixed with resultant depression, psychiatric disorders have been diagnosed, even resulting in admission to psychiatric wards. There are other reports of patients with osteomalacia being diagnosed with fibromyalgia, polymyalgia rheumatica, polymyositis, rheumatoid arthritis, ankylosing spondylitis, diffuse idiopathic skeletal hyperostosis, algodystrophy, osteitis fibrosa cystica, and multiple myeloma. The test patient was, at different stages in her workup, suspected of having a herniated lumbar intervertebral disk, a reaction to medication, complex regional pain syndrome, a parathyroid disorder, a viral infection, or a combination of these. She was seen by clinicians in multiple subspecialties, including podiatry, neurology, rheumatology, endocrinology, and orthopedic surgery. The first suggestion of either hypophosphatemia or oncogenic osteomalacia in the medical record by any clinician was made by a radiologist approximately 3 years after symptom onset and nearly 14 months after she initially sought care for this complaint.

A reasonable initial radiologic evaluation in a case of osteomalacia or other metabolic bone disease would include a skeletal survey, a bone densitometry evaluation, or both. Changes on radiographs are often subtle and initially missed. Radiographic evidence of osteomalacia includes diffuse decreased bone density; fractures of various ages with no history of appropriate trauma; a typical distribution of pseudofractures (bilateral and symmetric at the concave surfaces of bones, such as the medial proximal femora, medial proximal tibiae, pubic rami, ribs, and axillary margins of the scapulae); and, in certain cases, thickening of long bones because of subperiosteal deposition (enthesopathy).

The differential diagnosis for renal phosphate wasting disorders resulting in hypophosphatemic osteomalacia can be narrowed on the basis of age of onset and whether the loss of phosphate is isolated (as in oncogenic osteomalacia, XLH, and autosomal dominant hypophosphatemic rickets [ADHR]) or is seen in conjunction with other losses (as in Fanconi syndrome and renal tubular acidosis). XLH is the most common cause of hyperphosphaturia and hypophosphatemia, resulting

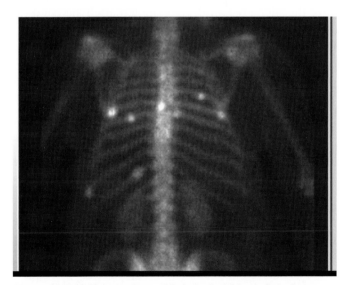

Figure 15-4. Multiple myeloma. Whole-body delayed-phase bone scan. Magnified view. Thorax. The image shows multiple foci of increased radiotracer uptake in the ribs and the thoracic spine. The eventual diagnosis was multiple myeloma, but a patient with osteomalacia could have similar findings, particularly in the ribs. Osseous metastatic disease also cannot be fully excluded on the basis of these imaging findings.

in the ineffective renal tubular reabsorption of phosphorus. One-third of cases are sporadic. This disorder has been traditionally termed vitamin D–resistant rickets in children because of the poor response to vitamin D supplementation.

As an important component of hydroxyapatite (the major substance composing bone mineral), inorganic phosphate is essential for skeletal mineralization; for multiple cellular functions, including glycolysis, gluconeogenesis, DNA synthesis, RNA synthesis, and cellular protein phosphorylation; as an element of cell membranes; and in intracellular regulatory roles. Dietary intake, intestinal absorption, and renal tubular filtration and reabsorption determine phosphate homeostasis. Dietary phosphate is primarily absorbed in the jejenum and ileum in proportion to food phosphate content. If phosphate intake is very low, then vitamin D metabolites have a role in increasing phosphate absorption through the gastrointestinal tract. Phosphate reabsorption occurs in the renal proximal tubules and is modulated by several peptide and steroid hormones. Growth hormones, insulinlike growth factor 1, insulin, epidermal growth factor, thyroid hormone, and 1,25-dihydroxyvitamin D stimulate renal phosphate reabsorption. PTH, PTH-related peptide, calcitonin, atrial natriuretic factor, and glucocorticoids inhibit this process. A prolonged deficiency of phosphorus and inorganic phosphate results in significant biological problems, including impaired mineralization of bone resulting in osteomalacia or rickets; abnormal erythrocyte, leukocyte, and platelet functions; impaired cell membrane integrity, which can result in rhabdomyolysis; and impaired cardiac output. Therefore, the maintenance of appropriate phosphorus homeostasis is critical for the well-being of the organism.

For the circulating paraneoplastic compound generally known as "phosphatonin" to result in the phenotype seen in hypophosphatemic osteomalacia, it must do each of the following: inhibit the enzyme 25-hydroxyvitamin D-1-α-hydroxylase, inhibit phosphorus reabsorption by the kidneys, be expressed by the tumor, be present at an increased concentration in the blood of patients with tumor-induced osteomalacia, and be present at a decreased concentration after tumor removal.

Through a variety of biochemical and molecular methods, at least four phosphate-regulating substances have been isolated from phosphate-wasting tumors associated with tumor-induced osteomalacia: fibroblast growth factor 23 (FGF-23), secreted frizzled related protein 4 (sFRP-4), matrix extracellular phosphoglycoprotein (MEPE), and fibroblast growth factor 7 (FGF-7).

Among these substances, the most information is available for FGF-23, which decreases the concentration of the protein Npt2a, a sodium-phosphorus cotransporter responsible for phosphorus reabsorption in the proximal renal tubules. FGF-23 is expressed by tumors associated with oncogenic osteomalacia, and its concentration in serum has been shown to decrease after removal of the neoplasm. In healthy people, a decreased level of phosphorus should result in a decreased level of FGF-23 (or any other hyperphosphaturic compound) to allow the increased reabsorption of phosphorus in the renal tubules. Therefore, in the presence of low phosphorus and 1,25-dihydroxyvitamin D levels, the normal or elevated levels of FGF-23 observed in oncogenic osteomalacia are not appropriate for the known biochemical feedback loop, meaning that FGF-23 is likely being secreted ectopically. When synthetic FGF-23 has been administered in clinical trials, hypophosphatemia and renal phosphate wasting have been shown. When the FGF-23 gene has been inactivated in some studies, hyperphosphatemia has resulted. Elevated FGF-23 levels have also been seen in XLH, fibrous dysplasia, and renal failure. In the test patient, FGF-23 levels decreased from 377 relative units per milliliter at 1 day after surgery to 98 relative units per milliliter (normal) at 2 months after surgery. In oncogenic osteomalacia, the serum phosphorus level is decreased, and the urine phosphorus level typically is increased. The serum calcium level is nearly always normal, and the PTH level is normal or slightly elevated. The 25-hydroxyvitamin D level is usually normal, but the level of active 1,25-dihydroxyvitamin D is decreased. In healthy people, a low level of 1,25-dihydroxyvitamin D is a powerful stimulus for an increase in the serum phosphorus level through the positive effects of PTH on the activity of the converting enzyme 1-α-hydroxylase; however, in oncogenic osteomalacia, this enzyme is inhibited by circulating phosphatonin. Because of the low level of 1,25-dihydroxyvitamin D, a vitamin D deficiency must be excluded first because it is the most common etiology of osteomalacia. The alkaline phosphatase level is increased in oncogenic osteomalacia. The level of alkaline phosphatase increases in disorders with bone formation with or without destruction but not in disorders with only bone destruction; this fact makes alkaline phosphatase useful in differentiating osteomalacia from osteoporosis, in which there is no new bone formation.

In an adult with a new onset of hypophosphatemic osteomalacia, tumor-induced osteomalacia should be the primary differential diagnosis, especially once dietary, genetic, or environmental causes have been excluded and there are no measurable losses of other substances in the urine. The primary goal of a clinical workup is to eliminate from the differential diagnosis the more malignant neoplasms that can result in hypophosphatemia through a paraneoplastic substance, such as breast, prostate, and small-cell lung carcinomas. Although these are less common causes of oncogenic osteomalacia, they are of significantly more immediate concern. The search for the inciting tumor should then focus on the more common (usually benign) etiologies, such as small mesenchymal tumors.

Once the inducing neoplasm has been removed, serum phosphorus levels, indexes of renal phosphate wasting, and circulating levels of 1,25-dihydroxyvitamin D return to normal within hours to days. In the test patient, for example, the phosphorus level was 1.3 mg/dL on the day of surgery and had increased to normal limits (2.9 mg/dL) by 4 days after surgery. The levels of 1,25-dihydroxyvitamin D were 13 pg/mL before surgery and 144 pg/mL after surgery. Biochemical markers of bone turnover, such as osteocalcin and alkaline phosphatase, take longer to normalize, and resolution of the radiographic changes of osteomalacia can take months. Symptoms nearly always resolve completely and quickly.

When the tumor is not found, therapy with oral neutral phosphorus and 1,25-dihydroxyvitamin D is instituted, just as it is for hypophosphatemic osteomalacia attributable to other etiologies. Patients show some improvement in symptoms and laboratory values with the medications but do not show complete resolution and have the added risk of developing tertiary hyperparathyroidism. Bypassing medical treatment in such cases can lead to patients becoming bedridden, with severe weakness and bone pain, and developing numerous fractures.

Compared with oncogenic osteomalacia, XLH usually results in less severe bone pain and proximal muscle weakness, a less significant increase in the alkaline phosphatase level, and less significant decreases in the serum 1,25-dihydroxyvitamin D and phosphorus levels. In fact, the level of 1,25-dihydroxyvitamin D in XLH is often normal. Oncogenic osteomalacia affects older patients and is progressive, whereas XLH typically appears early, usually in the second year of life **(Option (A) is incorrect)**.

Table 15-1 lists the differentiating factors for the most common forms of hypophosphatemic osteomalacia. The prevalence of XLH is approximately 1 in 20,000, with equal male and female distributions. Patients are often of short stature and have lower-extremity deformities, bone pain, and dental abscesses; in severe cases, cranial abnormalities and symptoms of spinal stenosis can occur as a result of short pedicles with superimposed calcification or ossification of the apophyseal ligaments and ligamentum flavum (Figure 15-5). Radiographs of children with XLH demonstrate typical findings of rickets, including metaphyseal cupping, fraying, and widening of and periosteal reaction adjacent to rapidly growing long bones, such as the ulna, radius, tibia, and distal femur (Figure 15-6). In adults, generalized osteopenia and pseudofractures can be seen in addition to lower-extremity bowing deformities (Figure 15-7). Older patients with XLH often have osteoarthrosis in the weight-bearing joints, especially the hips and ankles. Radiographs of patients with XLH can also demonstrate osteosclerosis and pronounced enthesopathy resulting in increased bone density in

the axial skeleton but decreased density peripherally (Figure 15-8). The pronounced enthesopathy worsens with age and can result in limited range of motion, joint dysfunction, and spinal facet or sacroiliac joint fusion. This final point can blur the differentiation from ankylosing spondylitis, although ankylosing spondylitis and the other seronegative spondyloarthropathies typically also show erosions and syndesmophytes (Figure 15-9). Further complicating the radiographic diagnosis in such cases is the fact that generalized enthesopathy can also be seen in diffuse idiopathic skeletal hyperostosis, fluorosis, and retinoid-induced hyperostosis. Diffuse idiopathic skeletal hyperostosis usually also shows ossification of the anterior longitudinal ligament. Fluorosis, in

Table 15-1. Differentiating factors for the most common forms of osteomalacia			
Factor	Nutritional hypophosphatemic osteomalacia	Oncogenic osteomalacia	X-linked hypophosphatemic osteomalacia
Population	Children, older people, populations with cultural or iatrogenic factors	Adults (usually new onset); rarely children or teenagers	Children (usually apparent by 2 years of age)
Serum calcium level	Decreased or low to normal	Normal	Normal
Serum 25-hydroxyvitamin D level	Decreased	Normal	Normal
Serum 1,25-dihydroxyvitamin D level	Decreased, normal, or increased	Decreased	Normal or slightly decreased
Serum PTH level	Increased	Normal or increased	Normal or slightly increased
Serum alkaline phosphatase level	Increased	Increased	Slightly increased
Urine calcium level	Decreased	Normal	Normal
Urine phosphate level	Normal	Normal	Normal
Renal phosphate clearance	Normal	Increased	Increased
Distinguishing characteristics	History	Tumor present Increased FGF-23 level Progressive if not treated	In children, radiographic findings typical of rickets In adults, osteosclerosis and pronounced enthesopathy resulting in increased bone density in the axial skeleton despite decreased bone density peripherally

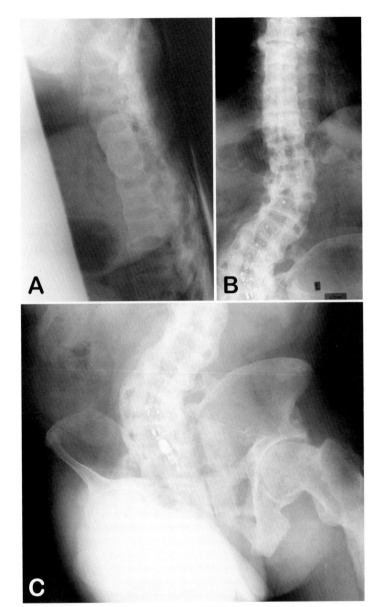

Figure 15-5. X-linked hypophosphatemia. Radiographs. Lateral view of the lumbar spine (A) and frontal views of the thoracolumbar and lumbar spine (B) and pelvis (C) in a patient with documented XLH show diffuse ligamentous ossification with short pedicles superimposed on scoliosis, resulting in spinal stenosis. Mild diffuse demineralization of the osseous structures is evident. Deformity of the proximal left femur, likely related to long-standing osteomalacia, can be seen. Radiopaque density throughout the course of the spinal canal represents residual myelogram iophendylate (Pantopaque) contrast from earlier interventions.

addition to the insufficiency fractures and short stature seen in osteomalacia, also shows osteophyte formation. Retinoid toxicity is only seen in patients with a history of retinoid use.

Fanconi syndrome is a rare dysfunction of the renal tubules with loss of phosphorus, amino acids, glucose, and bicarbonate into the urine, resulting in metabolic acidosis. Because of the large number of substances

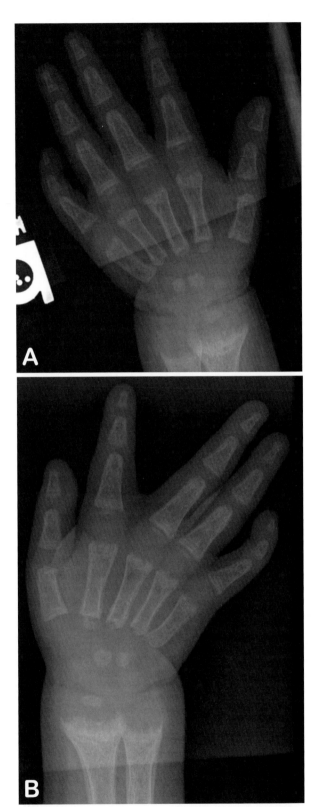

Figure 15-6. X-linked hypophosphatemia with findings typical of rickets. Radiographs. (A and B) Posteroanterior view. Hands. Images of the left (A) and right (B) hands in the same patient demonstrate cupping, fraying, and widening of the metaphyses of the distal radii, distal ulnae, metacarpal bones, and proximal phalanges. Also evident is a smooth periosteal reaction that is adjacent to the diaphyses of the radii, ulnae, and metacarpal bones and that is typical of rickets.

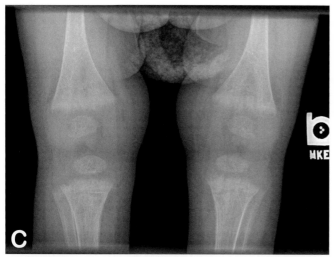

Figure 15-6 (continued). X-linked hypophosphatemia with findings typical of rickets. Radiographs. (C) Frontal view. Knees. The image of the knees in another patient shows a similar symmetric periosteal reaction and similar metaphyseal changes, again consistent with rickets.

whose reabsorption is affected, Fanconi syndrome is likely related to a malfunction in cellular energy metabolism instead of a defect involving each specific transporter. This malfunction in energy metabolism is itself induced by other abnormalities, such as cystinosis, galactosemia, and fructose intolerance. The clinical features include polyuria, polydipsia, dehydration, impaired growth, and bony deformities **(Option (B) is incorrect).**

Differentiating oncogenic osteomalacia from ADHR is often very difficult. ADHR affects males and females

equally and shows incomplete penetrance. When it presents in childhood, patients show the clinical and growth features described above for XLH. Adults show symptoms and radiographic features similar to those seen in patients with XLH and oncogenic osteomalacia, including bone pain, muscle weakness, and fractures. ADHR does not include the presence of a causative neoplasm **(Option (D) is incorrect).** Once patients are diagnosed with ADHR, treatment with oral vitamin D, phosphorus, and calcium as well as increased sun exposure has been shown to result in gradually increasing bone density on bone densitometry examinations performed every 6 months. This technique could presumably be used to decide when to decrease or stop phosphate supplementation to keep phosphorus levels in the low to normal range and to keep bone density normal, thereby decreasing the chances of a patient on therapy developing nephrocalcinosis and/or hyperparathyroidism.

Hypophosphatasia is a rare deficiency of alkaline phosphatase that has a wide spectrum of severity and that causes defective mineralization. This disorder affects males and females equally, with an incidence of 1 in 100,000. Patients have multiple stress fractures and diffuse changes of osteoarthrosis in the pelvis, lumbar spine, hips, knees, wrists, and hands **(Option (E) is incorrect).** Radiologically, flaring of the tibial metaphyses, cortical thinning, pseudofractures, and chondrocalcinosis can be seen. In children, bowed legs are common; adults typically show the findings of osteoarthrosis listed above. Normal levels of calcium, PTH, and inactive and active forms of vitamin D in serum are

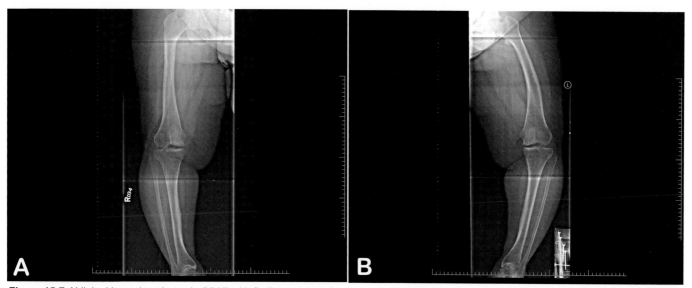

Figure 15-7. X-linked hypophosphatemia (XLH) with findings typical of osteopenia. Radiographs. Frontal view. Lower extremities. Standing images of the right (A) and left (B) lower extremities show osteopenia and severe genu varus deformity bilaterally in a 24-year-old woman; these findings can be seen in hypophosphatemic osteomalacia. This patient has a 5-year-old daughter who also has radiographic findings within the spectrum of hypophosphatemic osteomalacia, suggesting XLH.

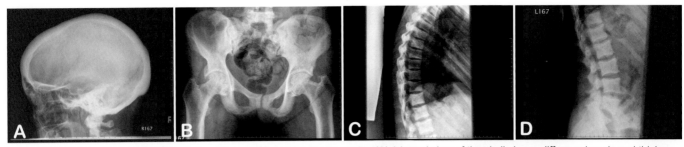

Figure 15-8. X-linked hypophosphatemia in a 55-year-old woman. Radiographs. (A) A lateral view of the skull shows diffuse sclerosis and thickening of the calvarium. (B) A frontal view of the pelvis shows diffuse sclerosis of the pelvic bones but resorptive changes in the femoral necks, pubic symphysis, and ischia, with resultant bowing of the femora and varus deformities of the hips; mild acetabular protrusion is also evident. (C and D) Lateral views of the thoracic spine (C) and lumbar spine (D) show diffuse multilevel vertebral sclerosis. Early enthesophyte formation is also evident in the upper and middle lumbar spine in panel D

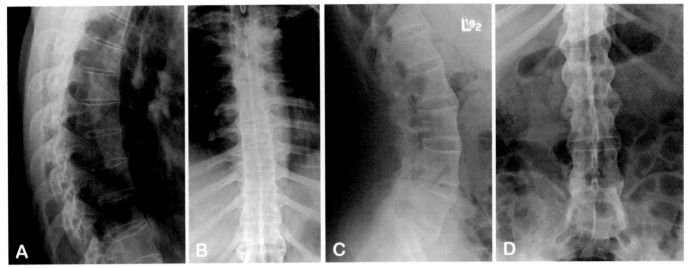

Figure 15-9. Ankylosing spondylitis. Radiographs. Spine. (A and B) Lateral (A) and frontal (B) views of the thoracic spine show the formation of syndesmophytes throughout the thoracic spine, resulting in diffuse ankylosis. (C and D) Lateral (C) and frontal (B) radiographs of the lumbosacral spine show similar findings of syndesmophytes and ankylosis in addition to fusion of both sacroiliac joints in a young male patient with confirmed ankylosing spondylitis.

present in the setting of decreased serum phosphorus and increased urinary phosphorus levels.

Question 69

Which *one* of the following is the BEST next step in the workup for a patient who has osteomalacia with low serum phosphate levels, evidence of renal phosphate wasting, no family history of a metabolic bone disorder, and no identifiable nutritional etiology?

(A) Whole-body delayed-phase bone scan
(B) Whole-body CT
(C) "Whole-body" MRI
(D) In-111 pentetreotide imaging

The appropriate order of the image-guided search for the inciting tumor in oncogenic osteomalacia is

debatable and has changed in recent years because of the advent and improvement of imaging techniques. The newest of these useful imaging methods is performed with Indium-111 pentetreotide (trade name: OctreoScan), which has been approved by the U.S. Food and Drug Administration for the imaging of neuroendocrine and other tumors with somatostatin receptors. These include pituitary tumors, pancreatic islet cell tumors, carcinoid tumors, medullary thyroid carcinomas, paragangliomas, pheochromocytomas, neuroblastomas, meningiomas, astrocytomas, malignant thymomas, breast cancers, small-cell lung cancers, and lymphomas. The accuracy of In-111 pentetreotide in the search for these tumors has ranged from 30% to 90%, depending on the specific tumor being investigated. Because many mesenchymal tumors have also been found to possess somatostatin receptors, the newer In-111–labeled somatostatin analogs (pentetreotide and octreotide) have been proposed for tumor localization in oncogenic osteomalacia **(Option (D) is correct).**

One limitation in the use of these substances is that In-111pentetreotide protocols at many institutions involve the acquisition of only planar images of the chest and abdomen (Figure 15-10). Such protocols can significantly limit the search for the common benign mesenchymal tumors that usually cause oncogenic osteomalacia because these tumors are more likely to occur in the extremities, in particular, the hands and feet; planar images of the extremities should be included when oncogenic osteomalacia is suspected. Additional assistance in localizing tumors can be provided by use of SPECT in addition to planar imaging. These radiolabeled somatostatin analogs, along with other metabolic markers under investigation, should be of great utility in the future.

During the workup to investigate a patient's symptoms, particularly generalized bone pain, a nuclear medicine bone scan with Tc-99m methylene diphosphonate (Figure 15-2C) can incidentally reveal a focus of soft-tissue uptake that correlates with the causative neoplasm. However, because the tumor is usually small and often only whole-body delayed-phase images are

obtained because of the nonspecific nature and generalized distribution of the complaints, the tumor can be missed unless a three-phase study with localized pool-phase images of a region of concern is performed **(Option (A) is incorrect).**

Whole-body CT has been used in the past but is generally now avoided because of the risks of excessive radiation exposure, which are of continually increasing concern to the medical community and public at large **(Option (B) is incorrect).**

Studies with "whole-body" MRI have also been undertaken—as survey studies. In 1996, Avila et al used axial short-T1 inversion recovery images of the cranium, thorax, and abdomen and coronal short-T1 inversion recovery images of the proximal upper and lower extremities. In 1999, Fukumoto et al divided all major bones into groups and screened them with T1- and T2-weighted images with the following sequences: axial sections of the skull and thorax, sagittal sections of the spine, and coronal sections of the upper and lower limbs. T1 sequences are more useful for evaluating osseous structures, and T2 sequences are better for soft-tissue masses. The inciting tumor is usually hypointense on T1-weighted images, hyperintense on T2-weighted images, or both. Although this technique

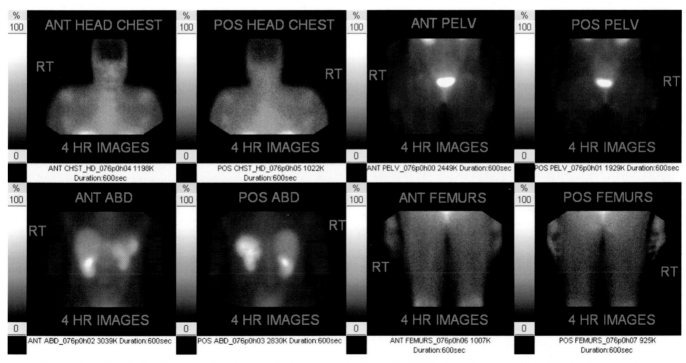

Figure 15-10. Tumor localization in oncogenic osteomalacia. In-111 pentetreotide scan. Static planar images. Chest, abdomen (ABD), pelvis (PELV), and thighs. The images show no abnormal focus of increased radiotracer uptake. In cases of suspected oncogenic osteomalacia, additional planar images of the remainder of the extremities would be useful in identifying an inconspicuous mesenchymal tumor. If a focus is found on planar images, then SPECT image acquisition would improve localization. ANT = anterior; POS = posterior; RT = right; HR = hour.

is expensive, it is often useful for finding the neoplasm and then definitively treating the patient's primary disorder to avoid the lifelong costs and complications of the medical treatments that are instituted when the tumor is not identified. Due to cost and time issues, such studies are done, by necessity, as surveys. As such, they do not include all of the possible anatomy, a fact that contributes to the risk that the tumor will not be in the field of view on any of the obtained sequences **(Option (C) is incorrect).**

No matter what imaging technique is used, the mass is most often located (in decreasing order of frequency) in the lower limbs (especially the soles of the feet), the head (nasopharynx, ethmoid air cells, mandible, paranasal sinuses, and skull), the upper limbs (the palms of the hands), and the abdominal wall.

Question 70

Which *one* of the following is the MOST commonly diagnosed tumor or process in a patient with oncogenic osteomalacia:

(A) Giant cell tumor of tendon sheath, bone, or soft tissues
(B) Angiofibroma
(C) Osteosarcoma
(D) Hemangiopericytoma
(E) Fibrous dysplasia

A wide range of tumors can cause oncogenic osteomalacia, but 84% of the tumors fall within a category known as phosphaturic mesenchymal tumors (mixed connective-tissue variants). This category includes masses with primitive stromal cells, variably prominent vessels with a hemangiopericyte pattern, osteoclastlike giant cells, focal areas of microcystic changes, osseous metaplasia, and poorly defined chondroid islands. Tumors in this category occasionally behave in a malignant fashion; for this reason, a wide margin at surgical excision is recommended. Approximately 50% of these inciting tumors are somewhat vascular.

Falling within this category and being the single most commonly diagnosed tumor causing osteomalacia is hemangiopericytoma **(Option (D) is correct).** When hemangiopericytomas occur in bone, they appear as lytic lesions in metaphyses of long or flat bones, usually in the lower extremities, vertebrae, pelvis, and skull. The appearance is similar to that of aneurysmal bone cysts. In soft tissues, hemangiopericytomas are slowly growing, well-circumscribed, painless tumors in muscles, often in the lower extremities, pelvis, and retroperitoneum.

Widely reported as the second most common etiology are giant cell tumors, which can arise from a tendon sheath, soft tissues, or bone **(Option (A) is incorrect).** Other causative neoplasms that are derived from mesenchymal tissues and that have been reported in the literature are hemangiomas (including the sclerosing type), mesenteric angiomas, angiofibromas **(Option (B) is incorrect),** fibromas (nonossifying and ossifying), fibrosarcomas, odontogenic maxillary tumors, osteoblastomas, malignant fibrous histiocytomas, chondromas, chondroblastomas, chondrosarcomas, and osteosarcomas, including the rare intracortical type **(Option (C) is incorrect).**

Often of more concern than these entities (most of which are benign) and vital to diagnose early are tumors that are epithelial in origin and that are more apt to behave in a malignant way. These include multiple myelomas, lymphocytic leukemias, breast carcinomas, small-cell lung carcinomas, and prostate carcinomas. Because of the potentially drastic results of metastatic spread, a workup to exclude each of these tumors should be undertaken once the suspicion of tumor-induced osteomalacia arises, even before the search for the more likely small, benign mesenchymal tumors is begun.

Still other causes of hypophosphatemic osteomalacia that are related not to a focal lesion but rather to a systemic or multifocal process have been described. These include neurofibromatosis type 2, melorheostosis, epidermal nevus syndrome, Paget disease, fibrous dysplasia **(Option (E) is incorrect),** and the use of tenofovir-containing highly active antiretroviral therapy for patients with AIDS. As evidenced by the study of Collins et al, in which 48% of patients with fibrous dysplasia had renal phosphate wasting and proteinuria, the presence of phosphatoninlike substances resulting in hypophosphatemia and subsequent osteomalacia is not unusual in these common disorders and clinical situations.

Question 71

Which *one* of the following is the gold standard for the diagnosis of osteomalacia?

(A) Radiographic skeletal survey
(B) Nuclear medicine bone scan
(C) Bone biopsy
(D) Bone densitometry

The gold standard for confirming osteomalacia is a bone biopsy, usually performed at the iliac crest, after double tetracycline labeling **(Option (C) is correct)**. In osteomalacia, a biopsy shows a disproportionately increased amount of osteoid versus mineralized bone. Tetracycline is normally deposited at the mineralization front and is incorporated into the bone as mineralization occurs, with the tetracycline moving away from the mineralization front and into the bone. Approximately 3 weeks before an iliac crest biopsy, oral tetracycline is administered at 25 mg/kg. A second, identical dose is given 1 week before the biopsy, and the distance between the two labels is measured; this value can be converted into the rate of mineralization (in micrometers per day). The distance between the two tetracycline labels is shorter in a patient with osteomalacia than in a healthy person; the two labels can be so close that they appear as an indistinct smear.

Radiographic skeletal surveys are useful for demonstrating the diffuse demineralization that is seen in osteomalacia (along with osteoporosis and many other diagnoses) and the pseudofractures that are classic in osteomalacia alone; however, these findings are too nonspecific to narrow the differential diagnosis in the way a confirmatory test should **(Option (A) is incorrect)**.

The results of a bone scan, as discussed above, are often positive for osteomalacia, with areas of increased radiotracer uptake that represent foci of active osteoblastic activity in response to decreased bone mineralization and developing pseudofractures. These foci of increased radiotracer uptake are nonspecific, however, and could also represent reparative areas in other forms of metabolic bone disease, foci of multiple myeloma or osseous metastatic disease, degenerative changes, or fractures (whether they be traumatic, pathologic, stress induced, or related to insufficiency). Obviously, a test that is unable to distinguish among so many diagnostic possibilities is not useful as a gold standard **(Option (B) is incorrect)**.

Bone mineral density measurements are very reliable in evaluating bone density and detecting bone demineralization. Studies have shown a statistical correlation between histology and bone mineral density measurements in several metabolic bone diseases, including osteomalacia and osteoporosis. Therein lies the problem, however: although bone densitometry is often sensitive for osteomalacia, it is not specific enough to act as a confirmatory test **(Option (D) is incorrect)**. However, bone density measurements are extremely useful in evaluating the success or failure of therapy once a diagnosis has been made.

Suggested Readings

HYPOPHOSPHATEMIC OSTEOMALACIA

1. Brandenburg VM, Ketteler M, Frank RD, et al. Bone pain with scintigraphy suggestive of widespread metastases—do not forget phosphate. Nephrol Dial Transplant. 2002;17:504–507.
2. Imanishi Y, Nakatsuka K, Nakayama T, et al. False-positive magnetic resonance imaging skeletal survey in a patient with sporadic hypophosphatemic osteomalacia. J Bone Miner Metab. 2003;21:57–59.
3. Jacobson JA, Kalume-Brigido M. Case 97: X-linked hypophosphatemic osteomalacia with insufficiency fracture. Radiology. 2006;240:607–610.
4. Kim S, Park CH, Chung YS. Hypophosphatemic osteomalacia demonstrated by Tc-99m MDP bone scan: a case report. Clin Nucl Med .2000;25:337–340.
5. Konishi K, Nakamura M, Yamakawa H, et al. Hypophosphatemic osteomalacia in von Recklinghausen neurofibromatosis. Am J Med Sci. 1991;301:322–328.
6. Linde R, Saxena A, Feldman D. Hypophosphatemic rickets presenting as recurring pedal stress fractures in a middle-aged woman. J Foot Ankle Surg. 2001;40:101–104.
7. Negri AL, Bogado CE, Zanchetta JR. Bone densitometry in a patient with hypophosphatemic osteomalacia. J Bone Miner Metab. 2004;22:514–517.
8. Quarles LD, Drezner MK. Pathophysiology of X-linked hypophosphatemia, tumor-induced osteomalacia, and autosomal dominant hypophosphatemia: a perPHEXing problem. J Clin Endocrinol Metab. 2001;86:494–496.
9. Reis-Filho JS, Paiva ME, Lopes JM. August 2003: 47-year-old female with a 7-year history of osteomalacia and hypophosphatemia. Brain Pathol. 2004;14:111–112, 115.
10. Ros I, Alvarez L, Guañabens N, et al. Hypophosphatemic osteomalacia: a report of five cases and evaluation of bone markers. J Bone Miner Metab. 2005;23:266–269.
11. Rowe PS. The molecular background to hypophosphataemic rickets. Arch Dis Child. 2000;83:192–194.
12. Scheinman SJ, Guay-Woodford LM, Thakker RV, Warnock DG. Genetic disorders of renal electrolyte transport. N Engl J Med. 1999;340:1177–1187.

HEREDITARY HYPOPHOSPHATEMIC RICKETS WITH HYPERCALCIURIA

13. Lorenz-Depiereux B, Benet-Pages A, Eckstein G, et al. Hereditary hypophosphatemic rickets with hypercalciuria is caused by mutations in the sodium-phosphate cotransporter gene SLC34A3. Am J Hum Genet 2006;78:193–201.
14. Chen C, Carpenter T, Steg N, Baron R, Anast C. Hypercalciuric hypophosphatemic rickets, mineral balance, bone histomorphometry, and therapeutic implications of hypercalciuria. Pediatrics. 1989;84:276–280.
15. Hochberg Z, Tiosano D. Disorders of mineral metabolism. In: Pescovitz OH, Eugster EA (eds.), Pediatric Endocrinology: Mechanisms and Management. Philadelphia, PA: Lippincott Williams & Wilkins; 2004:614–640.
16. Nishiyama S, Inoue F, Matsuda I. A single case of hypophosphatemic rickets with hypercalciuria. J Pediatr Gastroenterol Nutr. 1986;5:826–829.

ONCOGENIC OSTEOMALACIA

17. Ahn JM, Kim HJ, Cha CM, Kim J, Yim SG, Kim HJ. Oncogenic osteomalacia: induced by tumor, cured by surgery. Oral Surg Oral Med Oral Pathol Oral Radiol Endod. 2007;103:636–641.

18. Auethavekiat P, Roberts JR, Biega TJ, et al. Case 3. Oncogenic osteomalacia associated with hemangiopericytoma localized by octreotide scan. J Clin Oncol. 2005;23:3626–3628.

19. Avila NA, Skarulis M, Rubino DM, Doppman JL. Oncogenic osteomalacia: lesion detection by MR skeletal survey. AJR Am J Roentgenol. 1996;167:343–345.

20. Cai Q, Hodgson SF, Kao PC, et al. Brief report: inhibition of renal phosphate transport by a tumor product in a patient with oncogenic osteomalacia. N Engl J Med. 1994;330:1645–1649.

22. Carpenter TO. Oncogenic osteomalacia—a complex dance of factors. N Engl J Med. 2003;348:1705–1708.

22. Cheng CL, Ma J, Wu PC, Mason RS, Posen S. Osteomalacia secondary to osteosarcoma. A case report. J Bone Joint Surg Am. 1989; 71:288–292.

23. Clunie GP, Fox PE, Stamp TC. Four cases of acquired hypophosphataemic ('oncogenic') osteomalacia. Problems of diagnosis, treatment and long-term management. Rheumatology. (Oxford) 2000;39:1415–1421.

24. Collins MT, Chebli C, Jones J, et al. Renal phosphate wasting in fibrous dysplasia of bone is part of a generalized renal tubular dysfunction similar to that seen in tumor-induced osteomalacia. J Bone Miner Res. 2001;16:806–813.

25. Cukierman T, Gatt ME, Hiller N, Chajek-Shaul T. Clinical problem-solving. A fractured diagnosis. N Engl J Med. 2005; 353:509–514.

26. Reese DM, Rosen PJ. Oncogenic osteomalacia associated with prostate cancer. J Urol 1997;158:887.

27. Dowman JK, Khattak FH. Oncogenic hypophosphataemic osteomalacia mimicking bone metastases on isotope bone scan. Ann Rheum Dis. 2006;65:1664.

28. Econs MJ, Drezner MK. Tumor-induced osteomalacia—unveiling a new hormone. N Engl J Med. 1994;330:1679–1681.

29. Firth RG, Grant CS, Riggs BL. Development of hypercalcemic hyperparathyroidism after long-term phosphate supplementation in hypophosphatemic osteomalacia. Report of two cases. Am J Med. 1985;78:669–673.

30. Fukumoto S, Takeuchi Y, Nagano A, Fujita T. Diagnostic utility of magnetic resonance imaging skeletal survey in a patient with oncogenic osteomalacia. Bone. 1999;25:375–377.

31. Gonzales-Compta X, Mañós-Pujol M, Foglia-Fernandez M, et al. Oncogenic osteomalacia: case report and review of head and neck associated tumours. J Laryngol Otol. 1998;112:389–392.

32. Imel EA, Peacock M, Pitukcheewanont P, et al. Sensitivity of fibroblast growth factor 23 measurements in tumor-induced osteomalacia. J Clin Endocrinol Metab. 2006; 91:2055–2061.

33. Jan de Beur SM, Streeten EA, Civelek AC, et al. Localisation of mesenchymal tumours by somatostatin receptor imaging. Lancet. 2002;359:761–763.

34. Kumar R. Tumor-induced osteomalacia and the regulation of phosphate homeostasis. Bone. 2000;27:333–338.

35. MacGowan JR, Pringle J, Stamp TC. A severe case of acquired hypophosphataemic osteomalacia: the perils of a missed diagnosis. Rheumatology (Oxford). 2001;40:707–709.

36. Nguyen BD, Wang EA. Indium-111 pentetreotide scintigraphy of mesenchymal tumor with oncogenic osteomalacia. Clin Nucl Med. 1999;24:130–131.

37. Nuovo MA, Dorfman HD, Sun CC, Chalew SA. Tumor-induced osteomalacia and rickets. Am J Surg Pathol. 1989; 13:588–599.

38. Ogose A, Hotta T, Emura I, et al Recurrent malignant variant of phosphaturic mesenchymal tumor with oncogenic osteomalacia. Skeletal Radiol. 2001;30:99–103.

39. Reubi JC, Waser B, Laissue JA, Gebbers JO. Somatostatin and vasoactive intestinal peptide receptors in human mesenchymal tumors: in vitro identification. Cancer Res. 1996;56:1922–1931.

40. Reyes-Múgica M, Arnsmeier SL, Backeljauw PF, Persing J, Ellis B, Carpenter TO. Phosphaturic mesenchymal tumor-induced rickets. Pediatr Dev Pathol. 2000;3:61–69.

41. Rhee Y, Lee JD, Shin KH, Lee HC, Huh KB, Lim SK. Oncogenic osteomalacia associated with mesenchymal tumour detected by indium-111 octreotide scintigraphy. Clin Endocrinol (Oxford). 2001;54:551–554.

42. Sandhu FA, Martuza RL. Craniofacial hemangiopericytoma associated with oncogenic osteomalacia: case report. J Neurooncol. 2000;46:241–247.

43 Saville PD, Nassim JR, Stevenson FH, Mulligan L, Carey M. Osteomalacia in Von Recklinghausen's neurofibromatosis: metabolic study of a case. Br Med J. 1955;1:1311–1313.

44. Schapira D, Ben Izhak O, Nachtigal A, et al. Tumor-induced osteomalacia. Semin Arthritis Rheum. 1995;25:35–46.

45. Seufert J, Ebert K, Müller J, et al. Octreotide therapy for tumor-induced osteomalacia. N Engl J Med. 2001;345:1883–1888.

46. Siegel HJ, Rock MG. Occult phosphaturic mesenchymal tumor detected by Tc-99m sestamibi scan. Clin Nucl Med. 2002; 27:608–609.

47. Siegel HJ, Rock MG, Inwards C, Sim FH. Phosphaturic mesenchymal tumor. Orthopedics. 2002;25:1279–1281.

48. Stanbury SW. Tumour-associated hypophosphatemic osteomalacia and rickets. Clin Endocrinol 1972;1:1256–1266.

49. Stewart I, Roddie C, Gill A, et al. Elevated serum FGF23 concentrations in plasma cell dyscrasias. Bone. 2006;39:369–376.

50. Sundaram M, McCarthy EF. Oncogenic osteomalacia. Skeletal Radiol. 2000;29:117–124.

51. Vollbrecht JE, Rao DS. Images in clinical medicine. Tumor-induced osteomalacia. N Engl J Med. 2008;358:1282.

52. Weidner N. Review and update: oncogenic osteomalacia-rickets. Ultrastruct Pathol. 1991;15:317–333.

53. Weidner N, Santa Cruz D. Phosphaturic mesenchymal tumors. A polymorphous group causing osteomalacia or rickets. Cancer. 1987;59:1442–1454.

METABOLISM

54. Andress DL, Ozuna J, Tirschwell D,et al Antiepileptic drug-induced bone loss in young male patients who have seizures. Arch Neurol. 2002;59:781–786.

55. Bagga A, Bajpai A, Menon S. Approach to renal tubular disorders. Indian J Pediatr. 2005;72:771–776.

56. Berndt TJ, Schiavi S, Kumar R. "Phosphatonins" and the regulation of phosphorus homeostasis. Am J Physiol Renal Physiol 2005;289:F1170–F1182.

57. Blumsohn A. What have we learnt about the regulation of phosphate metabolism? Curr Opin Nephrol Hypertens. 2004; 13:397–401.

58. DiMeglio LA, White KE, Econs MJ. Disorders of phosphate metabolism. Endocrinol Metab Clin North Am.2000;29:591–609.

59. El-Desouki M, Al-Jurayyan N. Bone mineral density and bone scintigraphy in children and adolescents with osteomalacia. Eur J Nucl Med. 1997;24:202–205.

60. Murphey MD, Sartoris DJ, Quale JL, Pathria MN, Martin NL. Musculoskeletal manifestations of chronic renal insufficiency. RadioGraphics. 1993;13:357–379.

61. Reginato AJ, Falasca GF, Pappu R, McKnight B, Agha A. Musculoskeletal manifestations of osteomalacia: report of 26 cases and literature review. Semin Arthritis Rheum. 1999;28:287–304.

62. Resnick D. Bone and Joint Imaging. Philadelphia, PA: WB Saunders; 1996

63. Tejwani NC, Schachter AK, Immerman I, Achan P. Renal osteodystrophy. J Am Acad Orthop Surg. 2006;14:303–311.

FANCONI SYNDROME

64. Bickel H, Manz F. Hereditary tubular disorders of the Fanconi type and the idiopathic Fanconi syndrome. Prog Clin Biol Res. 1989;305:111–135.

65 Chan JS, Yang AH, Kao KP, Tarng DC. Acquired Fanconi syndrome induced by mixed Chinese herbs presenting as proximal muscle weakness. J Chin Med Assoc 2004;67:193–196.

66. Moxey-Mims M, Stapleton FB. Renal tubular disorders in the neonate. Clin Perinatol. 1992;19:159–178.

67. Mujais SK. Maleic acid-induced proximal tubulopathy: Na:K pump inhibition. J Am Soc Nephrol. 1993;4:142–147.

Case 16

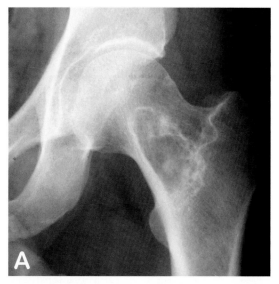

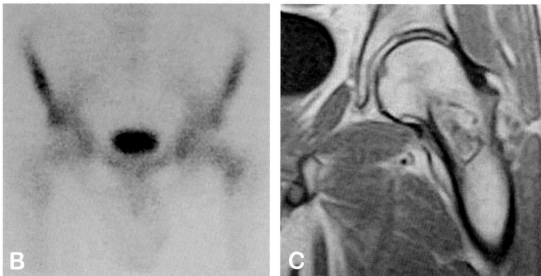

Figure 16-1. (A) Left femur. Radiograph. Anteroposterior position. (B) Pelvis. Technetium-99m MDP bone scan. Anteroposterior position. (C) Left femur. MR. T1-weighted (TR/TE; 650/25). Coronal plane.

Question 72

A 48-year-old man presented with a 2-month history of vague groin pain. You are shown an anteroposterior radiograph of his left femur, a corresponding image from a technetium-99m MDP bone scan, and an MR image (Figure 16-1). Which *one* of the following is the MOST likely diagnosis for the lesion shown in Figure 16-1?

(A) Fibrous dysplasia
(B) Nonossifying fibroma (fibroxanthoma)
(C) Intraosseous lipoma
(D) Osteoblastoma
(E) Lymphoma

Mark J. Kransdorf, M.D.

Intraosseous Lipoma

Question 72

Which *one* of the following is the MOST likely diagnosis for the lesion shown in Figure 16-1?

(A) Fibrous dysplasia
(B) Nonossifying fibroma (fibroxanthoma)
(C) Intraosseous lipoma
(D) Osteoblastoma
(E) Lymphoma

The anteroposterior radiograph of the proximal left femur (Figure 16-2A) shows a geographic, lytic lesion with a relatively thin sclerotic margin in the femoral neck and intertrochanteric region. There is no expansile remodeling. There is no periosteal reaction, but this is not seen in intertrochanteric area lesions. Globular areas of increased opacity are seen within the lesion, more readily at its periphery. A corresponding delayed anteroposterior image from a technetium -99m medylene-

diphosphonate (MDP) bone scan (Figure 16-2B) shows mildly increased tracer accumulation in the left intertrochanteric area.

The sclerotic margins noted on the radiograph are compatible with an indolent process. The internal matrix mineralization is characterized by focal areas of relatively homogeneously increased opacity, consistent with an osseous matrix. This constellation of findings is characteristic of an intraosseous lipoma **(Option (C) is correct)** with involutional change including calcification, fat necrosis, and reactive bone formation. The diagnosis was confirmed with MR imaging (Figure 16-2C), which showed large amounts of fat within the lesion. Subsequent surgery confirmed the nature of the internal matrix as lipomatous.

Fibrous dysplasia commonly involves the proximal femur. It is seen in as many as 28% of patients with monostotic disease. The matrix in fibrous dysplasia is

Figure 16-2 (same as Figure 16-1). Intraosseous lipoma. (A) Left femur. Anteroposterior radiograph. A geographic lytic lesion is seen in the intertrochanteric region (arrows). It has a relatively thin sclerotic margin, compatible with that of an indolent process. There is no sign of expansive bone remodeling. Areas of increased opacity can be seen within the lesion, most clearly around its periphery. (B) Pelvis. Technetium-99m MDP bone scan. Anteroposterior position. There is mildly increased tracer accumulation in the left femoral neck (arrows).

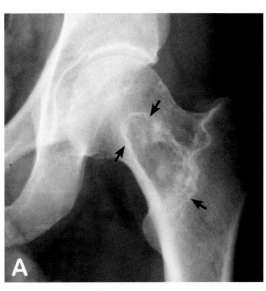

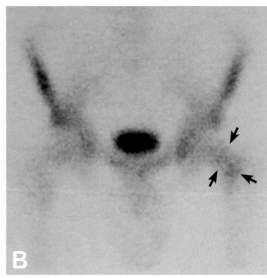

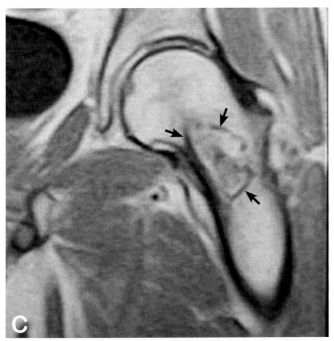

Figure 16-2 (continued). Intraosseous lipoma. (C) Left femur. MRI. T1-weighted (TR/TE; 650/25). Coronal plane. There is significant high signal in the femoral neck lesion (arrows), consistent with fat.

typically a more homogeneous hazy opacity, described as "ground glass." Equally important, scintigraphy will usually show markedly increased tracer accumulation **(Option (A) is incorrect)**.

Nonossifying fibroma is typically found in the metadiaphysis of long bones and is quite uncommon in the proximal femur. Lesions are usually lobulated and eccentric, causing mild expansile remodeling of the host bone. Nonossifying fibromas are unusual in older individuals, with the vast majority found in adolescents **(Option (B) is incorrect)**.

Osteoblastoma occurs in long bones in approximately one-third of cases, with the vast majority located in the diaphysis; the proximal femur is rarely affected. Lesions are usually osteolytic, with expansile remodeling; periosteal reaction is seen in about half of the cases. Mineralized matrix is identified on radiographs in less than 10 percent of cases **(Option (D) is incorrect)**.

Lymphoma typically shows a mixed osteolytic and osteoblastic pattern. Lesions show a much more aggressive pattern of bone destruction than is demonstrated in this current case **(Option (E) is incorrect)**.

Question 73

Regarding intraosseous lipoma:

(A) It is often perceived as a rare lesion.

(B) It is likely a congenital lesion.
(C) It is a precursor to liposarcoma.
(D) It is a simple histological diagnosis for the pathologist.
(E) Patients are invariably symptomatic.

While intraosseous lipomas are perceived as rare, they are likely more common than pathological series would indicate **(Option (A) is true)**. With the increased use of CT and MR imaging, intraosseous lipomas are being visualized with increasing frequency. Intraosseous lipomas are acquired lesions **(Option (B) is false)** (Figure 16-3). It is unclear if they are true neoplasms, reactive lesions, or the conglomeration of lipocytes replacing normal bone marrow elements. Liposarcoma of bone has been reported, but it is exceedingly rare, and there is no evidence to suggest a malignant potential for intraosseous lipoma **(Option (C) is false)**. Intraosseous lipomas may undergo varying amounts of involutional change, with prominent areas of cyst formation, fat necrosis, and dystrophic mineralization. Consequently, pathologists may confuse these lesions with bone infarcts **(Option (D) is false)**. Although reports vary, between 30% and 50% of patients are asymptomatic **(Option (E) is false)**. Microtrabecu-

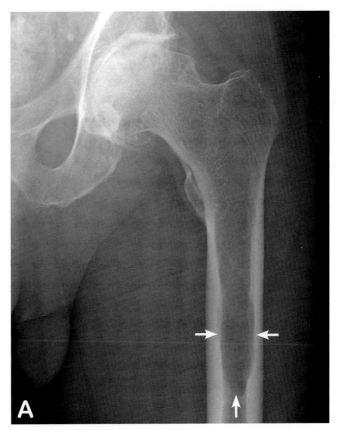

Figure 16-3. Left hip. Intraosseous lipoma. (A) Anteroposterior radiograph. There is a lytic lesion (arrows) in the proximal shaft of the left femur, scalloping the endosteal cortex. The proximal margin of the lesion is not well defined.

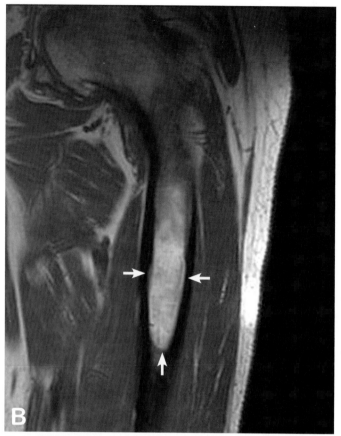

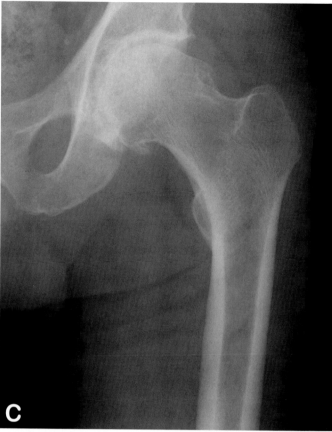

Figure 16-3 (continued). Intraosseous lipoma. (B) MRI. T1-weighted (TR/TE; 500/13). Coronal plane. The lesion (arrows) is a stage 1 intraosseous lipoma, containing high-signal-intensity fat. Note the scalloping of the medial and lateral femoral cortex. The diagnosis of intraosseous lipoma was confirmed at hip replacement surgery. (C) Anteroposterior radiograph. This image, obtained seven years earlier, shows no sign of the lesion. The patient was a 75-year-old man being evaluated for total hip arthroplasty.

lar fracture is suspected as the cause of pain when patients with intraosseous lipomas are symptomatic.

Question 74

Imaging findings in intraosseous lipoma:

 (A) Must show the lesion to be entirely adipose tissue
 (B) Must show the majority of the lesion to be adipose tissue
 (C) May show no or almost no adipose tissue in the lesion
 (D) May show cysts within the lesion
 (E) May show varying amounts of calcification/ossification

Milgram documented the involutional changes in intraosseous lipoma, highlighting the radiographic, gross, and histological features of the lesion at different stages of its evolution. Based on these involutional changes within the lesion, intraosseous lipomas can be separated into three distinct patterns: stage 1 shows no involutional changes (Figure 16-4); stage 2 shows partial secondary necrosis; and in stage 3 intraosseous

lipomas have complete or near-complete secondary necrosis. The imaging features in intraosseous lipoma will reflect these stages. Stage 1 lesions are completely radiolucent and fat-filled **(Option (A) is true)**. Stage 2 lesions will have variable amounts of internal fat and typically show areas of nonadipose tissue with calcification or ossification **(Option (B) is false)**. Stage 2 lesions will develop areas of infarction, necrosis, calcification, and ossification. Cyst formation is common within stage 2 lesions (Figure 16-5) and is a consequence of the involutional change **(Option (C) is true)**.

Stage 3 lesions are those in which there is complete or near-complete involutional change. Stage 3 lesions may show complete involution of the lipoma and therefore absence of any contained fat **(Option (D) is true)**.

While these changes can also be seen in stage 2 lesions, they are more prominent in stage 3 intraosseous lipomas **(Option (E) is true)**. Stage 3 lesions will contain varying amounts of calcification/ossification **(Option (E) is true)**.

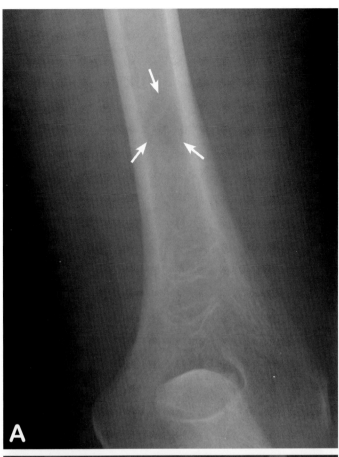

Question 75

Regarding intraosseous lipoma:

(A) It is most common in the calcaneus.
(B) It is almost invariably seen in children.
(C) Stage 3 lesions are the least common.
(D) The radiographic appearance is always specific for a benign mass.
(E) Calcaneal lesions typically have thin sclerotic margins with central calcification or ossification.

Approximately 60% of intraosseous lipomas occur in the long bones **(Option (A) is false).** Calcaneal lesions are commonly seen and account for about one-third of cases (between 10% and 35%). While children may be affected, most patients are in the 4th decade of life **(Option (B) is false).** Most series do not subdivide lesions into stages; however, stage 3 lesions probably

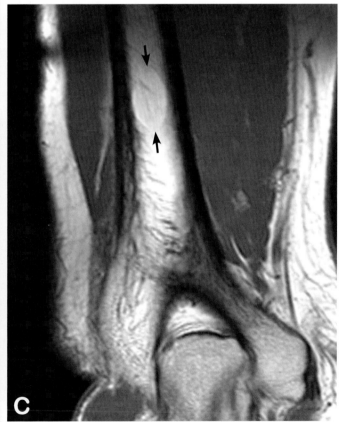

Figure 16-4. Stage 1 intraosseus lipoma. Humerus. (A) Radiograph. There is a lytic lesion (arrows) in the distal humerus. The inferior margin of the lesion is poorly delineated. (B) MRI. T1-weighted. Sagittal plane. The lesion (arrows) scallops the posterior cortex (arrows) and is responsible for the lucency identified on the radiograph. The lesion is of high signal intensity, and the anterior margin is not adequately differentiated from the adjacent marrow fat. (C) MRI. T1-weighted. Coronal plane. The margins of the lesion are better delineated in the coronal plane (arrows). The patient was a 65-year-old man being evaluated for multiple myeloma.

account for only 10% to 15% of cases **(Option (C) is true).**

The radiographic appearance of intraosseous lipoma is that of a geographic, osteolytic lesion. The margins typically, but not always, shows variable sclerosis. This is not always the case, however. Central ossification and calcification from involutional change may mimic other types of matrix. Expansile remodeling is most common in thin bones, such as the fibula, and is reported with variable prevalence (14% to 60%). While the radiographic appearance is usually that of a benign process, it is often not specific and may mimic malignancies such as myeloma and plasmacytoma **(Option (D) is false).** The exception to this is intraosseous lipoma in the anterior process of the calcaneus. In this location the lesion typically demonstrates a thin sclerotic margin, often with a central calcified or ossified focus (Figure 16-5) **(Option (E) is true).**

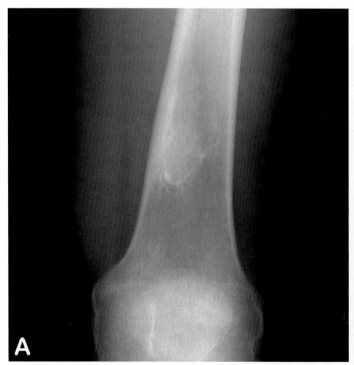

Figure 16-5. Stage 2 osseous lipoma. (A) Distal femur. Radiograph. Anteroposterior view. There is a rounded area of increased opacity with a rind of subtle sclerosis that represents the thin shell of bone surrounding the cyst. (B) MRI. T1-weighted (TR/TE; 623/17). Axial plane through the lesion. The central cyst (asterisk) has a thin calcified rind of decreased signal. Note surrounding lipomatous tissue, also with a thin surrounding margin (arrows), which is partially mineralized. (C) MRI. T2-weighted (TR/TE; 2230/83). Axial plane through the lesion. The central cyst (asterisk) shows a high signal intensity consistent with fluid. The margin of the lipoma (arrows) is more difficult to delineate. The patient was a 76-year-old woman being evaluated for knee pain.

Question 76

The differential diagnosis for the radiographic findings of intraosseous lipoma would include:

(A) Fibrous dysplasia
(B) Simple bone cyst
(C) Nonossifying fibroma (fibroxanthoma)
(D) Enchondroma
(E) Liposclerosing myxofibrous tumor (LSMFT)

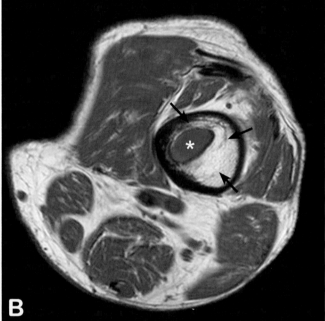

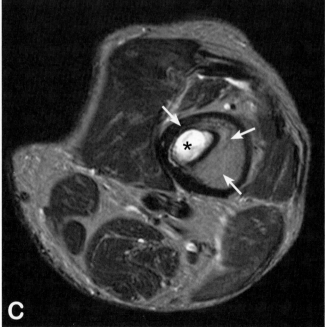

All of the listed lesions may have radiographic features that suggest an intraosseous lipoma **(Options (A) through (E) are true)**. A definitive diagnosis is usually made on CT or MR imaging by the identification of fat within the lesion. The diagnosis of stage 3 intraosseous lipoma (Figure 16-6) may be especially difficult to determine on imaging when involutional change involves the entire lesion. Extensive central calcification may mimic the mineralization within a cartilage cartilaginous tumor. Liposclerosing myxofibrous tumor (LSMFT) of bone is a benign fibro-osseous lesion that is characterized by a complex mixture of histologic elements. These may include lipoma, fibroxanthoma, myxoma, myxofibroma, fibrous dysplasia-like features, cyst formation, fat necrosis, ischemic ossification, and, rarely, cartilage. LSMFT occurs almost exclusively in the intertrochanteric region of the femur, with this location accounting for 85% of cases. An LSMFT can be distinguished from a lipoma on CT scan or MR imaging by the identification of fat within a lipoma. Distinguishing between LSMFT and classic fibrous dysplasia is more difficult and may not be possible in some cases. The relationship of LSMFT to fibrous dysplasia and intraosseous lipoma is not clear.

Question 77

Regarding intraosseous lipoma:

(A) Patients typically have multiple lesions.
(B) Upper extremity lesions are most common.
(C) Metaphyseal involvement is typical.
(D) MR imaging of Stage 2 lesions will often show cysts within lesions.
(E) Lesions are histologically identical to soft tissue lipoma.

In general, intraosseous lipomas are solitary lesions; multifocal involvement is rare **(Option (A) is false)**. Bilateral calcaneal involvement is an exception to this rule. The lower extremity is involved much more frequently (6:1 ratio) than the upper extremity (approximately 6:1) **(Option (B) is false)**. Long bone involvement is most common, with lesions typically located in the metaphysis **(Option (C) is true)**. Diaphyseal involvement is less common. Stage 2 lesions are most common, and cysts have been reported on MR imaging in as many as two-thirds of such patients **(Option (D) is true)**. Intraosseous lipomas are histologically identical to soft tissue lipomas **(Option (E) is true)**.

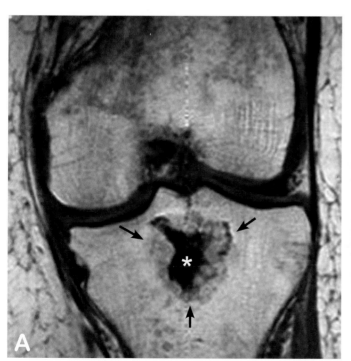
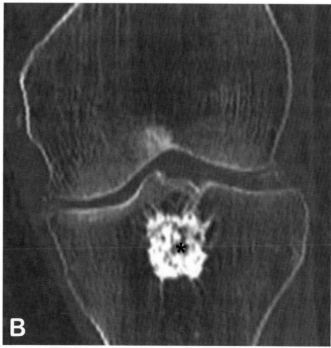

Figure 16-6. Stage 3 intraosseus lipoma. Knee (A) MRI. Coronal plane. There is a densely mineralized central mass (asterisk) within a lipomatous lesion (arrows). (B) CT. Coronal plane. The corresponding CT scan shows the densely mineralized central mass (asterisk), although neither the surrounding margin nor the lipomatous lesion is well defined.

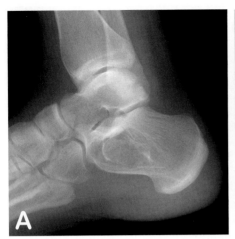
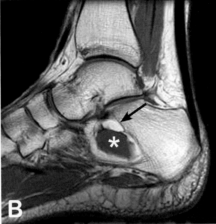
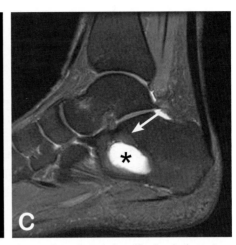

Figure 16-7. Ankle (A) Radiograph. Lateral view. There is a geographic lytic lesion with a thin sclerotic margin and central ossification in the anterior calcaneus. (B) MRI. T1-weighted. Sagittal plane. A central cyst (asterisk) has a rind of decreased signal representing a thin calcified rim. Note the surrounding high-signal lipomatous component (arrow). This is a stage 2 intraosseous lipoma. (C) MRI. T2-weighted, fat-suppressed, turbo spin-echo. The central cyst (asterisk) shows a high signal intensity consistent with fluid. The margin of the lipoma (arrow) is more difficult to delineate. The patient was a 37-year-old woman being evaluated for ankle pain.

Suggested Readings

1. Campbell RSD, Grainger AJ, Mangham DC, Beggs I, The J, Davies AM. Intraosseous lipoma: a report of 35 new cases and review of the literature. Skeletal Radiol. 2003;32:209–222.

2. Chung CB, Murphey M, Cho G, et al. Osseous lesions of the pelvis and long tubular bones containing both fat and fluid-like signal intensity: an analysis of 28 patients. Eur J Radiol. 2005;53:103–109.

3. Milgram JW, Intraosseous lipomas: radiologic and pathologic manifestations. Radiology. 1988;167:155–160.

4. Milgram JW. Intraosseous lipomas. A clinicopathologic study of 66 cases. Clin Orthop. 1988;231:277–302.

5. Mirra JM, Piero P. Tumors of fat. In: Mirra JM, ed. Bone Tumors. Clinical, radiologic and pathologic correlation. Philadelphia, PA: Lea & Febiger; 1989: 1479–1494.

6. Radl R, Leithner A, Machacek F, et al. Intraosseous lipoma: retrospective analysis of 29 patients. Int Orthop. 2004;28:374–378.

7. Ramos A, Castello J, Sartoris DJ, Greenway GD, Resnick D, Haghighi P. Osseous lipoma: CT appearance. Radiology. 1985;157:615–619.

8. Resnick D, Kyriakos M, Greenway GD. Tumors and tumor-like lesions of bone: imaging and pathology of specific lesions. In: Resnick D, ed. Bone and Joint Disorders, 4th ed. Philadelphia, PA: W.B. Saunders Company; 2002: 3763–4128.

Case 17

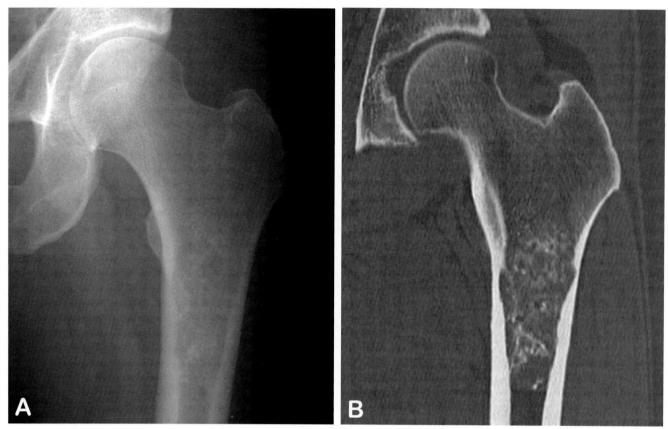

Figure 17-1. Left femur. (A) Radiograph. Anteroposterior view. (B) CT. Reformatted in coronal plane. No IV contrast.

Question 78

A 44-year-old man presented with increasing, vague groin pain of several months duration. You are shown a radiograph and a reformatted coronal CT, without contrast (Figure 17-1). Which *one* of the following is the MOST likely diagnosis for the lesion shown in Figure 17-1?

(A) Enchondroma
(B) Bone infarct
(C) Dedifferentiated chondrosarcoma
(D) Chondrosarcoma
(E) Fibrocartilagenous dysplasia

Mark J. Kransdorf, M.D.

Chondrosarcoma

Question 78

Which *one* of the following is the MOST likely diagnosis for the lesion shown in Figure 17-1?

(A) Enchondroma
(B) Bone infarct
(C) Dedifferentiated chondrosarcoma
(D) Chondrosarcoma
(E) Fibrocartilagenous dysplasia

The AP radiograph of the proximal right femur (17-2A) shows a geographic lytic lesion. The medial and lateral margins are well defined, without sclerosis. Note prominent scalloping of the endosteal cortical surfaces. The proximal and distal margins are not well seen. A

noncontrast reformatted coronal CT (17-2B) shows the full extent of the endosteal scalloping to better advantage. The pattern of mineralization within the mass is typical "arc-and-ring" calcification, representing intralesional foci of calcification and enchondral ossification. There is no expansile remodeling or periosteal new bone formation.

The pattern of mineralization shown on the test image is typical of that of a cartilaginous neoplasm. The primary differential in this case is between an enchondroma and a chondrosarcoma. The presence of deep endosteal scalloping (defined as involving more than two-thirds the thickness of the cortex) has been reported to increase the likelihood that a lesion is malignant by

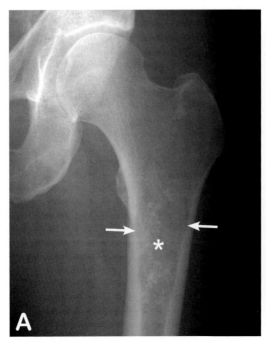
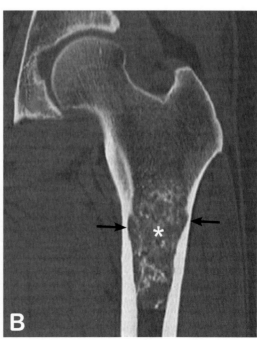

Figure 17-2 (Same as Figure 17-1). Left femur. (A) Radiograph. Anteroposterior view. The radiograph shows a geographic lytic lesion with well-defined medial and lateral margins scalloping the adjacent cortex (arrows) and chondroid matrix (asterisk). There is no sclerosis. The proximal and distal margins are not well seen. (B) CT. Reformatted in coronal plane. No IV contrast. The full extent of the endosteal scalloping (arrows) is better seen on CT. There is a typical "arc-and-ring" calcification pattern of mineralization (asterisk) within the mass.

more than 30 fold **(Option (D) is correct)**. The presence of periosteal new bone on radiographs, not seen in this case, has been reported to increase the likelihood of malignancy 30 fold, as well. While mild endosteal scalloping is not uncommon in long-bone enchondroma, being seen in almost two-thirds of cases, the degree of endosteal scalloping in this case is beyond that expected for an enchondroma **(Option (A) is incorrect)**.

A classic bone infarct is often included in the differential diagnosis for a cartilaginous lesion. The distinction can usually be made with confidence **(Option (B) is incorrect)**. The mineralization in a bone infarct is peripheral, occurring within the reactive interface, which forms at the periphery of the infarcted marrow. This is in contrast to the central mineralization typically found within a cartilaginous tumor. In addition to differences in the location of the mineralization, the pattern of mineralization is also different. Cartilage will demonstrate arc-and-ring, flocculent, and stippled calcifica-tions, while a bone infarct will show a serpentine rind of increased density (Figure 17-3).

Dedifferentiated chondrosarcoma accounts for approximately 10% of all chondrosarcomas, and represents a lesion in which a high-grade noncartilagenous sarcoma arises in association with a longstanding low-grade chondrosarcoma. Imaging findings vary with the relative proportions of the two components. As the high-grade noncartilaginous component increases in size, radiographs will show progressive bone lysis with decrease in cartilage matrix mineralization. When the dedifferentiated component is small, the areas of high-grade tumor are more difficult to identify; however, none are identified in the current case **(Option (C) is incorrect)**.

Fibrocartilagenous dysplasia is a term that is sometimes used for cases of fibrous dysplasia that contain benign cartilage nodules. These cartilage nodules typically occupy only a small portion of the lesion and

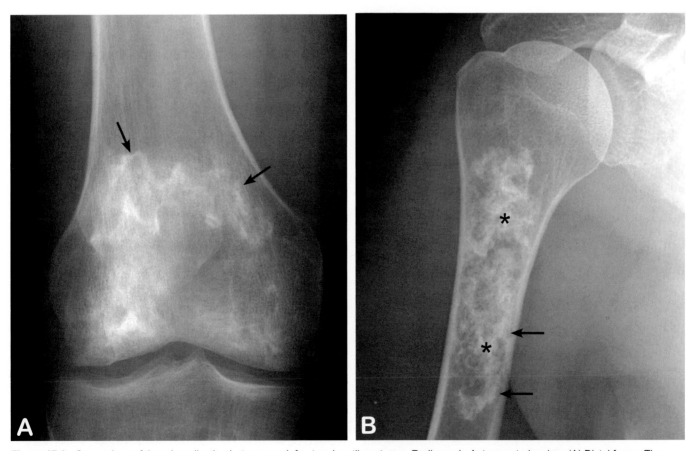

Figure 17-3. Comparison of the mineralization between an infarct and cartilage tumor. Radiograph. Anteroposterior view. (A) Distal femur. The image shows an intramedullary infarct in the distal femur of a 40-year-old man. Note the serpentine rind of mineralization (arrows). While it approaches the cortex, there is no mass effect or cortical scalloping. (B) Proximal humerus. The image shows an intramedullary enchondroma in the proximal humerus of a 56-year-old woman. Note multiple areas showing arc-and-ring mineralization (asterisks), as well as subtle endosteal scalloping (arrows) in the mid-aspect of the lesion. Identification of endosteal scalloping virtually excludes the diagnosis of an infarct.

may be seen in as many as 10% of cases. Typically, the imaging features of fibrous dysplasia will dominate in

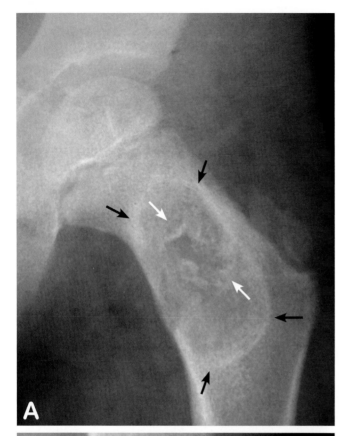

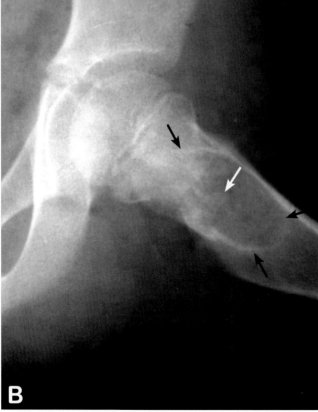

such cases (Figure 17-4) unlike the current unknown case, in which the features of a cartilage neoplasm dominate **(Option (E) is incorrect).** Rare cases of chondrosarcoma associated with fibrous dysplasia have been reported.

Question 79

Regarding intramedullary chondrosarcoma:

- (A) It is common in children.
- (B) Most patients will present with pain.
- (C) Pathologic fracture is not uncommon.
- (D) It is most common in the small bones of the hands.
- (E) Long bone involvement is usually limited to the diaphysis.

Conventional intramedullary chondrosarcoma is the most common type of primary chondrosarcoma. It has also been referred to as central chondrosarcoma. Patients with conventional chondrosarcoma most commonly present in the 4th to 5th decades of life **(Option (A) is false).** Clinical symptoms are usually nonspecific, with pain being the most frequent, occurring in at least 95% of patients **(Option (B) is true).** The pain is often insidious, progressive, and worse at night. Pain has often been present for months to years before the time of presentation. A palpable soft tissue mass or fullness has also been described in many patients. Pathologic fractures are not uncommon at initial presentation, and have been reported in from 3% to 17% of patients with conventional chondrosarcoma **(Option (C) is true).** The most common skeletal location for a conventional chondrosarcoma is the long tubular bones, accounting for approximately 45% of cases **(Option (D) is false).** The femur is the single most commonly affected long bone, representing approximately 20% to 35% of cases, followed in frequency by the tibia (5%). Chondrosarcoma of the long tubular bones most commonly involves the metaphysis, with this location accounting for approximately half the cases **(Option (E) is false).** About a third of cases occur in the diaphysis.

Figure 17-4. Fibrous dysplasia of the proximal femur. Left femur. Radiograph. There is a well-demarcated mass (black arrows) in the femoral neck. Histology showed small cartilage nodules of various sizes. (A) Anteroposterior view. An arc-and-ring pattern of mineralization can be seen (white arrows), representing cartilage calcification and enchondral ossification within nodules of cartilage. (B) Lateral view. Frog-leg positioning. The arc-and-ring pattern of mineralization (white arrow) is seen again, mixed with areas of ground glass opacity, typical of fibrous dysplasia. The patient was a 5-year-old boy.

Question 80

Regarding the distinction between enchondroma and chondrosarcoma:

(A) It is usually made easily based on percutaneous biopsy.
(B) It is usually made easily on clinical grounds.
(C) It is often a difficult distinction for pathologists.
(D) In general, chondrosarcomas are larger than enchondromas.
(E) Epiphyseal involvement is not a useful discriminating feature.

The percutaneous biopsy of cartilaginous lesions must always be undertaken with great care and should be planned with the surgeon who will perform the definitive surgery. Variations in the histological composition of the tumor make sampling errors a serious consideration. The small samples obtained during percutaneous biopsy often do not allow the pathologist to adequately assess entrapment and destruction of trabecular bone, which are hallmarks of chondrosarcoma **(Option (A) is false).**

Clinical information is important in the evaluation of musculoskeletal neoplasms. When a cartilage neoplasm is evaluated, the presence of associated pain increases the likelihood that the lesion is malignant. Unfortunately, juxtaarticular pain is not an uncommon clinical problem, and incidental lesions are frequently identified near joints. In a study of 57 patients with enchondromas of the proximal humerus presenting with pain, more than 80% had articular abnormalities on MR imaging that would explain their pain **(Option (B) is false).**

The microscopic distinction between enchondroma and chondrosarcoma can be difficult, even for experienced pathologists **(Option (C) is true).** In a recent study assessing interobserver reliability, 46 consecutive long bone cartilaginous lesions were evaluated by nine internationally recognized pathologists. Each lesion was classified as benign, low-grade malignant, or high-grade malignant. Kappa coefficient of interobserver reliability for pathologists on these lesions was 0.443, indicating only moderate agreement.

In general, chondrosarcomas tend to be larger than enchondromas **(Option (D) is true).** Although there is certainly overlap in size, lesions larger than 5-6 cm in diameter are much more likely to represent chondrosarcomas.

There is scant literature addressing epiphyseal cartilage lesions; however, the identification of cartilage extending from the diametaphysis into the epiphysis is an ominous feature. In a study specifically addressing the imaging distinction of enchondroma from chondrosar-

coma, 14 of 17 cases with an epiphyseal location were malignant **(Option (E) is false).**

Question 81

On radiographs of patients with long bone cartilage tumors:

(A) Chondrosarcomas usually demonstrate mineralization.
(B) In general, high-grade chondrosarcomas have more extensive matrix mineralization than low-grade chondrosarcomas.
(C) The presence of scalloping is more important than the depth of scalloping in determining malignancy.
(D) The longitudinal extent of scalloping is more important than the depth of scalloping in determining malignancy.
(E) The same criteria used for analyzing lesions of the small bones of the hands and feet can be used for assessing lesions of the long bones.

Mineralized chondroid matrix is seen in approximately 60% to 80% of cartilaginous tumors, typically demonstrating a ring-and-arc pattern of calcification **(Option (A) is true).** This pattern may coalesce to form a more radio-opaque, flocculent pattern of calcification. The image of cartilage matrix is characteristic and usually allows a confident radiologic diagnosis of cartilaginous tumor. In general, higher-grade chondrosarcomas contain relatively less extensive areas of matrix mineralization **(Option (B) is false).** The depth of endosteal scalloping, at its most prominent focus, is the best distinguishing feature between a benign long-bone enchondroma and a malignant chondrosarcoma **(Option (C) is false).** Endosteal scalloping depth greater than two-thirds the normal thickness of the long-bone cortex is strong evidence of chondrosarcoma. Longitudinal, endosteal scalloping in long-bone lesions, greater than two-thirds of the lesion's length, is also suggestive of a conventional chondrosarcoma, although it is not as distinctive a feature as the depth of scalloping **(Option (D) is false).** The imaging criteria that have been established for long-bone chondrosarcomas, particularly deep scalloping, are not readily applicable to the small bones of the hands and feet **(Option (E) is false).** While enchondromas in the small bones are common, chondrosaroma in these sites is quite rare.

Question 82

Regarding the imaging of intramedullary chondrosarcoma:

(A) Lesions generally do not show increased radionuclide accumulation on scintigraphy.

(B) CT is especially useful in determining the extent and depth of endosteal scalloping.

(C) The presence and pattern of mineralization on CT imaging is useful in distinguishing enchondroma from chondrosarcoma.

(D) The nonmineralized portions of low-grade chondrosarcoma will demonstrate a low attenuation on CT imaging.

(E) The nonmineralized portions will show peripheral and septal contrast enhancement on CT imaging.

In general, more than three-quarters of long bone chondrosarcomas will show radionuclide uptake greater than that of the anterior iliac crest. This is in contrast to long bone enchondromas, which show increased radiotracer activity in less than a quarter of cases **(Option (A) is false)**. In addition, a heterogeneous pattern of radionuclide uptake is also more common among conventional intramedullary chondrosarcomas.

CT imaging is ideal for evaluating the depth of endosteal scalloping. Reformatted long axis imaging is a useful adjunct in this regard and generally depicts the degree of scalloping more accurately than radiographs **(Option (B) is true)**. Long bone chondrosarcomas have focal areas of greater than two-thirds scalloping of the normal cortical thickness in 90% of cases, as opposed

to enchondromas, which demonstrate this finding in only 10%. The longitudinal extent of endosteal scalloping is also well depicted on CT scans. CT is very useful in identifying and characterizing matrix, especially when lesions are subtle or in areas with complex anatomy. Neither the presence nor extent of matrix mineralization, however, can help distinguish between a long bone enchondroma and a chondrosarcoma **(Option (C) is false)**. A temporal change in the pattern of mineralization, however, is important in identifying a change in biological behavior. Hence, an area with mineralized matrix that becomes lytic on follow-up examination is always suspicious for malignant transformation.

The nonmineralized intraosseous (and extraosseous) components of chondrosarcoma typically show a low attenuation on CT scans (reflecting the high water content of hyaline cartilage) and may mimic the attenuation of a cystic lesion **(Option (D) is true)**. Following the administration of contrast, CT may demonstrate mild peripheral rim as well as septal enhancement **(Option (E) is true)**. This pattern of enhancement is more readily seen at MR imaging. Higher-grade lesions may show higher CT attenuation, similar to that of muscle,

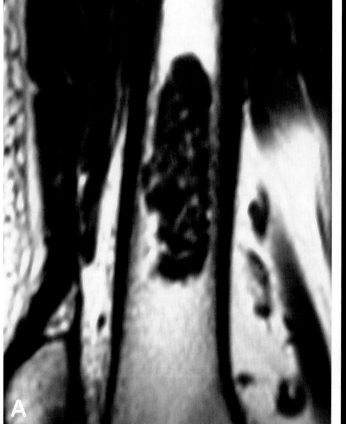
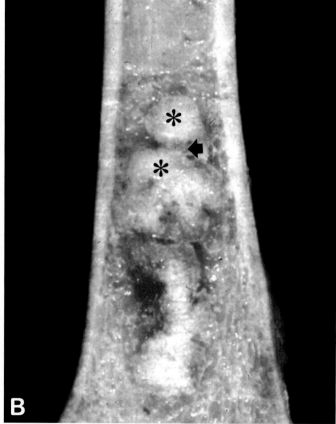

Figure 17-5. Enchondroma. Femur. MRI. T1-weighted. Sagittal plane. (A) Distal femur. There is fatty marrow extending between the nodules of cartilage within the tumor. (B) Tibia (different patient). Gross specimen. Fatty marrow (arrow) is extending between lobules of hyaline cartilage (asterisks).

and more prominent diffuse or nodular contrast enhancement, caused by increased cellularity and resultant reduced water content.

Question 83

Regarding the MR imaging of intramedullary chondrosarcoma:

(A) Identification of entrapped foci of yellow marrow on T1-weighted images within a cartilage lesion virtually excludes the diagnosis of chondrosarcoma.

(B) The nonmineralized hyaline cartilage within a chondrosarcoma may show a cyst-like signal intensity.

(C) The extent and depth of endosteal scalloping cannot be adequately assessed on MR imaging.

(D) The pattern of contrast enhancement on MR imaging can reliably distinguish enchondroma from chondrosarcoma.

(E) The rate of contrast enhancement on MR imaging has been accepted as a standard method to distinguish enchondroma from chondrosarcoma.

On T1-weighted MR images, hyaline cartilage tumors appear as focal masses with low to intermediate signal intensity. Areas of fatty marrow, demonstrating high signal intensity on T1-weighted MR images may be seen between the lobules of cartilage in cases of long bone intramedullary chondrosarcoma about 35% of the time. Such T1-weighted high signal areas are much more commonly seen among enchondromas (Figure 17-5), occurring in about 65% of cases **(Option (A) is false).**

The nonmineralized components of a chondrosarcoma have fluid-like signal intensity on MR images (Figure 17-6), reflecting the high water content of hyaline cartilage **(Option (B) is true).** Areas of matrix mineralization are common in intramedullary chondrosarcoma and have low signal intensity with all MR pulse sequences, giving the lesion a heterogeneous appearance, best appreciated on T2-weighted MR images.

Both the depth and extent of endosteal scalloping are well depicted by MR imaging, particularly with proton-density-weighted sequences **(Option (C) is false).** CT and MR imaging are both superior to radiography for evaluating scalloping.

Conventional intramedullary chondrosarcoma will typically demonstrate mild peripheral and septal contrast enhancement (Figure 17-7). It has been suggested

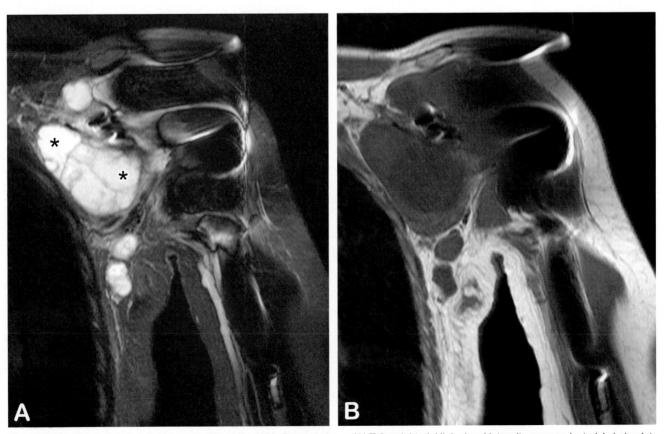

Figure 17-6. Recurrent chondrosarcoma. Shoulder. MRI. Coronal plane. (A) T-2 weighted. High signal intensity masses (asterisks) simulating cysts and representing nodules of hyaline cartilage of the recurrent tumor, extend into the axilla. (B) T1-weighted. On the T1-weighted image, the masses are low signal intensity within the recurrence, simulating cysts.

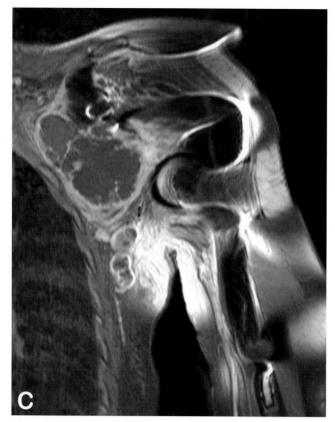

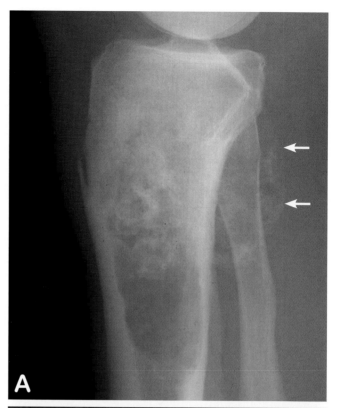

Figure 17-6 (continued). Recurrent chondrosarcoma. Shoulder. MRI. Coronal plane. (C) T1-weighted. IV contrast. Fat-suppression. The cyst-like masses show peripheral enhancement, an appearance that may also be seen in an abscess. The patient was a 48-year-old woman.

that this pattern of enhancement allows differentiation of intramedullary chondrosarcomas from enchondromas, which have peripheral enhancement only, but there is sufficient overlap of enhancement to preclude reliable distinction between low-grade intramedullary chondrosarcoma and enchondroma **(Option (D) is false).** The rate of contrast enhancement has also been suggested as a method of distinguishing between enchondroma and chondrosarcoma, with malignant lesions showing early enhancement. Although this technique has not been widely adopted, preliminary reports are encouraging. Fast-contrast-enhancement imaging has a sensitivity, specificity, and positive predictive value for chondrosarcoma of between 80% and 90%. While this technique may yet prove to be useful, at present it is not accepted as a reliable way to distinguish enchondroma and chondrosarcoma **(Option (E) is false).**

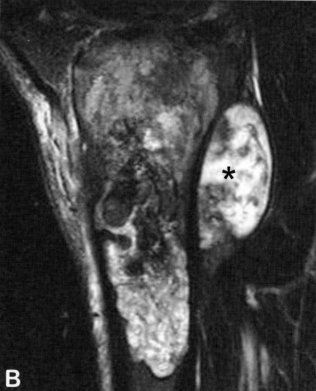

Figure 17-7. Chondrosarcoma of the proximal tibia. (A) Radiograph. Lateral view. A mass is seen in the proximal tibia. Its superior aspect is more mineralized, with a typical cartilaginous pattern. Note the extensive soft tissue extension posteriorly (arrows). (B) MRI. T2-weighted. Sagittal plane. The lesion has high signal intensity on this fluid-sensitive sequence. Note the posterior extension (asterisk). The signal intensity will vary with the amount of tumor mineralization, cellularity, and myxoid change.

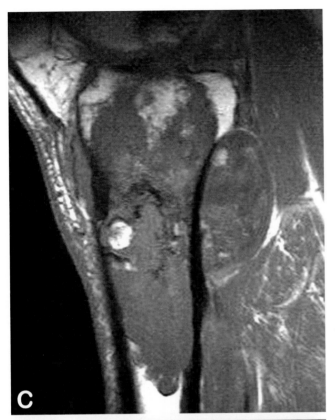

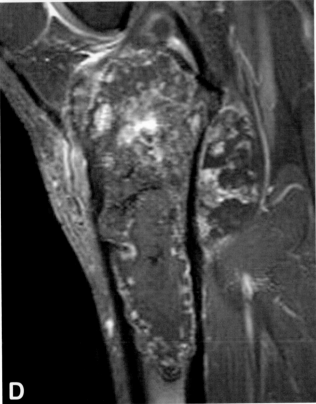

Figure 17-7 (continued). Chondrosarcoma of the proximal tibia. (C) MRI. T1-weighted. Sagittal plane. Note the fat within the lesion, seen as bright signal. (D) MRI. IV contrast. Sagittal plane. Following contrast administration the mass showed prominent areas of peripheral and septal enhancement. The patient was a 56-year-old man.

Suggested Readings

1. Brien EW, Mirra JM, Kerr R. Benign and malignant cartilage tumors of bone and joint: their anatomic and theoretical basis with an emphasis on radiology, pathology and clinical biology I. The intramedullary cartilage tumors. Skeletal Radiol. 1997; 26:325–353.

2. Geirnaerdt MJ, Hogendoorn PCW, Bloem JL, Taminiau AHM, van der Woude HJ, Cartilage tumors: fast contrast-enhanced MR imaging. Radiology. 2000;214:539–546.

3. Mirra JM. Intramedullary cartilage- and chondroid-producing tumors. In: Mirra JM, ed. Bone Tumors. Clinical, Radiologic and Pathologic Correlation. Philadelphia, PA: Lea & Febiger; 1989: 439–690.

4. Murphey MD, Walker EA, Wilson AJ, Kransdorf MJ, Temple T, Gannon HF. Imaging of primary chondrosarcoma: radiologic-pathologic correlation. RadioGraphics. 2003;23:1245–1278.

5. Murphey MD, Flemming DJ, Boyea SR, Bojescul JA, Sweet DE, Temple HT. Enchondroma versus chondrosarcoma in the appendicular skeleton: differentiating features. RadioGraphics. 1998;18:1213–1237.

6. Resnick D, Kyriakos M, Greenway GD. Tumors and tumor-like lesions of bone: imaging and pathology of specific lesions. In: Resnick D, ed. Bone and Joint Disorders, 4th ed. Philadelphia, PA: W.B. Saunders Company; 2002: 3763–4128.

7. SLICED Study Group. Reliability of histopathologic and radiologic grading of cartilaginous neoplasms in long bone. J Bone Joint Surg Am. 2007;89:2113–2123.

8. Unni KK. Dahlin's Bone Tumors. General Aspects and Data on 11,087 Cases, 5th ed. Philadelphia, PA: Lippincott-Raven; 1996: 71–108.

Case 18

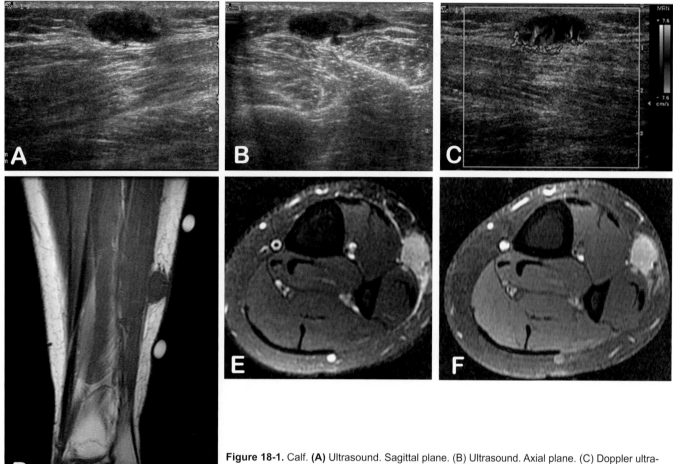

Figure 18-1. Calf. **(A)** Ultrasound. Sagittal plane. (B) Ultrasound. Axial plane. (C) Doppler ultrasound. Sagittal plane. (D) MRI. T1-weighted. Coronal plane. (E) MRI. T2-weighted. Axial plane. (F) MRI. Postcontrast. T1-weighted, fat-suppressed. Axial plane.

Question 84

A 19-year-old woman presented with a lump at the lateral aspect of the distal lower limb. It was slightly tender on palpation, and there was no redness or discoloration of the overlying skin. You are shown three ultrasound images and three MR images (Figure 18-1). Which *one* of the following is the MOST likely diagnosis?

(A)   Soft tissue sarcoma
(B)   Foreign body granuloma
(C)   Fibromatosis
(D)   Granular cell tumor
(E)   Hematoma

Cesare Romagnoli, M.D.

Soft Tissue Tumors

Question 84

Which *one* of the following is the MOST likely diagnosis?

(A) Soft tissue sarcoma
(B) Foreign body granuloma
(C) Fibromatosis
(D) Granular cell tumor
(E) Hematoma

Ultrasound shows a subcutaneous, solid nodule with lobulated contours (Figure 18-2A). Intense vascular flow is demonstrated by color Doppler ultrasound (Figure 18-2C) and power Doppler ultrasound (Figure 18-2G). Mild perinodular hyperechogenicity is present, consistent with edema. The nodule is not limited by the muscle fascia, and invasion of the underlying peroneal muscle is present (Figure 18-2B, 18-2C and 18-2D).

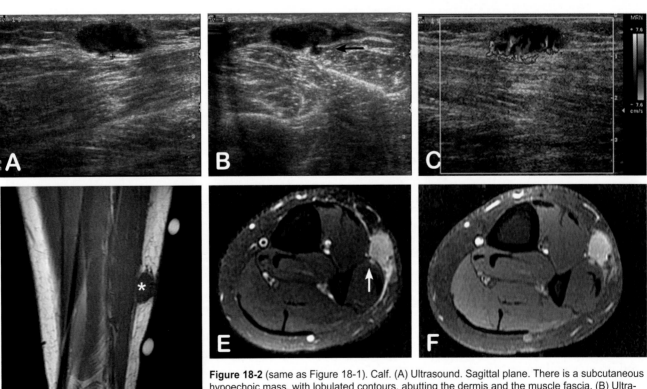

Figure 18-2 (same as Figure 18-1). Calf. (A) Ultrasound. Sagittal plane. There is a subcutaneous hypoechoic mass, with lobulated contours, abutting the dermis and the muscle fascia. (B) Ultrasound. Axial plane. A small nodule extends from the mass into the muscle belly of the underlying peroneal muscle, through a discontinuity of the fascia. (C) Doppler ultrasound. Sagittal plane. There is marked vascular flow to the mass, more so in its deeper aspect. (D) MRI. T1-weighted. Coronal plane. A subcutaneous nodule can be seen at the lateral aspect of the calf. It is homogeneously hypointense. (E) MRI. T2-weighted. Axial plane. There is a subcutaneous mass that is homogeneously hyperintense, extending along the fascia of the peroneal muscles. A small nodule extends from it into the muscle (arrows). (F) MRI. IV contrast-aided, T1-weighted, fat-saturated. Axial plane.

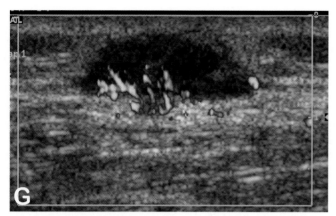

Figure 18-2 (continued). Marked enhancement of the subcutaneous mass is seen. The mass invades the underlying muscle fascia and the peroneal muscle. (G) Power Doppler ultrasound. Magnified image. Tumoral vessels extending into the underlying muscle are well seen.

On MR, the nodule has well defined but irregular contours. It is homogeneously hypointense on T1 (Figure 18-2D), and hyperintense on T2 (Figure 18-2E). Following IV gadolinium injection it shows diffuse, intense enhancement (Figure 18-2F). Again, it is seen to involve the adjacent peroneal muscle.

Due to the presence of deep muscle invasion, diffuse contrast enhancement, and intense vascular flow by Doppler ultrasound, malignancy should be considered. Biopsy confirmed the diagnosis of low-grade leiomyosarcoma **(Option (A) is correct).**

Soft tissue sarcomas can arise anywhere in the body. The most common sites of soft tissue sarcomas are the large muscles of the extremities, mediastinum and retroperitoneum. Subcutaneous soft tissue sarcomas are very rare, and the exact frequency is hard to assess. They are usually classified histologically as low-grade and high-grade. Low-grade sarcomas tend to be locally aggressive but without metastases, while high-grade sarcomas imply the presence or potential for disseminated metastases. However, this classification is often difficult and controversial.

Superficial leiomyosarcomas (cutaneous and subcutaneous) represent 2% or 3% of superficial soft tissue sarcomas. They are more common in the fifth to seventh decade of life but can happen at any age. Gender predominance is debated in the literature. The most typical location is the muscles within the hair-covered, extensor surface of the extremities. The cutaneous form of leiomyosarcoma produces changes in the overlying skin (such as discoloration, umbilication and ulceration), while the subcutaneous form produces only skin surface elevation. Both forms cause pain. Recurrence is relatively frequent (up to

50%), but metastases are not. However, distant spread of the disease is more common among the subcutaneous cases and those that penetrate the deep soft tissues than it is in the cutaneous forms. After recurrence, the probability of metastasis increases. Surgery is the treatment of choice. Radiotherapy has been used, but with poor results.

Benign soft tissue tumors are much more common than malignant soft tissue tumors, with a ratio of 100:1. Soft tissue sarcomas can occur at any age, but there is a certain preference for the fifth to seventh decades of life.

Granulomas may occur in response to relatively inert foreign bodies (e.g., suture, splinter, breast implant), forming so-called foreign-body granulomas. Granulomatous inflammation is a distinctive pattern of chronic inflammation characterized by aggregations of activated macrophages that have acquired an enlarged squamous-cell-like (called "epithelioid") appearance. Foreign body granulomas usually present as subcutaneous hypoechoic nodules, and can show some degree of vascular flow on Doppler ultrasound. The granulomas can abut the muscle fascia, but extension into the deep muscle is extremely unlikely **(Option (B) is incorrect).** Besides, in most cases the presence of a foreign body within the nodule is a very valuable clue to the diagnosis. Metal or glass foreign bodies are easily identified with radiography, while wooden foreign bodies (splinters) are usually missed (Figure 18-3A) by x-ray and can be better seen with sonography. The splinter is usually hyperechoic (Figure 18-3B), with well-defined contours and a specific form, such as a thorn (Figure 18-3C). Ultrasound can be used as a guide for removal of such foreign bodies under local anesthesia (Figure 18-3D), avoiding more aggressive surgery. CT and MRI are not needed for diagnosis and treatment in most cases.

Fibromatosis can present as superficial hypoechoic nodules, but the disease involves either the palmar aponeurosis (Dupuytren disease), or the plantar fascia (Ledderhose disease), or the penis (Peyronie disease). This is not the case with the test patient **(Option (C) is incorrect).**

Granular cell tumor is a relatively common disease, occurring more frequently in black people and women. Locations that are more frequent include subcutaneous tissue, submucosal tissue, and visceral structures. The tongue is the most common site, followed by chest wall and upper limbs. There is controversy about the histogenesis, but Schwann cells seem to be the most probable origin of granular cell tumors. His-

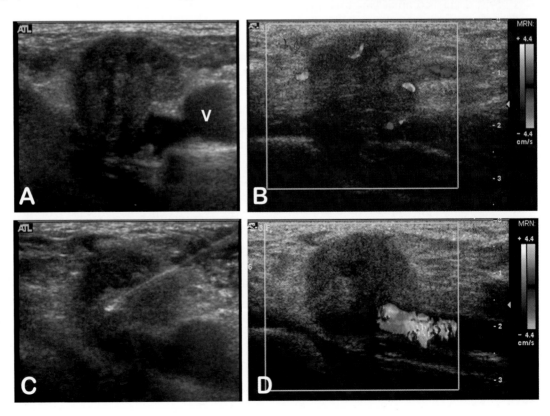

Figure 18-3. Foreign body in finger. (A) Radiograph. Lateral view. There is focal soft tissue swelling at the volar aspect of the base of the third finger. There is no evidence of abnormal opacities within the soft tissues. (B) Ultrasound. Axial view. An oval soft tissue mass can be seen, located within the subcutaneous tissue at the volar aspect of the third finger. Within the mass is an echogenic ring (arrow) with central hypoechogenicity and subtle posterior shadowing. (C) Ultrasound. Longitudinal plane, perpendicular to the mass in panel B. The central hyperechogenicity now has a triangular shape, strongly resembling a thorn. (D) Ultrasound. Longitudinal plane. Under ultrasound guidance, the foreign body is seen deep to the small echogenic forceps (arrows). Ultrasound allowed the foreign body to be carefully extracted, avoiding rupture of tissues.

Figure 18-4. Granular cell tumor. Left groin. Ultrasound. (A) Axial plane. There is a solid lobulated nodule abutting the femoral vessels (V = femoral vein). (B) Doppler. Longitudinal plane. Vascular flow is seen within the nodule. (C) Longitudinal plane. A linear echogenicity is seen extending into the mass from the reader's right. Its tip is seen within the mass, suggesting a successful biopsy. (D) Doppler. Longitudinal plane. Prior to biopsy, color Doppler was used to highlight the femoral artery (color-filled), so that it could be avoided during the procedure.

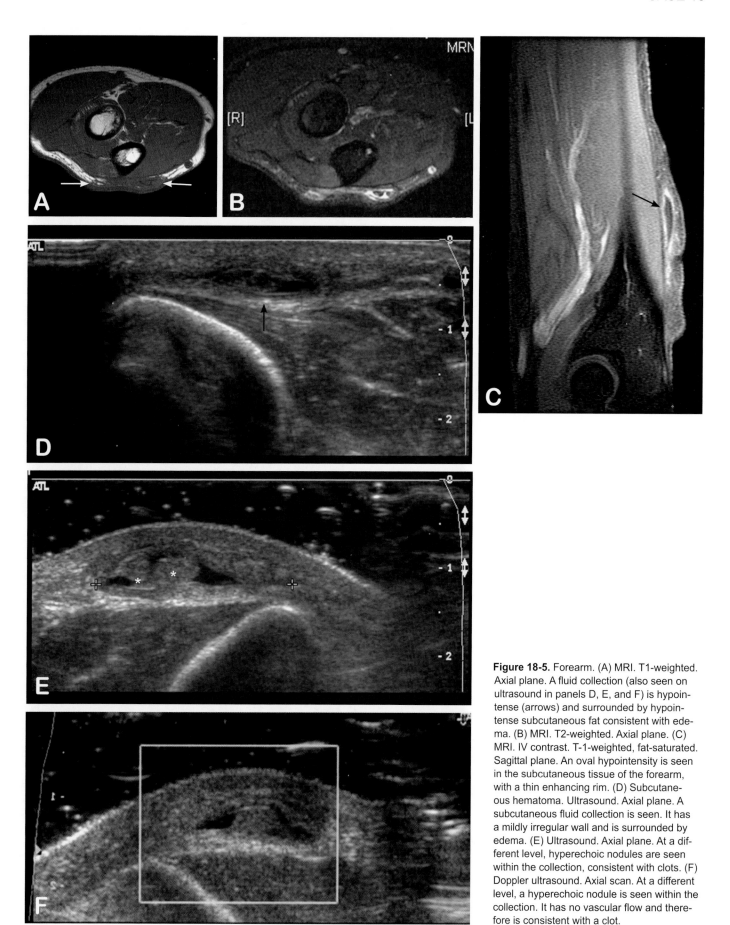

Figure 18-5. Forearm. (A) MRI. T1-weighted. Axial plane. A fluid collection (also seen on ultrasound in panels D, E, and F) is hypointense (arrows) and surrounded by hypointense subcutaneous fat consistent with edema. (B) MRI. T2-weighted. Axial plane. (C) MRI. IV contrast. T-1-weighted, fat-saturated. Sagittal plane. An oval hypointensity is seen in the subcutaneous tissue of the forearm, with a thin enhancing rim. (D) Subcutaneous hematoma. Ultrasound. Axial plane. A subcutaneous fluid collection is seen. It has a mildly irregular wall and is surrounded by edema. (E) Ultrasound. Axial plane. At a different level, hyperechoic nodules are seen within the collection, consistent with clots. (F) Doppler ultrasound. Axial scan. At a different level, a hyperechoic nodule is seen within the collection. It has no vascular flow and therefore is consistent with a clot.

tologically these tumors are formed by uniform round or polygonal cells, containing granules within their cytoplasm. They often occur in close association with peripheral nerves. Malignancy is very rare, but cases have been described, representing about 1% of the total number of granular cell tumors.

On sonography, these masses are typically well-defined nonspecific hypoechoic nodules which show no evidence of extension into surrounding structures (Figure 18-4A). Doppler ultrasound shows mild vascular flow (Figure 18-4B). The test case images are not consistent with these findings **(Option (D) is incorrect)**. Imaging findings are usually not specific, and ultrasound-guided biopsy is usually required (Figure 18-4C). Doppler can be useful to help define adjacent vascular structures during a biopsy procedure (Figure 18-4D).

On MRI, granular cell tumors are slightly hypointense on T1- and heterogeneously hyperintense on T2-weighted sequences. Following contrast injection, those nodules show homogeneous enhancement. On CT, nonspecific solid nodules with homogeneous contrast enhancement are demonstrated.

Hematomas are commonly found in the subcutaneous tissue. A subcutaneous fluid collection is usually demonstrated, sometimes containing a fluid-fluid level, due to sedimentation of the cellular component **(Option (E) is incorrect)**. In most cases, a history of previous trauma is very helpful in confirming the diagnosis, but sometimes the patient is not able to recollect any trauma. This is the case for the patient in Figure 18-5 who had an MRI study to assess a lump in the left elbow. No bruise was seen on the adjacent skin, and the patient stated that the lump had decreased in size during the last two weeks. An elongated, subcutaneous fluid collection is demonstrated that is hypointense on T1-weighted MRI (Figure 18-5A). On T2-weighted (Figure 18-5B) sequences, the lesion is mostly hyperintense with a few hypointense foci, an appearance consistent with clots. A thin, regular, mildly enhancing rim is seen following intravenous injection of gadolinium (Figure 18-5C). On sonography a mildly echogenic fluid collection is present that corresponds to the one seen on MRI (Figure 18-5D). It is surrounded by some subcutaneous edema. Echogenic foci within the collection likely represent clots (Figure 18-5E). Mild vascular flow is demonstrated at the edge of the collection by Doppler ultrasound (Figure 18-5F).

Most subcutaneous hematomas are self-limiting, but occasionally they can become chronic and even begin to grow slowly. The mechanism is thought to be secondary to the disruption of capillaries in the dermis, and therefore the disruption of the drainage of

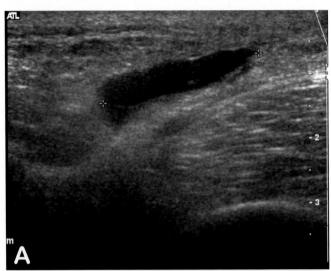

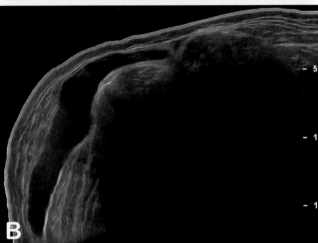

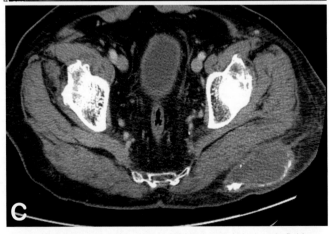

Figure 18-6. Morel-Lavallee lesion. (A) Ultrasound. A chronic fluid collection abuts the muscle aponeurosis at the lateral aspect of the hip (so-called Morel-Lavallee lesion). (B) Ultrasound. A large chronic subcutaneous fluid collection abutting the aponeurosis of the quadratus lumborum muscle is another example of the Morel-Lavallee lesion. (C) CT. The image shows the presence of a subcutaneous fluid collection with a calcific wall, abutting the underlying muscle aponeurosis. It is surrounded by subcutaneous fat stranding, suggesting infection.

blood lymph and debris into the perifascial plane. This occurrence is more likely in areas where the dermis has a richer vascular plexus, such as the peritrocanteric area (so called "Morel-Lavallee lesions") (Figure 18-6A). However the same abnormality can also be seen in other locations, such as the abdominal wall (Figure 18-6B). Lesions at these sites can last many years, without causing serious trouble, although occasionally complications such as infection and abscess formation can be seen, (Figure 18-6C-E).

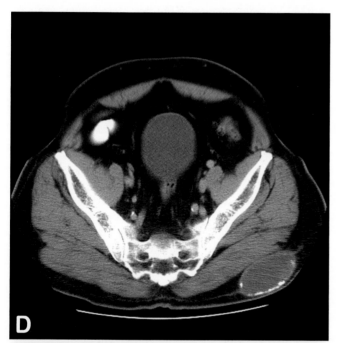

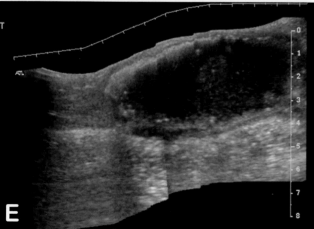

Figure 18-6 (continued). Morel-Lavallee lesion. (D) CT. A scan taken seven years earlier showed a similar fluid collection, confirming the chronic nature of the lesion. Note, however, the lack of perilesional subcutaneous edema. (E) Ultrasound. The presence of a fluid collection with an irregular debris-containing wall is confirmed on this image. Ultrasound-guided biopsy confirmed the presence of pus.

Question 85

Regarding fibromatosis:

(A) It can cause metastasis.
(B) The superficial form is more aggressive than the deep form.
(C) Palmar fibromatosis causes retraction more often than plantar fibromatosis.
(D) Plantar fibromatosis is a synonym for plantar fasciitis.
(E) Palmar fibromatosis and plantar fibromatosis are often bilateral.

The term fibromatosis represents a group of diseases showing fibroblastic proliferation. They can be locally aggressive with a tendency to recur after surgery, but they do not metastasize **(Option (A) is false).** The histology seen in fibromatosis can vary with the phase of the disease. In an early phase lesions appear more cellular, with uniform, proliferating fibroblasts. In a later phase, abundant, dense collagen predominates. Cases of fibromatosis are divided into superficial and deep forms (See Table 18-1). Superficial forms also show predominantly abundant and dense collagen.

Table 18-1. Classification of Fibromatosis	
Superficial	*Deep*
Palmar	Extra-abdominal (aggressive)
Plantar	Abdominal (desmoid)
Penile	Intra-abdominal - mesenteric - pelvic - Gardner's syndrome

Deep fibromatosis tends to grow faster and recurs more often after resection, while superficial fibromatosis has a less aggressive pattern **(Option (B) is false).**

Plantar fibromatosis (Ledderhose disease) is a superficial fibromatosis and is relatively common. Contracture is possible, but less common than with cases of superficial palmar or penile fibromatosis **(Option (C) is true).** On sonography, plantar fibromatosis presents with elongated, hypoechoic nodules (Figure 18-7A) that involve the plantar fascia. It can be easily distinguished from plantar fasciitis, which involves the plantar fascia at its insertion into the calcaneus (Figure 18-7B), while plantar fibromatosis involves the distal and medial aspect of the plantar fascia (Figure 18-7C) **(Option (D) is false).** Usually, Doppler ultrasound fails to show vascular flow (Figure 18-7D).

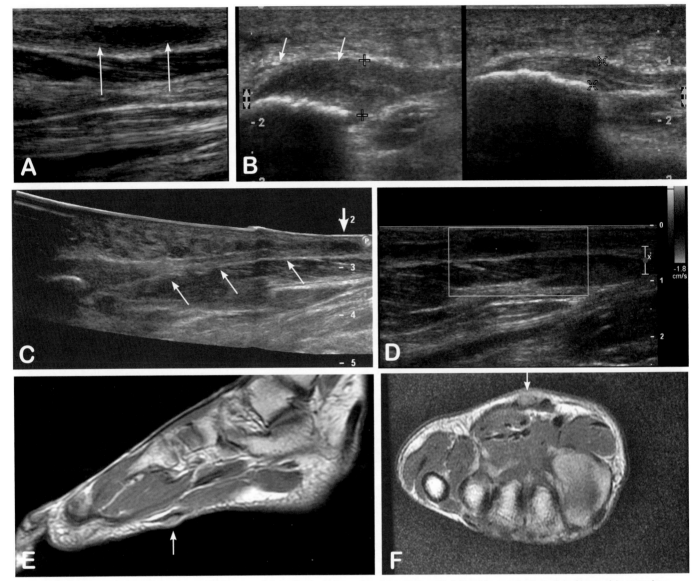

Figure 18-7. Plantar fibromatosis. Foot. (A) Ultrasound. Longitudinal plane. An elongated, well-defined hypoechoic nodule (arrows) is seen between the intrinsic muscles of the foot and the skin. (B) Plantar fascitis in another patient. Ultrasound. Axial plane. There is thickening and hypoechogenicity of the plantar fascia at the calcaneal insertion (arrows) on the left. Compare this with the normal side on the reader's right. (C) Plantar fibromatosis. Ultrasound, Longitudinal plane. An extended view shows the location of the nodule (large arrow) within the distal portion of the plantar fascia (thin arrows) (D) Plantar fibromatosis. Doppler ultrasound. Longitudinal plane. (E) Plantar fibromatosis. MRI. T1-weighted. Sagittal plane.This sequence shows the fibromatosis nodule in the distal medial plantar fascia and adjacent subcutaneous tissues. An elongated nodule of intermediate signal (arrow) is located at the superficial aspect of the plantar fascia. (F) Plantar fibromatosis. MRI. T2-weighted. Axial plane.This sequence shows the flat fibromatosis nodule in the distal medial plantar fascia and adjacent subcutaneous tissues. The small mass (arrow) is noted to be slightly hyperintense compared to muscle.

On MRI, the nodules are usually of low to intermediate signal intensity on T1 and T2 (Figure 18-7E and 18-7F), with possible central hyperintensity on fat-saturated, fast-proton-density, or inversion-recovery sequences. Contrast enhancement is variable. The nodules can be single or multiple, and are often bilateral **(Option (E) is true).**

Question 86

Regarding subcutaneous lipomas:

(A) They represent the most common subcutaneous mass.
(B) At least two-thirds of superficial lipomas have a characteristic ultrasound pattern and do not require further workup.
(C) Marked vascular flow on Doppler virtually excludes the diagnosis of lipoma.
(D) Follow up of subcutaneous lipomas is recommended to rule out malignant transformation.

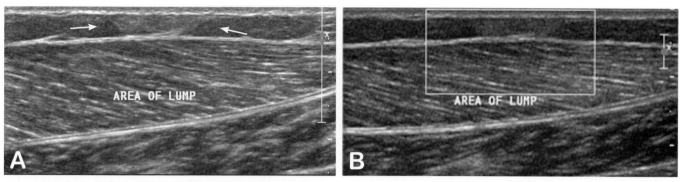

Figure 18-8. Subcutaneous lipoma. Calf. Ultrasound. (A) Longitudinal plane. A well-defined, subcutaneous, hyperechoic oval nodule is seen. (B) Doppler ultrasound. No vascular flow is visible within the nodule. This was a lipoma.

Subcutaneous lipomas are very common. Although their precise incidence is not known, because most lesions are not reported or treated, they are thought to represent at least 50% of subcutaneous masses **(Option (A) is true).** On ultrasound they are soft, compressible masses. Subcutaneous lipomas are usually oval or elongated, oriented along the axis of the skin. About a third of them are homogeneously hyperechoic (Figure 18-8A), with faint or absent flow on Doppler ultrasound (Figure 18-8B). Another third are hypoechoic to the surrounding fat, with irregular septations, resembling muscle (Figure18-8A). The rest have mixed, nonspecific echogenicity **(Option (B) is true).**

On CT, subcutaneous lipomas have a homogeneous fatty density. If they are not well encapsulated they can be difficult to distinguish from the surround-

ing subcutaneous fat (Figure 18-9B). On MR, subcutaneous lipomas typically are diffusely hyperintense on T1 and hypointense on T2. The signal drops with fat suppressed sequences. Most lipomas show little, if any, enhancement following intravenous injection of iodine contrast or gadolinium. Most superficial lipomas show mild or no vascular flow on Doppler ultrasound (Figure 18-8B). There are important exceptions to this rule, however, because a few subtypes, such as spindle cell lipomas, may show intense vascular enhancement in the nonadipose component of the tumor (Figure 18-10A to Figure 18-10D) **(Option (C) is false).**

Despite the fact that sporadic reports of malignant transformation can be found, this possibility is considered either extremely rare or nonexistent, and follow-up is not thought necessary **(Option (D) is false).**

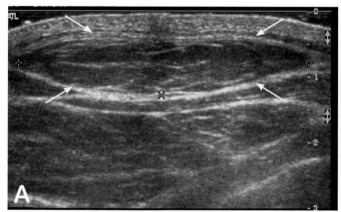
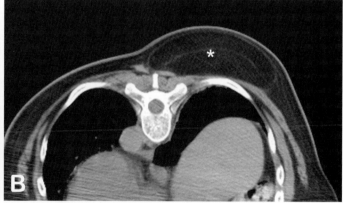

Figure 18-9. Subcutaneous lipoma. Neck. (A) Ultrasound. Axial plane. There is an elongated, biconvex nodule, hypoechoic to the subcutaneous fat, with irregular septations. Note the resemblance to the underlying muscle. It proved to be a lipoma despite being hypoechoic. (B) Subcutaneous lipoma in a different patient. CT. Axial plane. A subcutaneous mass is seen on the right posterior chest wall, producing bulging of the overlying skin. It has fat (negative Hounsfield unit) density with a few thin septations. There is faint demarcation with the surrounding subcutaneous fat.

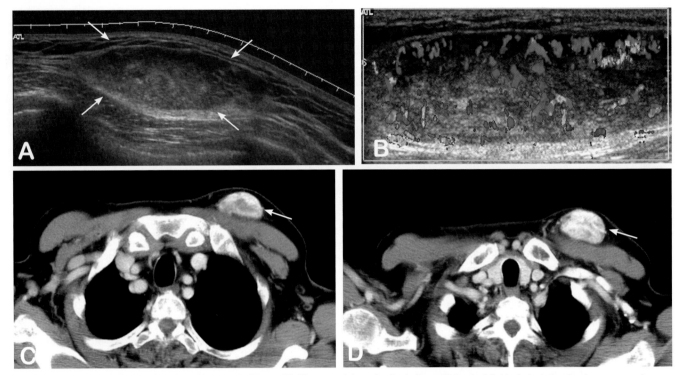

Figure 18-10. Spindle cell lipoma of the chest wall. Chest. (A) Ultrasound. Longitudinal plane. Extended field of view. A subcutaneous oval mass with heterogeneous echotexture is seen (arrows). (B) Doppler ultrasound. Longitudinal plane. Intense vascular flow is seen with the mass. (C) CT. Upper chest/low neck area. IV contrast. A mass in the left chest wall shows intense, heterogenous contrast enhancement.

Question 87

Regarding benign/malignant characterization of subcutaneous nodules:

(A) Subcutaneous benign nodules are 5 times more common than subcutaneous malignant nodules.
(B) Absence of fat in a mass virtually excludes liposarcoma.
(C) Posterior enhancement of a subcutaneous nodule on ultrasound is not a reliable sign that it is benign.
(D) Malignant peripheral nerve sheath tumors are 10 times more common in patients with neurofibromatosis 1 than in the general population.
(E) Neurofibromatosis 1 is associated with numerous neoplasms, including gastrointestinal stromal tumors.

Benign soft tissue tumors are much more common than malignant ones, in a ratio of 100:1 **(Option (A) is false).**

Liposarcoma is the second most common soft tissue malignancy, after malignant fibrous hystiocytoma. From an imaging perspective it is useful to divide liposarcomas into two categories: well-differentiated and dedifferentiated. The presence of fat varies according to histologic grade. A high-grade tumor may have so little fat that it cannot be detected by the usual imaging techniques. Twenty-two to fifty percent of dedifferentiated liposarcomas fail to show any fat on MR studies **(Option (B) is false).** However, dedifferentiated liposarco-

mas are much more common in the retroperitoneum and mediastinum, and quite rare in a subcutaneous location.

Posterior enhancement is a common finding in ultrasound imaging **(Option (C) is true).** It is typically seen posterior to cysts whose fluid content does not affect sound transmission. Consequently there is sound (echogenicity) seen posterior to a cyst. Posterior enhancement or prominent through transmission can also be seen posterior to masses made up of many small cells (such as some lymphomatous nodes). It is not a reliable sign for a benign lesion, because the small cells may be either benign or malignant **(Option (C) is true).** This increased through transmission consists of a bright zone of echoes deep to objects or lesions, which attenuates sound less than the surrounding tissue. Since less power of the ultrasound beam is spent going through the lesion, more echos are seen originating from the deeper structures. The ultrasound machine normally compensates for the rapid decline of the amplitude of echoes in deeper structures with the so-called "time compensation gain." When the decline does not happen due to lack of significant reflection or refraction within the lesion, the time compensation gain further amplifies the amplitude of the echoes arising from structures located deep to the lesion.

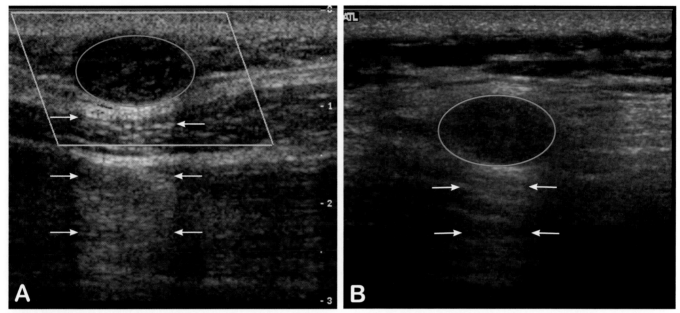

Figure 18-11. (A) Inclusion cyst. Ultrasound. Longitudinal plane. A subcutaneous, hypoechoic nodule (oval) shows prominent through transmission, related to its homogeneous sebaceous content. (B) In a different patient, a subcutaneous hypoechoic nodule (oval) abutting the muscle aponeurosis also shows through transmission. It was proven to be metastatic melanoma by ultrasound-guided biopsy.

This artifact is often seen in cystic anechoic lesions, usually increasing the confidence in a benign diagnosis. However, any homogeneous tissue that lacks interfaces able to change sound velocity can cause the same artifact (Figure 18-11A-B). Therefore solid masses (both benign and malignant) may also be associated with this artifact **(Option (C) is true)**.

Neurofibromatosis 1 (NF1) is a common genetic disease, with the genetic abnormality located in chromosome 17. The pattern of inheritance is autosomal dominant, but it is believed that the majority of cases are the consequence of new mutations. The malignant transformation of neurofibromas is a feared complication of NF1. Malignant peripheral nerve sheath tumors are ten times more common in patients with NF1 than in the general population **(Option (D) is true)**. However, malignant transformation of neurofibromas not associated with NF1 is rare.

Multiple neurofibromas and, above all, plexiform neurofibromas are the specific abnormality of neurofibromatosis 1. Neurofibromas localized in the dermis and subcutaneous tissue can be very numerous, are easily recognizable clinically, and are called fibroma molluscum (Figure 18-12A).

NF1 is associated with a long list of other findings and abnormalities, including café-au-lait spots, Lisch nodules (iris hamartoma) and osseous abnormalities such as scoliosis and kyphosis. It is also associated with tumors such as optic glioma, astrocytoma, glioblastoma multiforme, rhabdomyosarcoma, Triton tumor, pheochromocytoma, carcinoid, nephroblastoma gastrointestinal stromal tumor **(Option (E) is true)** and juvenile chronic myeloid leukemia. Figure 18-12B illustrates the case of a patient with NF1 and multiple intraperitoneal nodules consistent with neurofibromas. The largest nodule has a quite different echotexture (Figure 18-12C) compared to the other nodules, with a round central hypoechogenicity. On CT the same nodule was homogeneously enhancing (Figure 18-12D). This nodule was biopsied under ultrasound guidance to rule out malignant transformation, and the pathologist confirmed the presence of gastrointestinal stromal tumor (GIST).

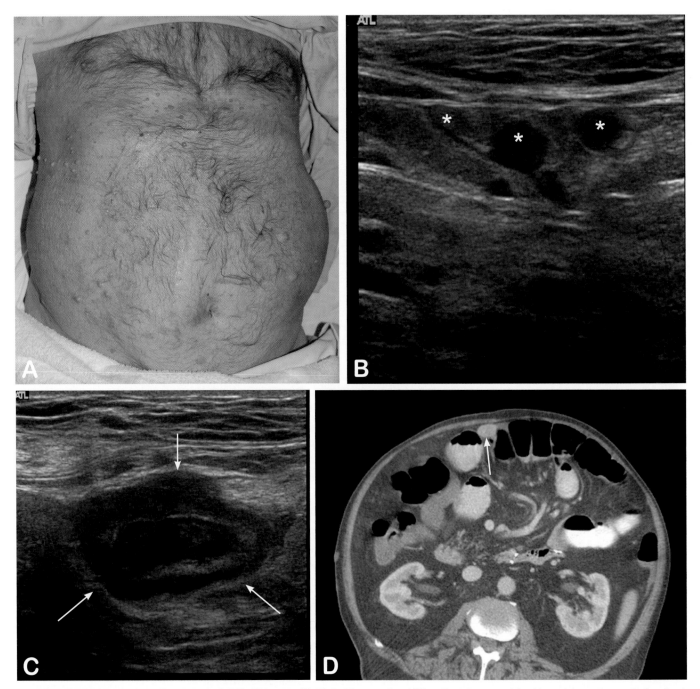

Figure 18-12. Findings in neurofibromatosis (NF1). Abdomen. (A) Clinical image of an NF1 patient. Innumerable skin nodules are seen in the chest and abdomen, consistent with fibroma molluscum. (B) Ultrasound. There are round hypoechoic nodules within the preperitoneal fat, consistent with small neurofibromas. (C) Ultrasound. The largest nodule shows a bulls-eye echotexture with a round central hypoechogenicity. (D) CT. The same nodule was homogeneously enhancing. This nodule when biopsied under ultrasound guidance proved to be a gastrointestinal stromal tumor (GIST).

Suggested Readings

1. Berquist TH. Musculoskeletal Imaging Companion, 2nd ed. Wolters Kluwer Health. Philadelphia, PA: Lippincott Williams and Wilkins; 2006.
2. Blacksin MF, Ha D. Superficial soft tissue masses of the extremities. RadioGraphics. 2006;26:1289–1304.
3. Enzinger FM, Weiss SW. Soft Tissue Tumors, 2nd ed. St. Louis, MO: Mosby; 1988.
4. Gaskin CM, Helms CA. Lipomas, Lipoma variants and well-differentiated liposarcomas (atypical lipomas): Results of MRI evaluations of 126 consecutive fatty masses. AJR Am J Roentgenol. 2004;182:733–739.
5. Jacobson JA, Powell A, Craig JG, et al. Wooden foreign bodies in soft tissue: detection at US. Radiology. 1998;206:45–48.
6. Kaplan PA, Helms CA, Dussault R, Anderson MW, Major NM. Muscoloskeletal MRI. Philadelphia, PA: Saunders; 2001.
7. Kransdorf MJ, Murphey MD. Imaging of Soft Tissue Tumors, 2nd ed. Philadelphia, PA: Lippincott Williams & Wilkins; 2006.
8. Kumar V, Cotran RS, Robbins SL. Basic Pathology, 6th ed. Philadelphia, PA: WB Saunders Company; 1997.
9. Levy A, Patel N, Abbot R, Dow N, Miettinen M, Sobin L. Gastrointestinal stromal tumors in patients with neurofibromatosis: imaging features with clinicopathologic correlation. AJR Am J Roentgenol. 2004;183:1629–1636.
10. Mellado JM, Perez del Palomar L. Long-standing Morel-Lavallee lesions of the trochanteric region and proximal thigh: MRI features in five patients. AJR Am J Roentgenol. 2004;182:1289–1294.
11. Middleton WD, Kurtz AB, Hertzberg BS, Ultrasound. The Requisites. 2nd ed. St. Louis, MO: Mosby; 2004.
12. Stoller DW, Atlas of Magnetic Resonance Imaging in Orthopedics and Sport Medicine, 3rd ed. Baltimore, MD: Lippincott Williams & Wilkins; 2007.
13. Torreggiani WC, Munk PL, Al-ismail K, et al. Granular cell tumour of the deltoid muscle. J HK Coll Radiol. 2001;4:160–163.
14. van Holsbeeck MT, Introcaso JH, Musculoskeletal Ultrasound, 2nd ed. St. Louis, MO: Mosby; 2001.

Case 19

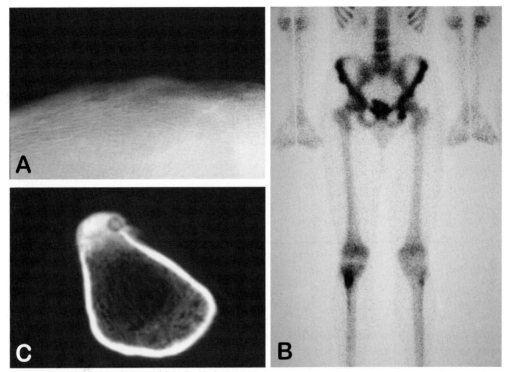

Figure 19-1. (A) Right knee. Cross-table radiograph. Right knee. Coned-down lateral view at the level of the tibial tuberosity. (B) Delayed phase technetium bone scan centered over the lower extremity. (C) CT. Right knee (proximal tibia).

Question 88

A 20-year-old man presented with knee pain. You are shown a lateral radiograph of his right knee (Figure 19-1A), a technetium bone scan delayed image (Figure 19-1B), and an unenhanced axial CT scan (Figure 19-1C). Which *one* of the following is the MOST likely diagnosis?

(A)   Cortical abscess
(B)   Stress fracture
(C)   Cortical hemangioma
(D)   Osteoid osteoma

Geert M. Vanderschueren, M.D., Ph.D.

Osteoid Osteoma

Question 88

Which *one* of the following is the MOST likely diagnosis?

(A) Cortical abscess
(B) Stress fracture
(C) Cortical hemangioma
(D) Osteoid osteoma

An osteoid osteoma typically consists of a small intracortical lucency (which may be calcified), the so-called nidus, surrounded by reactive sclerosis. It is typically seen in patients less than 20 years of age. There is a male predilection, with a male/female ratio of 2:1. Intraarticular lesions, however, may result in reactive synovitis but only a little bone formation, thus making radiographic diagnosis difficult. The location of the nidus is diaphyseal or metaphyseal, and only rarely epiphyseal. There is a predilection for the lower extremity, i.e. the femur and tibia.

A patient with osteoid osteoma typically presents with pain that is most severe at night and responds well to salicylates or other nonsteroidal antiinflammatory drugs. Prostaglandins, probably produced by the nidus, cause this pain by acting on unmyelinated sensory nerves in the region.

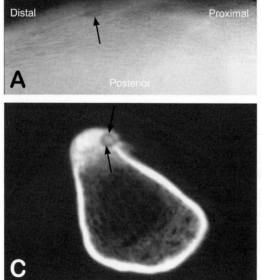

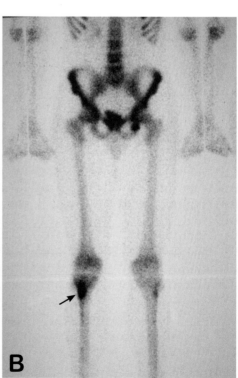

Figure 19-2 (same as 19-1). Right knee. (A) Cross-table radiograph. Lateral view. Coned-down image at the level of the tibial tuberosity. The image demonstrates a faint oval radiolucency (arrows) in the tibial tuberosity, with surrounding sclerosis. No definite intralesional calcification is appreciated. (B) Delayed-phase technetium bone scan. Increased uptake is identified in the region of the right tibial tuberosity (arrow). (C) CT. Axial plane at the proximal tibia. There is an intracortical lucency with surrounding sclerosis to the reader's left, and intralesional calcification noted as increased radiodensity (arrows). Findings are consistent with an osteoid osteoma of the tibial tuberosity.

Clinical suspicion for osteoid osteoma is typically confirmed by additional imaging, i.e., radiographs, scintigraphy or thin-slice (1-2 mm) CT. Radiographic criteria for the diagnosis of osteoid osteoma are the presence of a lucent nidus (varying in size from a few mm to 1.5 cm), surrounding reactive sclerosis, and, often, periosteal reaction (Figure 19-2A). The nidus may exhibit central calcification. Osteoid osteoma displays prominent activity on both immediate and delayed-phase bone scintigrams (Figure 19-2B). A "double density" sign may be present, representing the focally increased activity of the nidus, surrounded by an area of less intense activity. The radiographic features of osteoid osteoma are better displayed on thin-slice CT than on conventional radiographs, because the nidus is more clearly differentiated from the surrounding sclerosis on thin-slice cross-sectional imaging (Figure 19-2C). The test case is an osteoid osteoma **(Option (D) is correct).**

The role of magnetic resonance imaging (MRI) in the diagnosis of osteoid osteoma remains controversial (Figure 19-3). Early experience with MRI has shown that for cases in which the nidus is not identified, the presence of secondary marrow edema, joint effusion and reactive soft tissue changes/soft tissue edema may lead to an erroneous diagnosis of malignancy. Chronic osteomyelitis and intracortical abscess occur at all ages, and without a sex predilection. There is diffuse cortical thickening on radiographs, due to endosteal and periosteal bone apposition. A central lucency may be present on radiographs. The tibia is one of the more common locations, perhaps secondary to its immediately subcutaneous location, which predisposes it to traumatic implantation of bacteria. In addition, the rather poor blood supply, particularly of the anterior cortex of the tibia, facilitates chronic infection. Diagnosis often relies on tissue cultures (Figure 19-4). Magnetic resonance imaging (MRI) may be helpful to exclude associated soft tissue abscesses **(Option (A) is incorrect).**

Insufficiency fractures occur when normal stress is placed upon abnormal bone. Figure 19-2 shows a circular radiolucency rather than the linear radiolucency of a fracture **(Option (B) is incorrect).** Radionuclide bone scans often show focally increased uptake and may show unsuspected bilateral involvement. Stress fractures also occur at all ages and without sex predilection. The weight-bearing lower extremity is most commonly affected, with the tibia, fibula, tarsal navicular and metatarsals being the most common sites. Radiographs reveal cortical thickening. A linearly oriented fracture line may be seen (Figure 19-5). There are two types of stress fractures: fatigue fractures and insufficiency fractures. Fatigue

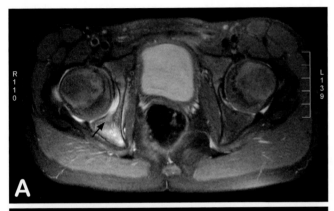

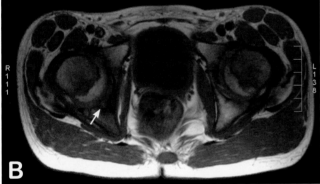

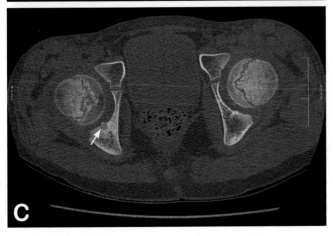

Figure 19-3. Osteoid osteoma. Axial plane through the lower pelvis. (A) MRI. T2-weighted. Fat-suppressed. There is bone marrow edema seen as high-intensity signal in the acetabulum, particularly posteriorly. A nidus is not definitely seen or separable from the edema. The MRI was performed because both conventional radiographs and bone scintigraphy (not shown) were inconclusive. (B) MRI. T1-weighted. An arrow points to a somewhat high-intensity posterior acetabular area surrounded by low-intensity signal. This is consistent with a partially calcified nidus. For cases in which the nidus is not clearly identified on MRI, the presence of reactive bone marrow and soft tissue edema may lead to an erroneous diagnosis of malignancy. (C) CT. Axial plane. A circular radiolucency (arrow) is surrounded by sclerosis. The nidus, which is partially calcified, is best seen on this CT image. The patient was a 10-year-old boy.

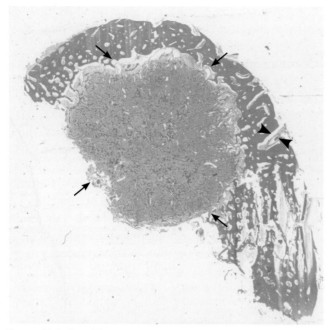

Figure 19-4. Osteoid osteoma. Pathologic specimen. The nidus (arrows) comprises a network of woven bone and osteoid embedded in a highly vascular stroma. The zone of reactive sclerosis (thickened bone surrounding the nidus) contains ecstatic blood vessels (arrowheads).

fractures are frequently seen in runners and occur when abnormal stress is placed on normal bone.

The intracortical hemangioma is a rare lesion **(Option (C) is incorrect).** Radiographically, it presents as a well-defined lucency that may be associated with cortical thickening or periostitis. Intracortical hemangioma typically demonstrates internal bone septation ("wire-netting" appearance) on radiographs, CT and MRI. Figure 19-2 demonstrates a nidus with central calcification, but without internal bone septations, going against the diagnosis of intracortical hemangioma.

Question 89

This 25-year-old woman (Figure 19-6 in the Test section) presented with left hip pain. The diagnosis of osteoid osteoma was made based upon clinical and radiological criteria. Thermocoagulation was performed successfully through a lateral approach (two electrode positions were used, corresponding to the "double track" present after thermocoagulation). The electrode is placed in different positions

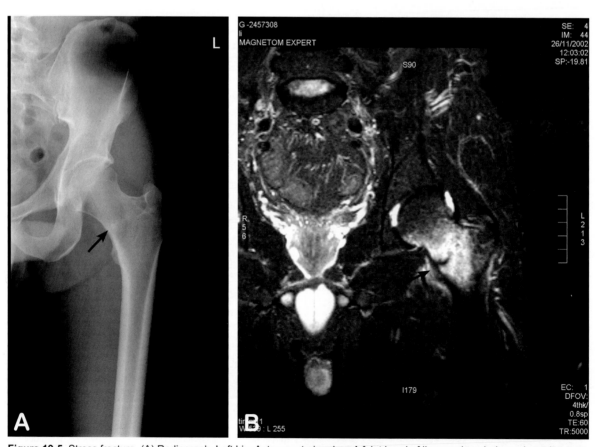

Figure 19-5. Stress fracture. (A) Radiograph. Left hip. Anteroposterior view. A faint band of linear sclerosis (arrow) can be seen medially in the lower left femoral neck. (B) MRI. Inversion-recovery, T2-weighted. The image reveals a linearly oriented stress fracture (arrow), with surrounding bone marrow edema. There is a small left hip joint effusion. The patient is a 50-year-old man who is an avid long-distance runner and complained of left hip pain.

across the osteoid osteoma to ensure complete ablation. Which *one* of the following is the MOST likely routine heating time for the thermocoagulation of an osteoid osteoma per electrode position?

(A) Four minutes at 90° C
(B) Two minutes at 90° C
(C) Four minutes at 150° C
(D) Ten minutes at 45° C

Thermocoagulation is generally performed under general anesthesia, with a routine heating time of four minutes (at 90°C) per electrode position **(Option (A) is correct)**. Some authors prefer a heating time of six minutes. A heating time of two minutes per electrode position is insufficient and may be the cause of treatment failure **(Option (B) is incorrect)**. A temperature above the boiling point of water (100° C) is considered inappropriate for thermocoagulation **(Option (C) is incorrect)**. During thermocoagulation the cytotoxic temperature threshold is 50° C, so a heating temperature of 45°C would be insufficient to produce thermonecrosis **(Option (D) is incorrect)**. A contraindication for thermocoagulation is the presence of a cardiac pacemaker. Potential complications are bleeding, nerve injury, and skin necrosis.

The first application of CT-guided thermocoagulation in the treatment of peripheral osteoid osteomas was described by Rosenthal et al in 1992. A short description of the thermocoagulation procedure in eight steps and recommendations (where applicable) follow:

1. *Localization and planning:* The procedure is performed under CT guidance. For a lesion greater than 1 cm, more than one electrode position is recommended, preferably with overlap of treatment zones. Sometimes entrance through the opposite normal cortex is recommended to avoid neurovascular structures in the proximity of the osteoid osteoma. Accurate measurement and localization of the lesion size prior to the procedure is therefore critical (Figure 19-7A).

2. *Placement of the grounding pad:* The pad should be positioned close to the planned skin entry to allow the shortest current path through the patient. A large grounding pad reduces the risk of skin burns at the site of the grounding pad.

3. *Superficial entry with use of tenting:* This technique minimizes the displacement of the needle by overlying tissues.

4. *Drilling:* This is performed with a drill inserted through a penetration cannula (Figure 19-7B).

5. *Biopsy:* In cases with an atypical radiological appearance (e.g., a diameter > 15 mm), intramedullary location or postsurgical changes obscuring the original lesion, or atypical clinical criteria (e.g., no nocturnal pain or no typical response to nonsteroidal anti-inflammatory drugs), a biopsy is recommended. Where Brodie's abscess is suspected, histology as well as cultures should be obtained.

6. *Thermocoagulation cannula and electrode placement:* Generally, the tip of the electrode should be positioned in the center of the lesion. The penetration cannula should be withdrawn at least 1 cm above the bare tip of the electrode, to prevent contact between the current and the penetration cannula; otherwise, tissue burns or loss of current may result. More than one electrode positioning may be necessary for complete tumor ablation. This is particularly true if the tumor tissue extends 5 mm beyond the electrode tip.

7. *Electrode connection:* If, after the electrode connection to the radiofrequency generator, the tissue resistance exceeds 1000 Ohm (200 to 600 Ohm is considered normal), there will be an inadequate circuit. Current would need to be excessively increased in order to achieve the desired temperature of 90°C. Possible causes may be an equipment fault or more commonly a "dry tip," an accumulation of dry debris at the electrode tip that can cause increased resistence and impede current flow. This can be avoided by flushing the thermocoagulation cannula with normal saline.

8. *Radiofrequency thermocoagulation:* Routine heating is performed at 90°C during a four-minute interval per electrode position. Current intensity is one of the most important variables influencing the size of the treatment zone. Only if appropriately applied current is used during thermocoagulation, can a treatment zone of the desired (predicted) and necessary size be obtained. If the current is too low, an undersized treatment zone will result. This occurs when the temperature at the electrode tip fails to reach 90° C for the four minutes duration of treatment. If the current is too high or applied too rapidly, a suboptimally small treatment zone or an irregularly shaped treatment zone of unpredictable size may result.

Note that during thermocoagulation, while entering the nidus, a physiologic reaction (increase of blood pressure, heart rate, and frequency of respiration) may occur.

For osteoid osteomas close to joints a transarticular approach should be avoided in order to minimize the risk of infection and reduce the risk of inadvertent heating of the joint cartilage. Damage to the growth plate in children should always be avoided during the thermocoagulation procedure.

In cases of superficial osteoid osteomas (e.g. the anterior surface of the tibia, metacarpals or metatarsals) the bone-penetration cannula should be withdrawn at least 1 cm above the surface skin in order to avoid skin burns.

At the end of the procedure, immediately after the needle system is removed, CT is routinely performed to check for possible acute complications (e.g. hematoma). CT can also be used to confirm whether the nidus was truly "hit," since the individual needle tracks are visualized after the procedure (Figure 19-7C). The mean procedure time is about 90 minutes, starting from the moment general anesthesia is initiated.

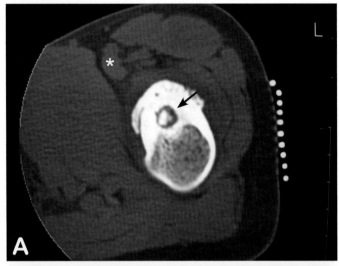

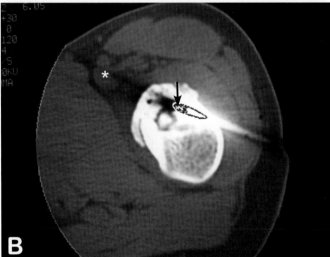

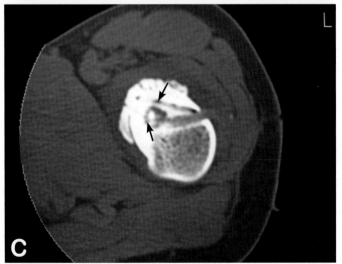

Question 90

In this 19-year-old woman successful thermocoagulation of an osteoid osteoma in the right mid-tibia was performed. Axial CT images before, during, and 12 months after successful thermocoagulation are shown (Figure 19-8 in the Test section). Select the *one* MOST appropriate answer to the question below.

After successful thermocoagulation for osteoid osteoma with a routine noncooled tip (5mm exposed tip) the likelihood of advanced bone healing (complete to nearly complete ossification of the nidus) on CT scan 6 to12 months later, is:

    (A)   0 percent for successfully treated patients
    (B)   20 percent of successfully treated patients
    (C)   50 percent of successfully treated patients
    (D)   75 percent of successfully treated patients

After routine thermocoagulation with a noncooled 5 mm exposed tip (and a heating time of four minutes at 90° C), complete ossification of the nidus is seen in approximately 50% of successfully treated cases (**Option**

Figure 19-7 (same as Figure 19-6). CT-guided thermocoagulation of an osteoid osteoma. CT. Left proximal femur (lesser trochanter). Axial plane. (A) The image demonstrates a ±1-cm large intracortically located osteoid osteoma (arrow), with surrounding sclerosis and intralesional calcification. Skin markers were placed laterally in order to localize the lesion prior to the thermocoagulation procedure. The femoral neurovascular bundle (asterisk) is located anteromedially relative to the lesion. (B) The image shows the left proximal femur during the "drilling" portion of the procedure prior to thermocoagulation, with the drill (arrow) in place. A lateral approach was chosen to avoid the femoral neurovascular bundle (asterisk) located anteromedially. (C) This image depicts the osteoid osteoma immediately after the thermocoagulation procedure. CT is always performed immediately afterwards to check for acute complications (e.g. hematoma) and to confirm that the nidus was hit. CT shows the electrode track(s) that remain after the procedure. On this post-treatment scan two different electrode tracks were visualized (arrows), one immediately anterior to the nidus, the other through the posterior portion of the (calcified) nidus. This osteoid osteoma was successfully treated.

(C) is correct) (Options (A), (B), and (D) are incorrect). Lindner et al reported a complete ossification of the nidus in 53% (8/15) of such patients treated successfully. In their study the CT follow-up was performed only once, six months after the procedure.

Similar results were reported by Vanderschueren et al. They observed the presence of advanced bone healing (the presence of complete ossification or a minimal residual nidus rest) in 37% (13/35) of patients at ≤ 12 months and 58% (16/28) of those successfully treated patients at > 12 months after CT. This ossification mainly occurred within the first year, since no significant progression of ossification after the first year was observed (p = 0.07). Interestingly, all patients with complete ossification of the nidus had osteoid osteomas that were located within the cortex. In patients with an endosteal or an intramedullary nidus the highest degree of bone healing observed was the presence of a minimal nidus rest. No patient had complete ossification. This relationship between intraosseous location and bone healing was statistically significant (p = 0.03). Lindner et al also reported that osteoid os-

teomas located within the cortex had a greater tendency to ossify after successful thermocoagulation than did those located in other intracortical locations. Ossification rates of less than 50% after successful routine thermocoagulation have been reported in the literature. The lowest percentage of complete ossification (19% of patients at 12-month CT follow-up) observed after successful thermocoagulation of osteoid osteoma was reported by Papagelopoulos et al. The 16 intraarticular osteomas included in that study were all confined to the intraarticular hip region, however, while Lindner et al and Vanderschueren et al treated patients with osteoid osteomas at various locations.

The largest reported fraction of complete ossification (75%) of the nidus after successful thermocoagulation was reported by Martel et al in 24 of 32 patients successfully treated and imaged on follow-up CT scan after 12 months. They used a cooled instead of a noncooled tip, however. This difference in thermocoagulation technique may explain the higher percentage of complete ossification in their study. From a theoretical perspective (Pinto et al) we know that a routine 5-mm

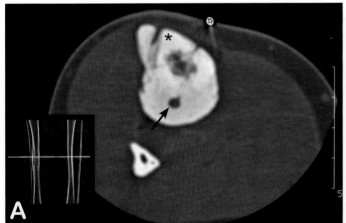

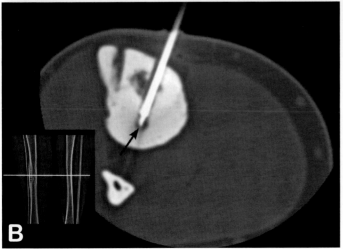

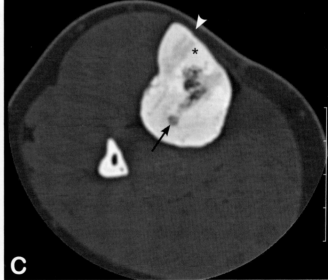

Figure 19-9 (same as Figure 19-8). Osteoid osteoma thermocoagulation. Right tibia. CT. Axial plane through the right mid-tibia. (A) The scan demonstrates postsurgical changes (asterisks) after failed surgery. A 5-mm intracortical nidus that was missed during the previous surgery is identified more posteriorly (arrow). Marked reactive sclerosis surrounds this lesion. An anteroposterior scout view (inserted in the lower left-hand corner) demonstrates the actual scan level. (B) Another scan demonstrates the same lesion seen in panel A during the "drilling and milling" portion of the procedure prior to thermocoagulation, with the presence of a drill (arrow) whose end is inserted in the nidus through a penetration cannula. (C) A follow-up CT scan of the same lesion 12 months after the procedure shows nearly complete filling in of the nidus. The nidus (arrow) is only faintly identified, consistent with nearly complete ossification. The site of previous surgery (asterisks) now demonstrates complete bony bridging at its margin (arrowhead).

noncooled tip creates a spherical treatment zone of focal osteonecrosis of approximately 1 cm in diameter. Martel et al used a cooled electrode with an active tip of 10 mm. The treatment zone for that technique would be expected to be larger due to the longer size of the active tip and the infusion of saline, which allows greater heat transmission. This larger treatment zone and thus larger area of thermal injury may have caused more inflammation and secondary ossification, and might, therefore, have contributed to the higher degree of ossification.

Vanderschueren et al observed advanced bone healing (nearly complete to complete ossification of the nidus) only in their cases of successful thermocoagulation, seeing it in 46% of 63 patients. It was not seen in any of the 23 patients that had unsuccessful procedures (p < 0.001) **(Option (A) is incorrect).**

Since absence of ossification of the nidus was observed equally as often in patients with good response to treatment as in those with poor response, CT follow-up after thermocoagulation is of limited value in the selection of candidates for repeat thermocoagulation. Persistence or recurrence of clinical symptoms remains the most important parameter to diagnose residual or recurrent disease, because CT and MRI cannot reliably identify residual or recurrent tumor after thermocoagulation for osteoid osteoma. The potential role of scintigraphy in the detection of recurrent or residual tumor after thermocoagulation of osteoid osteoma has not yet been fully explored.

Thermocoagulation for osteoid osteoma causes fewer severe complications than surgery. Complications after surgical resection of osteoid osteoma (Figure 19-8) include fracture (especially in the lower limb), infection, and, in the spine, postoperative instability and even neurovascular injury (vertebral artery rupture). Complication rates of up to 46% (10/22 patients) have been reported after surgical en-bloc resection for osteoid osteoma.

Thermocoagulation is performed under CT guidance, which allows for accurate imaging of the nidus during the entire procedure. Therefore geographical misses (as reported after surgery) do not tend to occur after thermocoagulation.

Thermocoagulation causes no structural bone weakening and therefore no increased fracture risk. Because of its nondestructive and minimally invasive nature, as well as its low procedure-related morbidity, thermocoagulation is easily repeatable in case of treatment failure. The reported success rates after surgery for osteoid osteoma range between 90% and 100% in three large series, with between 88 and 104 patients

treated. Lindner et al reported a comparable primary success rate of 95% (55/58 patients) after CT-guided thermocoagulation for osteoid osteoma. Only one complication (skin burn) was observed in that series. Vanderschueren et al treated 97 consecutive patients with osteoid osteoma at different locations. Response was good after one session of thermocoagulation in 74 of 97 patients (76%). Patients with persistent symptoms did well after repeated thermocoagulation with a good response in 10 of 12 patients. The results of repeated thermocoagulation, however, were poor in patients with recurrent symptoms, with a good response in only 5 of 10 patients. The overall success rate after one or two thermocoagulation procedures combined was 92% (89 of 97 patients). Complications were observed in 2% (2 of 97) of patients. These included hardware failure (a broken biopsy needle tip, which had to be removed surgically) and skin necrosis.

The largest series (126 procedures) of osteoid osteoma treated by thermocoagulation was reported in 2003 by Rosenthal et al. The primary clinical success rate was 89% (112/126 procedures). Two anesthesia-related (aspiration and cardiac arrest) and two minor procedure-related complications (cellulitis and sympathetic dystrophy) were observed in this series.

One disadvantage of thermocoagulation is the relative lack of histological proof, due to the small amount

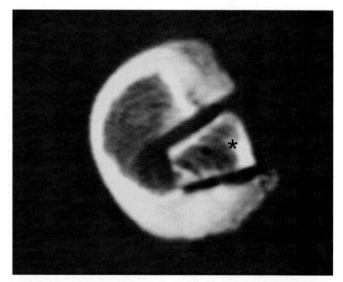

Figure 19-8. Osteoid osteoma treatment with bone graft. CT. Axial plane through the right mid-femur. The image demonstrates placement of a bone graft after surgical resection of an osteoid osteoma. The bone graft (asterisk) was harvested from the iliac crest. No signs of graft incorporation are identified in this image obtained 3 weeks after surgery. Surgical bone loss greatly increases the risk of fracture, especially in weight-bearing bones such as the femur. In the spine, surgical bone loss may lead to instability.

of tissue sampled during biopsy. Although the diagnosis of osteoid osteoma was confirmed after surgery in up to 100% of cases, the highest diagnostic confirmation rate reported after thermocoagulation was only 75% (Rosenthal 2003). Thus, the use of the clinical and radiological criteria described in Question 1 to differentiate osteoid osteoma from other lesions such as intracortical abscess remains of paramount importance.

Another percutaneous CT-guided technique to treat osteoid osteomas is laser ablation. Like thermocoagulation, laser ablation causes heat-induced thermonecrosis, but the principles of heat formation differ. Gangi et al treated 114 patients with osteoid osteomas at various locations by this technique. The primary success rate in this series was comparable to thermocoagulation (95% or 108/114 patients) and only one temporary and self-limiting complication occurred in one patient (reflex sympathetic dystrophy in a patient treated for a carpal lesion).

CT-guided percutaneous resection is an emerging surgical technique used for the treatment of osteoid osteoma and consists of extracting the nidus of the osteoid osteoma percutaneously under CT guidance. Sans et al treated 38 patients with a presumed diagnosis of osteoid osteoma by this technique. The cure rate was 84% (32/38 patients) for all patients and 88% (28/32 patients) for patients with a histologically confirmed diagnosis of osteoid osteoma. The complication rate after percutaneous resection of osteoid osteoma, however, was high (24% or 9/38 patients) compared to CT-guided thermocoagulation. Complications included fracture, chronic osteomyelitis, hematoma, skin burns, and post-procedural nerve irritation. The hospitalization period after percutaneous resection was comparable to surgery (mean of five days), and patients were able to bear weight on the extremity at a mean of 30 days. By comparison, thermocoagulation generally requires no overnight hospital stay, and patients are able to resume their normal activities soon after the procedure.

Several authors reported on risk factors that may impede a favorable clinical outcome after thermocoagulation for osteoid osteoma. Cribb et al found a statistically significant relationship between treatment failure and a nondiaphyseal location of the osteoid osteoma (p < 0.01).

They attributed this to the fact that diaphyseal lesions are more contained by surrounding sclerosis, which makes them easier to treat by heat ablation than nondiaphyseal lesions. In 2003, Rosenthal et al observed that thermocoagulation performed as the initial treatment had a significantly higher success rate than procedures performed after a different treatment failed (91% versus 60% success rate) (p < 0.001).

Vanderschueren et al observed that parameters associated with an increased risk for thermocoagulation treatment failure were younger age (the reason for this was unclear) and a smaller number of electrode positions used during thermocoagulation. Patients with lesions of 10 mm or greater tended to have a higher risk for unsuccessful treatment. The study concluded that multiple needle positions reduce the risk of treatment failure in all patients and should especially be used in large (10 mm or greater) lesions or lesions that are difficult to engage. The treatment zone can be increased by using multiple electrode positions, by increasing the size of the noninsulated tip or by using a cooled tip. However, the use of a cooled tip for the thermocoagulation of osteoid osteomas is not recommended because of safety considerations. A cooled tip not only creates a larger treatment zone, but it also makes the size of the treatment zone difficult to predict. This applies especially to osteoid osteomas of the spinal canal, because of the risk of thermal injury to the myelum or exiting nerve roots.

In conclusion, CT-guided thermocoagulation has become an established technique for the safe and effective treatment of nonspinal osteoid osteomas. The risk for unsuccessful treatment after thermocoagulation for osteoid osteoma may be reduced by using multiple needle positions, especially in large (≥ 10-mm) lesions or in lesions that are difficult to engage.

As an aside, thermocoagulation treatment is a promising palliative technique to relieve pain in patients with metastatic bone disease. External beam radiation therapy (RT) is considered the current standard of care for cancer patients who present with localized bone pain. Unfortunately, patients with recurrent pain are often not eligible for further RT. Analgesics remain the only alternative treatment, since surgery, chemotherapy, hormonal therapy, or the use of radiopharmaceuticals are usually not therapeutic options in such cases.

Selection of patients for palliative thermocoagulation requires that they have significant pain and that the pain is limited to a few osteolytic metastases. Thermocoagulation of bone metastases that are within 1 cm of critical structures (including bowel, bladder, spinal cord or motor nerves) should be avoided to prevent thermal damage to these structures.

Thermocoagulation for bone metastasis can cause a significant reduction in pain, without causing major complications, as has been demonstrated by several studies. Large multicenter trials are now being devised to evaluate the efficacy of pain reduction after thermocoagulation in patients with metastatic bone disease.

Suggested Readings

IMAGING APPEARANCE, HISTOPATHOLOGICAL APPEARANCE AND DIFFERENTIAL DIAGNOSIS OF OSTEOID OSTEOMA

1. Brukner P, Bradshaw C, Khan KM, White S, Crossley K. Stress fractures: a review of 180 cases. Clin J Sport Med. 1996; 6:85–89.

2. Gaeta M, Minutoli F, Pandolfo I, Vinci S, D'Andrea L, Blandino A. Magnetic resonance imaging findings of osteoid osteoma of the proximal femur. Eur Radiol. 2004; 14:1582–1589.

3. Greenspan A. Benign bone-forming lesions: osteoma, osteoid osteoma, and osteoblastoma. Clinical, imaging, pathologic, and differential considerations. Skeletal Radiol. 1993;22:485–500.

4. Helms CA, Hattner RS, Vogler JB, III. Osteoid osteoma: radionuclide diagnosis. Radiology. 1984;151:779–784.

5. Levine SM, Lambiase RE, Petchprapa CN. Cortical lesions of the tibia: characteristic appearances at conventional radiography. Radiographics. 2003;23:157–177.

6. O'Connell JX, Nanthakumar SS, Nielsen GP, Rosenberg AE. Osteoid osteoma: the uniquely innervated bone tumor. Mod Pathol. 1998;11:175–180.

THERMOCOAGULATION OF OSTEOID OSTEOMA

7. Bitsch RG, Rupp R, Bernd L, Ludwig K. Osteoid osteoma in an ex vivo animal model: temperature changes in surrounding soft tissue during CT-guided radiofrequency ablation. Radiology. 2006;238:107–112.

8. Bruneau M, Cornelius JF, George B. Osteoid osteomas and osteoblastomas of the occipitocervical junction. Spine. 2005; 30:E567–E571.

9. Cantwell CP, O'Byrne J, Eustace S. Current trends in treatment of osteoid osteoma with an emphasis on radiofrequency ablation. Eur Radiol. 2004;14:607–617. Epub 2003 Dec 9

10. Cantwell CP, O'Byrne J, Eustace S. Radiofrequency ablation of osteoid osteoma with cooled probes and impedance-control energy delivery. AJR Am J Roentgenol. 2006;186:S244–S248.

11. Cribb GL, Goude WH, Cool P, Tins B, Cassar-Pullicino VN, Mangham DC. Percutaneous radiofrequency thermocoagulation of osteoid osteomas: factors affecting therapeutic outcome. Skeletal Radiol. 2005;34:702–706.

12. Dupuy DE, Hong R, Oliver B, Goldberg SN. Radiofrequency ablation of spinal tumors: temperature distribution in the spinal canal. AJR Am J Roentgenol. 2000;175:1263–1266.

13. Goldberg SN, Gazelle GS, Solbiati L, Rittman WJ, Mueller PR. Radiofrequency tissue ablation: increased lesion diameter with a perfusion electrode. Acad Radiol. 1996;3:636–644.

14. Lindner NJ, Ozaki T, Roedl R, Gosheger G, Winkelmann W, Wortler K. Percutaneous radiofrequency ablation in osteoid osteoma. J Bone Joint Surg Br. 2001;83:391–396.

15. Martel J, Bueno A, Ortiz E. Percutaneous radiofrequency treatment of osteoid osteoma using cool-tip electrodes. Eur J Radiol. 2005;56:403–408.

16. Osti OL, Sebben R. High-frequency radio-wave ablation of osteoid osteoma in the lumbar spine. Eur Spine J. 1998;7:422–425.

17. Papagelopoulos PJ, Mavrogenis AF, Kyriakopoulos CK, et al. Radiofrequency ablation of intra-articular osteoid osteoma of the hip. J Int Med Res. 2006;34:537–544.

18. Pinto CH, Taminiau AH, Vanderschueren GM, Hogendoorn PC, Bloem JL, Obermann WR. Technical considerations in CT-guided radiofrequency thermal ablation of osteoid osteoma: tricks of the trade. AJR Am J Roentgenol. 2002;179:1633–1642.

19. Rosenthal DI, Alexander A, Rosenberg AE, Springfield D. Ablation of osteoid osteomas with a percutaneously placed electrode: a new procedure. Radiology. 1992;183:29–33.

20. Rosenthal DI, Springfield DS, Gebhardt MC, Rosenberg AE, Mankin HJ. Osteoid osteoma: percutaneous radio-frequency ablation. Radiology. 1995;197:451–454.

21. Rosenthal DI. Percutaneious Radiofrequency treatment of osteoid osteomas. Semin Musculoskelet Radiol. 1997;1:265–272.

22. Rosenthal DI, Hornicek FJ, Wolfe MW, Jennings LC, Gebhardt MC, Mankin HJ. Percutaneous radiofrequency coagulation of osteoid osteoma compared with operative treatment [see comments]. J Bone Joint Surg Am. 1998;80:815–821.

23. Rosenthal DI, Hornicek FJ, Torriani M, Gebhardt MC, Mankin HJ. Osteoid osteoma: Percutaneous treatment with radiofrequency energy. Radiology. 2003;229:171–175. Epub 2003 Aug 27

24. Rosenthal DI, Marota JJ, Hornicek FJ. Osteoid osteoma: elevation of cardiac and respiratory rates at biopsy needle entry into tumor in 10 patients. Radiology. 2003;226:125–128.

25. Vanderschueren GM, Taminiau AH, Obermann WR, Bloem JL. Osteoid osteoma: clinical results with thermocoagulation. Radiology. 2002;224:82–86.

26. Vanderschueren GM, Taminiau AH, Obermann WR, van den Berg-Huysmans AA, Bloem JL. Osteoid osteoma: factors for increased risk of unsuccessful thermal coagulation. Radiology. 2004;233:757–762.

27. Vanderschueren GM, Taminiau AH, Obermann WR, van den Berg-Huysmans AA, Bloem JL, van Erkel AR. The healing pattern of osteoid osteomas on computed tomography and magnetic resonance imaging after thermocoagulation. Skeletal Radiol. 2007;36:813–821. Epub 2007 May 11

28. Woertler K, Vestring T, Boettner F, Winkelmann W, Heindel W, Lindner N. Osteoid osteoma: CT-guided percutaneous radiofrequency ablation and follow-up in 47 patients. J Vasc Interv Radiol. 2001;12:717–722.

SURGERY OF OSTEOID OSTEOMA

29. Campanacci M, Ruggieri P, Gasbarrini A, Ferraro A, Campanacci L. Osteoid osteoma. Direct visual identification and intralesional excision of the nidus with minimal removal of bone [see comments]. J Bone Joint Surg Br. 1999;81:814–820.

30. Sluga M, Windhager R, Pfeiffer M, Dominkus M, Kotz R. Peripheral osteoid osteoma. Is there still a place for traditional surgery? J Bone Joint Surg Br. 2002;84:249–251.

31. Yildiz Y, Bayrakci K, Altay M, Saglik Y. Osteoid osteoma: the results of surgical treatment. Int Orthop. 2001;25:119–122.

CT-GUIDED LASER ABLATION AND CT-GUIDED PERCUTANEOUS RESECTION OF OSTEOID OSTEOMA

32. Gangi A, Gasser B, de Unamuno S, et al. New trends in interstitial laser photocoagulation of bones. Semin Musculoskelet Radiol. 1997;1:331–338.

33. Gangi A, Alizadeh H, Wong L, Buy X, Dietemann JL, Roy C. Osteoid osteoma: percutaneous laser ablation and follow-up in 114 patients. Radiology. 2007;242 :293–301. Epub 2006 Nov 7

34. Sans N, Galy-Fourcade D, Assoun J, et al. Osteoid osteoma: CT-guided percutaneous resection and follow-up in 38 patients. Radiology. 1999;212:687–692.

THERMOCOAGULATION OF BONE METASTASES

35. Callstrom MR, Charboneau JW. Percutaneous ablation: safe, effective treatment of bone tumors. Oncology (Williston Park). 2005;19:22–26.

36. Callstrom MR, Charboneau JW, Goetz MP, et al. Image-guided ablation of painful metastatic bone tumors: a new and effective approach to a difficult problem. Skeletal Radiol. 2006;35:1–15. Epub 2005 Oct 5

37. Callstrom MR, Charboneau JW, Goetz MP, et al. Painful metastases involving bone: feasibility of percutaneous CT- and US-guided radio-frequency ablation. Radiology. 2002;224:87–97.

38. Goetz MP, Callstrom MR, Charboneau JW, et al. Percutaneous image-guided radiofrequency ablation of painful metastases involving bone: a multicenter study. J Clin Oncol. 2004;22:300–306.

39. Simon CJ, Dupuy DE. Percutaneous minimally invasive therapies in the treatment of bone tumors: thermal ablation. Semin Musculoskelet Radiol. 2006;10:137–144.

Index